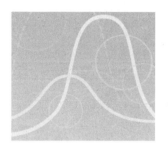

Statistical Methods
for Health Care Research

FIFTH EDITION

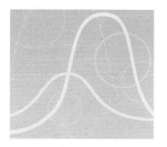

Statistical Methods for Health Care Research

FIFTH EDITION

Barbara Hazard Munro, PhD, FAAN
Dean and Professor
William F. Connell School of Nursing
Boston College
Chestnut Hill, Massachusetts

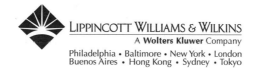

LIPPINCOTT WILLIAMS & WILKINS
A **Wolters Kluwer** Company
Philadelphia • Baltimore • New York • London
Buenos Aires • Hong Kong • Sydney • Tokyo

Senior Acquisitions Editor: Margaret Zuccarini
Managing Editor: Helen Kogut
Editorial Assistant: Carol DeVault
Production Editor: Danielle Michaely
Director of Nursing Production: Helen Ewan
Managing Editor/Production: Erika Kors
Art Director: Carolyn O'Brien
Senior Manufacturing Manager: William Alberti
Compositor: TechBooks
Printer: R.R. Donnelley—Crawfordsville

5th Edition

9 8 7 6 5 4 3 2 1

Library of Congress Cataloging-in-Publication Data
Munro, Barbara Hazard.
Statistical methods for health care research / Barbara Hazard Munro.—5th ed.
  p. ; cm.
Includes bibliographical references and index.
ISBN 0-7817-4840-2 (alk. paper)
1. Nursing—Research—Statistical methods. 2. Medical care—Research—Statistical methods. I. Title.
[DNLM: 1. Health Services Research—methods. 2. Statistics. WA 950 M968s 2005]
RT81.5.M86 2005
610'.7'27—dc22
          2004007098

LWW.com

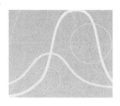

Contributors

Karen J. Aroian, PhD, RN, CS, FAAN
Professor of Nursing Research
College of Nursing
Wayne State University
Detroit, Michigan

Jane Karpe Dixon, PhD
Professor, Doctoral Program
School of Nursing
Yale University
New Haven, Connecticut

Mary E. Duffy, PhD, FAAN
Professor & Director, Center for Nursing Research
School of Nursing
Boston College
Chestnut Hill, Massachusetts

Barbara S. Jacobsen, MS
Professor (Retired)
The University of Pennsylvania School of Nursing
Philadelphia, Pennsylvania

Anne E. Norris, PhD, RN, CS
Associate Professor
School of Nursing
Boston College
Chestnut Hill, Massachusetts

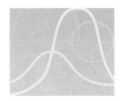

Reviewers

Denise Côté-Arsenault, PhD, RN
Associate Professor of Nursing
Syracuse University
Syracuse, New York

Karen K. Badros, EdD, CRNP
Professor of Nursing
Salisbury University
Salisbury, Maryland

Vera Brancato, EdD, MSN, RN, BC
Associate Professor of Nursing
Kutztown University
Kutztown, Pennsylvania

Anne Folta Fish, PhD, RN
Associate Professor
University of Missouri-St. Louis
St. Louis, Missouri

Stephen D. Krau, PhD, RN, BSN, BA, MSN, MA
Professor and Coordinator of Continuing Education
Middle Tennessee State University
Murfreesboro, Tennessee

Sarah Newton, PhD, RN
Associate Professor
Oakland University School of Nursing
Rochester, Michigan

Linn Stranak, PhD
Professor and Department Chair
of Physical Education, Wellness and Sport
Union University
Jackson, Tennessee

Donald E. Stull, PhD
Associate Professor
University of Maryland School of Nursing
Baltimore, Maryland

Laura Talbot
Johns Hopkins University
Baltimore, Maryland

Mary A. (Sandy) Wyper, PhD, RN
Associate Professor
Ursuline College
Pepper Pike, Ohio

Nashat Zuraikat, PhD, RN
Graduate School Coordinator
Indiana University of Pennsylvania
Indiana, Pennsylvania

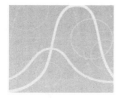

Preface

The purpose of the first edition of Statistical Methods for Health Care Research was to acquaint the reader with the statistical techniques most commonly reported in the research literature of the health professions. We attempted to make the book user-friendly by keeping mathematical symbolism to a minimum and by using computer printouts and examples from the literature to demonstrate specific techniques. In the second edition, we further reduced mathematical equations, moved from mainframe to personal computer examples, and added new techniques such as logistic regression. In the third edition, we added a dataset for use with the exercises at the end of the chapters. In the fourth edition, we incorporated suggestions from students and reviewers to clarify complex statistical procedures.

Once again, in this fifth edition, we have updated the examples from the literature and included additional content primarily in the area of preparing data for statistical analyses. We believe that it is essential that one spend time preparing the data prior to running statistical analyses. We, therefore, have added a section on the principles for preparing data for analyses and included more detail on carrying out data transformations. We also have expanded the sections on handling outliers and dealing with missing data.

The concepts of sensitivity and specificity are now part of data analyses. We have added an introductory section on these concepts, and, in the chapter on logistic regression, we demonstrate how to interpret the printout in terms of sensitivity and specificity.

The statistical software has been updated using SPSS version 12.0. The exercises at the end of each chapter are based on the database provided on a CD-ROM in the back of the book. Each year, our students add additional cases to the database, and we encourage you to have your students add cases for their use, as well. We continue to underplay the role of mathematical calculations, assuming that readers will be using a personal computer for statistical analyses.

As a support for instructors, we have produced PowerPoint presentations for each chapter.

TEXT ORGANIZATION

We have organized the text into two sections:

Section I includes three chapters that present content essential to Understanding the Data. Content includes organizing and displaying data, univariate descriptive statistics, inferential statistics, hypothesis testing, and dealing with missing data and outliers.

Section II presents 14 chapters that address Specific Statistical Techniques including nonparametric techniques, *t* tests, one-way and multifactorial analysis of variance, analysis of covariance, repeated measures analysis of variance, correlation, regression, canonical correlation, logistic regression, factor analysis, confirmatory factor analysis, path analysis, and structural equation modeling.

Once again, we would like to thank the users and reviewers of the first four editions who made very helpful suggestions for this fifth edition. The students at Boston College, The University of Pennsylvania, and Yale University who have taken courses taught by authors of this text have most definitely played a role in the continuing development of this text, and we thank them too.

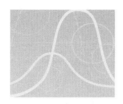

Contents

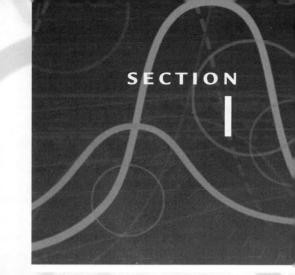

Understanding
the Data

Organizing and Displaying Data

Mary E. Duffy
Barbara S. Jacobsen

Objectives for Chapter 1

After reading this chapter, you should be able to do the following:

1. Discuss the nature, purpose, and types of statistics.
2. Discuss variables, levels of measurement, and their relationship to statistical analysis.
3. Discuss principles of data handling.
4. Interpret a frequency distribution created by a computer program.
5. Organize data into a table.
6. Interpret data presented in a chart.

Research is the systematic study of one or more problems, usually posed as research questions germane to a specific discipline. Quantitative research uses specific methods to advance the science base of the discipline by studying phenomena relevant to the goals of that discipline. Quantitative research methods include experiments, surveys, correlational studies of various types, and some commonly encountered procedures such as meta-analysis and psychometric evaluations (Knapp, 1998).

Usually when researchers collect data to answer specific quantitative research questions, they want to draw conclusions about a broader base of people, events, or objects than those actually included in the particular study. For example, a researcher may want to draw conclusions about how effective a telephone-delivered coaching intervention delivered by Registered Nurses (RNs) is in relieving postoperative distress in patients having knee surgery in a same-day, ambulatory surgical setting. Yet the researcher selects only a specific number of these patients to study, not the total group of knee surgery patients. The larger group of patients the researcher wants to draw conclusions about is called the *population*; the term *parameter* is used when describing the characteristics of the population. The group of patients the researcher actually studies is called the *sample*; the term *statistic* is used to describe the characteristics of this group. In most studies, the population parameters are not known and must be estimated from the sample statistics (Norusis, 2002).

THE NATURE OF STATISTICS

Statistics is a branch of applied mathematics that deals with collecting, organizing, and interpreting data using well-defined procedures. Researchers use a variety of techniques to gather these data, which become the observations used in statistical analyses. Thus, the raw materials of research are data, gathered from a sample that has been selected from a population. Applying statistics to these data permits the researcher to draw conclusions and to understand more about the sample from whence the data were obtained.

The purpose of statistics is threefold: to describe and summarize information, thereby reducing it to smaller, more meaningful sets of data; to make predictions or to generalize about occurrences based on observations; and to identify associations, relationships, or differences between the sets of observations. When our goal is to summarize data, we take a large mass of unorganized bits of information and reduce them to smaller sets that describe the original data without sacrificing critical elements. If our goal is to make predictions or to generalize about occurrences of data, we use statistics as an inferential measuring tool. This permits us to state the degree of confidence we have in the accuracy of the measurements we make in a specific research context. When we want to identify associations, relationships, or differences between variables of interest, we are using knowledge about one set of data to infer or predict characteristics about another set of data. Each statistical technique discussed in this book serves one or more of these purposes.

There are two main types of statistics: descriptive and inferential. *Descriptive statistics* are used to describe or characterize data by summarizing them into more understandable terms without losing or distorting much of the information. Summary tables, charts, frequencies, percentages, and measures of central tendency are the most common statistics used to describe basic sample characteristics. In contrast, *inferential statistics* consist of a set of statistical techniques that provide predictions about population characteristics based on information in a sample from that population. The primary focus of most research is the parameters of the population under study; the sample and statistics describing it are important only insofar as they provide information about the population parameters. Thus, an important aspect of statistical inference involves reporting the likely accuracy, or degree of confidence, of the sample statistic that predicts the value of the population parameter (Agresti & Finlay, 1997).

VARIABLES AND THEIR MEASUREMENT

Data are the raw materials of research. The most common way a researcher acquires data is to design a study that will answer a specific research question. The researcher then attempts to answer the question by collecting information (data) about the characteristics of interest in the study, usually people, events, or objects. Once collected, the data must be organized, examined, and interpreted using well-defined procedures. Almost all quantitative studies involve data that are entered into a computer-based statistical spreadsheet for subsequent data analysis. The logistics and time required to collect data, enter it into a statistical spreadsheet, and prepare it for data analysis are often greatly underestimated and poorly understood. Davidson (1996) recommends taking control of the structure and flow of your data from the beginning. Hopefully, this will help eliminate faulty data leading to faulty conclusions.

In research, the specific characteristics of interest are commonly called variables. *A variable* is a characteristic being measured that varies among the persons, events, or objects being studied. Measurement, in the broadest sense, is the assignment of numerals to objects or events according to a set of rules (Stevens, 1946). For example, the length of a piece of paper can be measured by following a set of rules for placing a graduated straightedge (eg, a ruler) and then reading the numeral that corresponds to the concept of the paper's length. This definition can be broadened to include the assignment of numerals to abstract, intangible concepts such as resilience, self-esteem, and health status. After determining a method of measurement for the concept, it is then called a variable (ie, a measured characteristic that takes on different values). Stevens (1946) noted four types of measurement scales for variables: nominal, ordinal, interval, and ratio. When analyzing data, the first task is to be aware of the type of measurement scale for each of the variables, because this knowledge helps in deciding how to organize and display data.

Nominal Scales

This type of scale, the lowest form of measurement, allows the researcher to assign numbers that classify characteristics of people, objects, or events into categories. Sometimes nominal variables are called *categorical* or *qualitative*. These numeric values are usually assigned to the categories as labels for computer storage, but the choice of numerals for those labels is absolutely arbitrary. Some examples follow:

Variables	*Values*
Group Membership	1 = Experimental
	2 = Placebo
	3 = Routine
Gender	0 = Female
	1 = Male
Adherence to Scheduled Appointment	0 = Did not keep appointment
	1 = Kept appointment

Ordinal Scales

In this case, the characteristics are placed in categories *and* the categories are ordered in some meaningful way (ie, the assignment of numerals is not arbitrary). Ordinal measures can be ranked from high to low. The distance between the categories, however, is unknown. Summated rating scales, as exemplified by the popular Likert scale, are examples of ordinal scales. For example, an RN who works in long-term care could rank patients on their ability to carry out activities of daily living (ADLs): 3 = fully able to perform all ADLs, 2 = partially able to perform ADLs, or 1 = not able to perform any ADLs independently. For the record, however, it is irrelevant how many ADLs fall into each category. Some other examples follow:

Variables	Values
Socioeconomic status	1 = Low
	2 = Middle
	3 = High
Health Status	1 = Very Poor
	2 = Poor
	3 = Fair
	4 = Good
	5 = Excellent
Pain Intensity	0 = No pain
	1 = Minor/Little Pain
	2 = Moderate Pain
	3 = Severe Pain

Interval Scales

For this type of scale, the distances between these ordered category values are equal because there is some accepted physical unit of measurement. Because the units are in equal intervals, it is possible to add and subtract across an interval scale. You can say that the difference between 5 and 10 is the same amount (5) as the difference between 75 and 80. An interval scale provides information about the rank ordering of categories and the magnitude of the difference between different values on the scale. Interval variables may be *continuous* (ie, in theory, they may take on any numerical value within the variable's range), or they may be discrete (ie, takes on only a finite number of values between two points). A good example of interval-level measurement is the Fahrenheit scale of temperature.

Ratio Scales

The fourth and most precise level of measurement consists of meaningfully ordered characteristics with equal intervals between them and the presence of a zero point that is not arbitrary but is determined by nature. Blood pressure, pulse rate, and weight are examples of ratio variables. With ratio scales, all mathematical operations (addition, subtraction, multiplication, division) are possible. Thus, one can say that a 200-pound man is twice as heavy as a 100-pound man. The distinction between interval and ratio variables is interesting, but for the purposes of this text, these two types of variables are handled the same way in analyzing data when the assumptions underlying the statistical test are met.

Measurement Scale Considerations

Researchers need to be very clear about the measurement levels of their study variables, particularly when it comes to classifying variables as either ordinal, interval, or ratio (Burns & Grove, 2001). When measuring variables derived from psychosocial scales, psychological inventories, or tests of knowledge, there may be differences of opinion as to the variable's level of measurement. Many of these scales have arbitrary zero points as determined by the test developer, and they have no accepted unit of measurement comparable to a standard ruler measurement of inches and feet. Technically, these variables are ordinal in nature, but in practice, researchers often think of them as interval- or ratio-level scales. This has been a controversial issue in the research literature for years. Gardner (1975) reviewed the early literature on this conflict, and Knapp (1990) has commented on more recent literature. In his original article on measurement (1946) and in a later article (1968), Stevens noted that treating ordinal scales as interval or ratio scales may violate a technical canon, but in many instances the outcome had demonstrable use. More recently, Knapp (1990, 1993) and Wang, Yu, Wang, and Huang (1999) pointed out that such considerations as measurement perspective, the number of categories that make up an ordinal scale, the concept of *meaningfulness*, and keeping in mind the relevancy of measurement scales to permissible statistics may be important in deciding whether to treat a variable as ordinal or interval. We recommend these articles for further reading on this topic.

It is usually best to gather data at the highest level of measurement for research variables because this permits the researcher to perform more mathematical operations and gain greater precision in measurement. However, interval or ratio variables can be converted to ordinal or nominal variables. For example, diastolic blood pressure, as measured by a sphygmomanometer, is a ratio variable. However, for research purposes, if blood pressure is recorded as either controlled or uncontrolled, then it is a nominal variable. In this case, there is a physiologic basis for such a dichotomous division. But when no such reason exists, converting interval or ratio variables to lower-level nominal or ordinal variables can be unwise because it results in a loss of information. Cohen (1983) detailed the amount of degradation of measurement as a consequence of dichotomization and urged researchers to use all of the original measurement information.

PRINCIPLES OF DATA HANDLING

Traditionally, very little has been written about the principles of getting research data ready for statistical analysis. In recent years, however, the principles of data handling have begun to be written about. Davidson (1996) delineates major principles of statistical data handling to fill the gap between getting data into the computer and running statistical tests. These principles are based on his view that data handling has certain universal concepts that apply no matter what the data-gathering context or the computer software used. We encourage you to read Davidson's book for a full listing of his principles. We have listed below those principles that relate directly to data collection, input, manipulation, and debugging.

> **Atomicity Principle**: You cannot analyze below the data level that you observe. For example, you gather information about study participants' ages by asking them to circle the number that best reflects their chronological age. For example,
>
> 1. 21–25 years
> 2. 25.1–29.9 years
> 3. 30–39.9 years
> 4. 40 or more years
>
> This age variable is measured at the nominal (categorical) level, the lowest form of measurement. Had you asked for participants' ages using a higher form of measurement (ie, What is your age in years?_____), you would be able to manipulate the age variable to produce measures of central tendency, including respondents' average age, standard deviation, and variance. With the lower-level nominal-level age data, the frequency and related percent of persons falling within the stated categories are the best information about age available to you.
>
> **Appropriate Data Principle**: You cannot analyze what you do not measure. If you want to know a respondent's age but do not gather such information, then you can't use age as a variable in subsequent analyses. Adhering to this principle requires that you anticipate what variables might be needed to explain the results of your data analyses.
>
> **Social Consequences Principle**: Data about people are about people. Data can have social consequences. Suppose you are gathering information on how effective (ie, efficacy) a specific nonpharmocologic pain management intervention is in relieving pain in patients with chronic headaches. You find that the intervention does not significantly differ from the standard method of giving nonsteroidal anti-inflammatory drugs (NSAIDS) every 4 hours as needed. Thus, it would not be appropriate, and possibly unethical, to counsel them to use the nondrug intervention rather than take a dose of NSAIDS that works.
>
> **Data Control Principle**: Take control of the structure and flow of your data. Even if you are not going to be the person who enters data into a statistical or other computer program, you should take responsibility for developing and monitoring the procedure for the layout of each respondent's data record (ie, a codebook for how data will be entered into the program; data entry and data manipulations such as recoding variable levels and computing new variables).

Data Efficiency Principle: Be efficient in getting your data into a computer, but not at the cost of losing crucial information. For example, do not hand-total respondents' scores on a 10-item self-esteem scale and then enter only the total score as the measure of their self-esteem in each electronic respondent's data record. By so doing, you are not able to determine the internal consistency reliability of the self-esteem scale because you chose not to enter the items that formed the self-esteem scale score into respondents' data records. Thus, you have sacrificed scientific rigor in favor of efficient data entry.

Change Awareness Principle: Data entry is an iterative process. Keep a list of the changes you have to make (computations), the values you will have to change (recoding), and the problems you will have to solve (debugging), but try to use the computer to do as much computing and debugging as possible.

Data Manipulation Principle: Let the computer do as much work as possible. Instruct it to do tasks such as recoding, variable computation, dataset catenation (linking), dataset subsetting, data merging, and similar tasks that would, frankly, waste your time. Let the computer manipulate your data for you.

Original Data Principle: Always save a computer file of the original, unaltered data. In this way, if you make a mistake in manipulating data through improper recoding of variables or computing new variables, you will have the original data file to use to rectify any mistakes.

Kludge Principle: Sometimes the best way to manipulate data is not elegant and seems to waste computer resources. A kludge is sometimes justifiable; the end CAN justify the means. (In information technology, a kludge [*pronounced clue-j*] is an awkward or clumsy patching together of a series of computer commands to make the data do what you want.)

Default Principle: Know your software's default settings. Know whether these settings meet your needs. In particular, be aware of the default handling of missing values in your software. Not being aware of such settings can produce study results that are inaccurate. For example, the SPSS computer program has a default option that prints only the results of data analyses in the output unless the user specifies that a log of what commands were used to compute the analyses is set prior to running the analysis. The same thing applies to recoding variables and/or computing scores from several item variables. Not setting this option can result in not knowing what, if any, mistakes were made in undertaking data analyses.

Complex Data Structure Principle: If your software can accommodate complex data structures (eg, hierarchical relational databases), then you might benefit from using that software feature. Alternatively, you might prefer a kludge (eg, copying the same information to each record). The choice is yours as to how best to achieve your data entry purpose.

Software's Data Relations Principle: Know whether your software can perform the following four relations and, if so, what commands are necessary for it to do so: subsetting (Can subgroups be formed from the larger dataset?), catenation (Can two subgroups of data be joined to form one larger dataset?), merging (Can two separate datasets of cases and/or variables be joined together to form one larger dataset?), and relational database construction (Can two separate datasets be joined together in a hierarchical fashion?).

Software's Sorting Principle: Know how to perform a sort in your software and whether your software requires a sort before a by-group analysis or before merging. For example, prior to merging two datasets containing the same cases but different variables, the variable on which you will match cases (normally, the subject identification code) may need to be sorted in an ascending (smallest to highest numbers) or descending (largest to smallest numbers) order in both data files. Thus, the larger dataset variables will be matched to the correct participant data record.

Impossibility/Implausibility Principle: Use the computer to check for impossible and implausible data. This should be done routinely by computing frequencies and measures of central tendency (eg, descriptive statistics) on all study variables and examining them for mistakes and/or bugs. If found, correct them immediately and then save the dataset.

Burstein's Data Sensibility Principle: Run your data all the way through to the final computer analysis and ask yourself whether the results make sense. Be prepared to decide that they do not, and hence, be prepared to treat the analysis not as final, but as another debugging step. You need to know your data as completely as possible so as not to be surprised by unexpected findings.

Extant Error Principle: Data bugs exist. Even if you have corrected one or more mistakes in your dataset, it is still possible that you missed something. Thus, always maintain an attitude of healthy skepticism when examining your data analysis results. And don't be surprised if you find another bug that needs fixing.

Manual Check Principle: Nothing can replace another pair of eyes to check over a dataset. Either check your data entry, input, and manipulation yourself, or get somebody else to do it. Determine the criticality of your dataset before expending human resources to check it manually. Highly critical datasets require manual checking regardless, possibly a priori, certainly a posteriori. Ideally, all datasets require manual checking. You should debug data by computer (Impossibility/Implausibility Principle) before you check it manually so that manual checking is easier.

Error Typology Principle: Debugging includes detection and correction of errors. To ease correction, try to classify each error as you uncover it. The two most common types of error are entry errors and logic errors. An entry error, a mistake in typing one or more responses correctly, is quite common and, once detected, is simple to fix. Locate the respondent's identification number, then retrieve the original data record and correct the mistake. In contrast, a logic error may be less detectable and more serious. For example, suppose the scoring instructions for computing a total score for a health status measure (10 items measured on a 5-point Likert scale) directs you to reverse-score (ie, make 1 = 5, 2 = 4, 3 = 3, 4 = 2, 5 = 1) one or more items prior to adding them together. You neglect to reverse-score these items and just add the items together, forming a health-status score. The resulting sum is incorrect because some of the items are not correctly recoded prior to being tallied.

In summary, Davidson's principles summarize the key dilemmas faced by researchers and the decisions they may have to make as they work with data destined for statistical analyses. The thing to keep in mind is to avoid the worst-case scenario: that of finding yourself with data that are inappropriate for the intended statistical analyses that will achieve study aims. Thus, it is extremely important from the earliest possible moment to foresee the form of statistical analysis that is intended to achieve study aims.

UNIVARIATE ANALYSES

As our society has grown more dependent on statistics and other numeric information, the need to present data in an appropriate way has become extremely important. As the first step, researchers should examine each variable separately, whether those variables are demographic, prognostic, group membership, or outcomes. Univariate analyses are helpful in cleaning and checking the quality of data that have been entered into a statistical computer program. The data values for each variable in the dataset must be examined visually or via computer. If the data indicate that a pregnant woman is 86 years old, then an error most likely occurred in data entry for that variable in that individual case. The researcher can then locate the individual case identification number in the dataset, check the original test information, correct the data entry error, and save the new information in the data file.

Univariate analyses are also helpful in examining the variability of data, describing the sample, and checking statistical assumptions before performing more complex analyses. In some cases, data analysis may end here if the research questions can be answered solely by univariate analyses.

PRESENTING DATA

A set of data can be presented in a table or in a chart. Tables offer two main advantages: They condense data into a form that can make them easier to understand (Morgan, Reichert, & Harrison, 2002); and they show many details in summary fashion. But tables have one major disadvantage: Because the reader sees only numbers, the table may not be readily understood without comparing it with other tables. In contrast, charts speak directly to the reader; despite their lack of exact details, charts are very effective in giving the reader a picture of differences and patterns in a set of data (Wallgren et al., 1996). They are often a very effective way to describe, explore, and summarize a set of numbers (Morgan et al., 2002; Tufte, 1983).

Tables

When data are organized into values or categories and then described with titles and captions, the result is called a *statistical table*. A researcher begins to construct a table by tabulating data into a frequency distribution—that is, by counting how often each value or category occurs in a variable or set of variables.

For nominal and ordinal variables, the categories should be listed (in some natural order if possible) and then the frequencies indicated for each category. Table 1-1 is an example of such a table, as produced by a computer, for the nominal variable of marital status. It is helpful to state the percentage in each category. Then the reader can quickly see that the majority of subjects in this sample were widowed (53.5%). The Percent column displays the percentage in each category, calculated on the total number of cases, including those with missing data on this variable. The next column, Valid Percent, provides the percentage of cases in each category based on the number of cases with no missing data. The Cum. Percent column refers to cumulative percentages, again with missing values excluded. By summing the valid percents (14.1%, 53.5%, 14.5%, and 12.4%), the cumulative percentage of 94.6% was formed, indicating that all but 5.4% of persons in this sample were either married or formerly married (ie, widowed, divorced, separated combined).

For interval or ratio variables, an ordered array of values (Table 1-2) is usually the first step in constructing a table. This frequency distribution table might be termed a *working table*. If the difference between the maximum and the minimum

TABLE 1-1 *Example of Frequency Distribution Produced by SPSS 12.0 for Windows: Marital Status in a Sample of 246 Older Black Women**

Program

FREQUENCIES VARIABLES = MARITAL

Output

MARITAL Marital Status

Value Label	Value	Frequency	Percent	Valid Percent	Cum. Percent
Married	1	34	13.8	14.1	14.1
Widowed	2	129	52.4	53.5	67.6
Divorced	3	35	14.2	14.5	82.2
Separated	4	30	12.2	12.4	94.6
Never married	5	13	5.3	5.4	100.0
Total				100.0	
System missing		5	2.0		
Total		246	100.0		

*Data from Wood, R. Y. (1997). The development and testing of video breast health kits for older women. National Cancer Institute Small Business Innovation Research (SBIR) Phase II R43 CA 63935-02.

value exceeds 15, the researcher may want to group the data into classes or categories before forming the final table (this also may be true for some ordinal variables). In Table 1-2, the ages of older women go from 60 to 105, with a range of 45 (ie, $105 - 60 = 45$). Therefore, grouping the values in a meaningful way will make the data more comprehensible.

As the next step, the computer printout for Table 1-3 shows a frequency distribution for the same data, with the values grouped into 3 classes, each containing those women whose age fit within the category of young-old, old-old, and oldest-old, a common method of grouping older persons. The young-old group contained 173 older women between the ages of 60 and 74.9 years; the old-old group had 50 older women between the ages of 75 and 84.9 years; and the oldest-old group had

TABLE 1-2 *Example of Frequency Distribution (Condensed) Produced by SPSS 12.0 for Windows: Age of Older Black Women in Sample**

Program

FREQUENCIES VARIABLES = AGE

Output

AGE Older Women's Age

Value Label	Frequency	Value Label	Frequency
60	14	78	7
61	13	79	5
62	15	80	2
63	13	81	6
64	11	82	6
65	19	83	1
66	11	84	4
67	13	85	3
68	7	86	3
69	9	87	4
70	5	88	6
71	22	89	1
72	4	90	1
73	8	92	1
74	9	94	1
75	5	98	1
76	4	100	1
77	10	105	1

*Data from Wood, R. Y. (1997). The development and testing of video breast health kits for older women. National Cancer Institute Small Business Innovation Research (SBIR) Phase II R43 CA 63935-02.

TABLE 1-3 *Example of Frequency Distribution (Condensed) Produced by SPSS 12.0 for Windows: Age Groups of Older Black Women in Sample**

Program

RECODE AGE (60 through 74.9 = 1) (75 through 84.9 = 2) (85 through 105 = 3) INTO RECAGE.
EXECUTE.

Output

RECAGE Older Women's Recoded Age Group

Value Label	Value	Frequency	Percent	Valid Percent	Cum. Percent
Young-Old Women (60–74.9 years)	1	173	70.3	70.3	70.3
Old-Old Women (75–84.9 years)	2	50	20.3	30.3	90.7
Oldest-Old Women (85–105 years)	3	23	9.3	9.3	100.0

*Data from Wood, R. Y. (1997). The development and testing of video breast health kits for older women. National Cancer Institute Small Business Innovation Research (SBIR) Phase II R43 CA 63935-02.

23 women 85 or more years. Again, it is most helpful to know the percentage falling into each group. The groupings fall in the expected direction with the youngest young-old group being far more numerous than the oldest-old group. By looking at the "Cum. Percent" column, the reader can quickly see that almost 91% of the sample were less than 85 years old.

By using the Recode command in a computer program, the researcher can easily form this new nominal level group (RECAGE) variable from the original interval level (AGE) variable. When creating such a variable, it is wise to create the new variable by using the *Recode into a Different Variable* command rather than to permanently change the original variable by recoding into the same variable. It is best to preserve the variable in its original form.

Computer programs can also group variable values automatically; however, some programs have defaults for the interval width and the number of classes produced, resulting in an inconveniently constructed table. Most statistical programs let the researcher control the choice of interval and the number of classes. Using a multiple of five for the interval width is helpful because it is easier to think about numbers that are divisible by five.

Authorities differ on their recommendations for the number of classes. Glass and Hopkins (1996) suggest there should be at least ten times as many observations as classes until there are between 20 and 30 intervals. Freedman et al. (1991) suggest 10 to 15 classes; Ott and Mendenhall (1990) suggest 5 to 20; and Freund (1988) suggests 6 to 15 classes. Thus, it is up to the researcher to determine the number of intervals in a frequency distribution of a variable. Usually, the clustering that best depicts the important features of the distribution of scores for the intended audience should be the major consideration. Too few or too many classes will obscure important features of a frequency distribution. Some detail is lost by grouping the values, but information is gained about clustering and the shape of the distribution.

The final presentation of the data from Table 1-3 depends on the format requirements of each journal or of the dissertation or thesis. If a table is included, it should be mentioned in the text of the research report. The discussion of a table should reinforce the major points for which the table was developed (Burns & Grove, 2001). Researchers should comment on the important patterns in the table as well as the major exceptions (Chatfield, 1988), but should not rehash every fact in the table.

Suggestions for the Construction of Tables for Research Reports

The specific content of a table will vary depending on the statistical analysis you are summarizing and/or the hypothesis you are testing. It is wise to use a table only to highlight major facts. Most of the tables examined by researchers while analyzing their data do not need to be published in a journal. If a finding can be described well in words, then a table is unnecessary. Too many tables can overwhelm the rest of a research report (Burns & Grove, 2001).

The table should be as self-explanatory as possible. The patterns and exceptions in a table should be obvious at a glance once the reader has been told what they are (Ehrenberg, 1977). With this goal in mind, the title should state the variable, when and where the data were collected (if pertinent), and the size of the sample. Headings within the table should be brief and clear. Find out the required format for tables in the research report. If the report is being submitted to a particular journal, examine tables in recent past issues. Follow the advice about table format for publication in a manual of style, such as the *Publication Manual of the American Psychological Association* (APA, 2001). Rudestam and Newton (1992) also suggest that tables should be numbered as whole numbers, such as Table 1, Table 2, and the like. They recommend not using a chapter number-table number form like Table 2.1 or Table 2.2. However, in a book chapter or a dissertation, table titles need to conform to the publisher's or university's requirements. If the data being presented in the table are not original, notes, including the data source, should be included.

Morgan and colleagues (2002) offer several principles that should guide table construction:

1. Don't try to do too much in a table. Model tables after published exemplars of similar research to find the right balance for how much a table should contain.
2. Use white space effectively so as to make the layout of the table pleasing to the eye and aid in comprehension and clarity.
3. Make sure tables and text refer to each other; but not everything displayed in a table needs to be mentioned in the text.
4. Use some aspect of the data to order and group rows and columns. This could be size (largest to smallest), chronology (first to last), or to show similarity or invite comparison.

5. If appropriate, frame the table with summary statistics in rows and columns to provide a standard of comparison. Remember when making a table that values are compared down columns more easily than across rows.
6. It is useful to round numbers in a table to one or two decimal places because they are more easily understood when the number of digits is reduced.
7. When creating tables for publication in a manuscript, they should be double-spaced unless contraindicated by the journal.

Charts

Although there are many different kinds of charts, most are based on several basic types that are built with lines, areas, and text. These include bar charts, histograms, pie charts, scatter plots, line charts, flow charts, and box plots. Charts can quickly reveal facts about data that might be gleaned from a table only after careful study. They are often the most effective way to describe, explore, and summarize a set of numbers (Tufte, 1983). Charts, the visual representations of frequency distributions, provide a global, bird's-eye view of the data and help the reader gain insight.

Choosing which type of chart to use in a given situation depends on what we wish to convey. When drawing a chart, Wallgren et al. (1996) suggest three things should be considered: data structure, variable type, and measurement characteristics. The researcher should ask these questions:

- Do the data represent one point in time, indicating *cross-sectional data*, or do they represent several points in time, called *time series data*?
- What type of variable do we wish to illustrate?
  - Is the variable *qualitative*, consisting of words, or *quantitative*, consisting of numbers?
  - If quantitative, is the variable *discrete*, which can take on only certain values, or *continuous*, which can take all the numbers in a range?
- What level of measurement is the variable of interest?

Answering these questions will help the researcher choose the type of chart that best illustrates a variable's characteristics.

BAR CHART

A bar chart, the simplest form of chart, is used for nominal or ordinal data. When constructing such charts, the category labels usually are listed horizontally in some systematic order, and then vertical bars are drawn to represent the frequency or percentage in each category. A space separates each bar to emphasize the nominal or ordinal nature of the variable. The spacing and the width of the bars are at the researcher's discretion, but once chosen, all the spacing and widths should be equal. Figure 1-1 is an example of a bar chart for ordinal data. If the category labels are lengthy, it may be more convenient to list the categories vertically and draw the bars horizontally, as in Figure 1-2.

Bar charts also make it easier to compare univariate distributions. Two or more univariate distributions can be compared by means of a cluster bar chart (Fig. 1-3). Current computer graphics, statistics, and spreadsheet programs offer

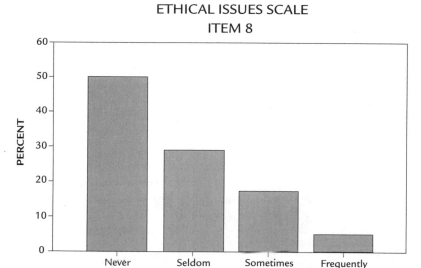

FIGURE 1-1. Degree of frequency that nurses experience the ethical issue of acting against their personal or religious beliefs. (Data from Fry, S., & Duffy, M. [2000]. *Ethics and Human Rights in Nursing Practice: A Study of New England Registered Nurses.* Chestnut Hill, MA: Nursing Ethics Network & The Center for Nursing Research, Boston College.)

many tempting patterns for filling in the bars. The legend explaining Figure 1-3 is outside the chart to avoid clutter (Cleveland, 1985). Wallgren et al. (1996) recommend filling bars with either shading of various depths or simple dot or line patterns, avoiding complex patterns, slanting lines in different directions, or a combination of horizontal and vertical lines in the same chart.

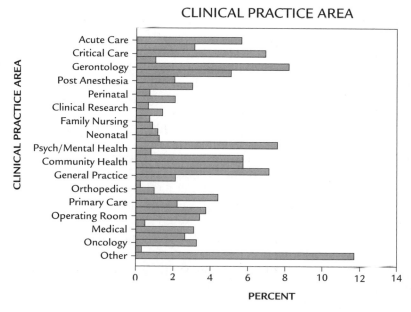

FIGURE 1-2. Major clinical practice area of registered nurses working in the six New England states in 1997 (N = 2,090). (Data from Fry, S., & Duffy, M. [2000]. *Ethics and Human Rights in Nursing Practice: A Study of New England Registered Nurses.* Chestnut Hill, MA: Nursing Ethics Network & The Center for Nursing Research, Boston College.)

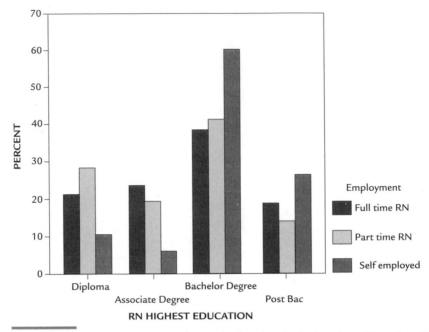

FIGURE 1-3. Employment status by RN highest level of education. (Data from Fry, S., & Duffy, M. [2000]. *Ethics and Human Rights in Nursing Practice: A Study of New England Registered Nurses.* Chestnut Hill, MA: Nursing Ethics Network & The Center for Nursing Research, Boston College.)

PIE CHART

The pie chart, an alternative to the bar chart, is simply a circle that has been partitioned into percentage distributions of qualitative variables. Simple to construct, the pie chart has a total area of 100%, with 1% equivalent to 3.6° of the circle. Figure 1-4 is an example of a pie chart displaying RNs' need for ethics and human rights education.

When constructing a pie chart, Wallgren et al. (1996) recommend the following:

- Use the pie chart to provide overviews: readers find it difficult to get precise measurements from a circle.
- Place the different sectors in the same order as would be found in the bar chart, beginning either in an ascending or a descending order. Retain the order between the variables.
- Use the percentages corresponding to each category rather than the absolute frequency of each category.
- Read the pie chart by beginning at the 12 o'clock position and proceeding clockwise.
- Use no more than six sectors in a given pie chart; clarity is lost with more than six sectors.

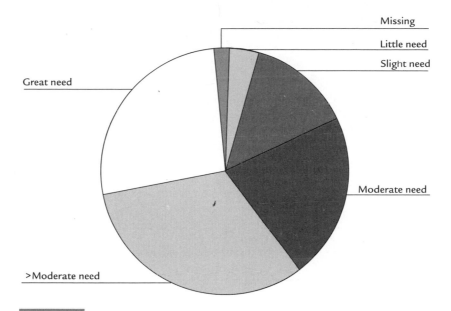

FIGURE 1-4. New England RNs' reported need for ethics and human rights education. (Data from Fry, S., & Duffy, M. [2000]. *Ethics and Human Rights in Nursing Practice: A Study of New England Registered Nurses.* Chestnut Hill, MA: Nursing Ethics Network & The Center for Nursing Research, Boston College.)

- Use a low-key shading pattern that does not detract from the meaning of the pie chart.
- If using more than one pie chart, give the number on which the percentages are based for each circle.
- Make sure the sum of the pie chart sectors equals 100%.

HISTOGRAM

Histograms, appropriate for interval, ratio, and sometimes ordinal variables, are similar to bar charts, except the bars are placed side by side. The bar length represents the number of cases (frequency) falling within each interval. Histograms are often used to represent percentages instead of, or in addition to, frequencies because percentages are more meaningful than simple number counts. Therefore, each histogram has a total area of 100%.

The first decision is to select the number of bars. With too few bars, the data will be clumped together; with too many, the data will be overly detailed. Figure 1-5 shows how the choice for the number of bars affects the appearance of a histogram. The top chart presents a jagged appearance; the bottom chart clumps the data into only four bars and makes the data seem skewed. The middle chart, with 10 bars, presents a smoother appearance.

Computer programs are handy for a preliminary chart of a variable, but the researcher should be aware of built-in defaults and should think about the adjustments

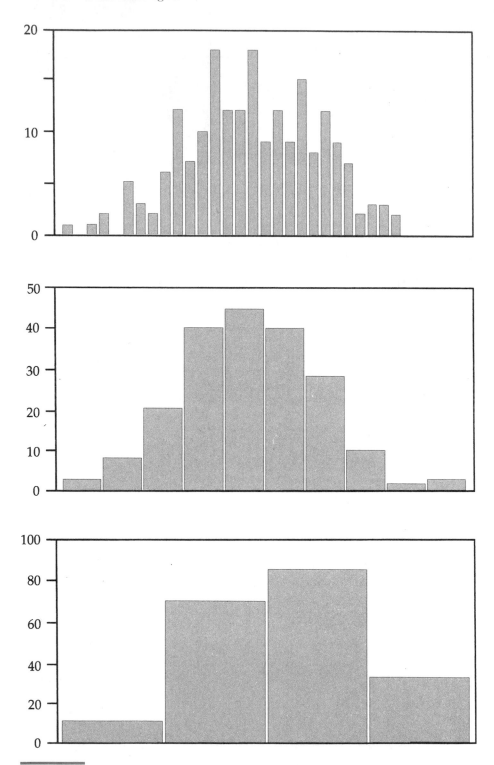

FIGURE 1-5. Illustration of the importance of the number of bars when designing a histogram for a set of data.

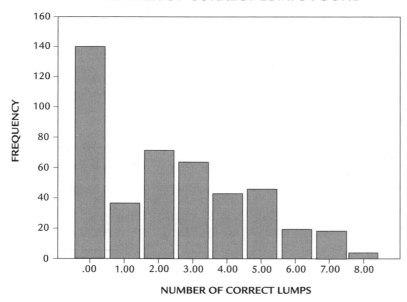

FIGURE 1-6. Number of correct breast lumps identified by older Black women (*N* = 246). (Data from Wood, R. Y. [1997]. The development and testing of video breast health kits for older women. National Cancer Institute Small Business Innovation Research (SBIR) Phase II R43 CA 63935-02.)

that are necessary. The advice given in the previous section for constructing frequency distributions for interval or ratio variables is helpful here. For example, if the difference between the maximum and minimum values exceeds 15, the researcher should consider grouping the data. The interval and the starting point should be divisible by five. Most histograms have 5 to 20 bars.

For interval or ratio variables that are discrete, the numerals representing the values should be centered below each bar to emphasize the discrete nature of the variable. Figure 1-6 illustrates a histogram for the discrete variable of number of correct lumps identified by older Black women. For continuous variables, the numerals representing the values should be placed at the sides of the bars to emphasize the continuous nature of the distribution.[1] Figure 1-7 depicts a histogram for the continuous variable of number of cigarettes smoked per day for a national sample of community-dwelling adults. Tick marks are placed outside the data region to avoid clutter (Cleveland, 1985).

Once the number of bars has been determined, the next decision concerns the height of the vertical axis. If the chart is horizontal, Tufte (1983) recommends a height of approximately half the width. Other authorities, such as Schmid (1983), recommend a height approximately two thirds to three fourths the width. The reason for these recommendations is the different effect that can be produced by altering the height of a chart. Figure 1-8 shows the different impressions that can be created for

[1]The grouping interval of "25 to 29" has a lower limit of 25 and an upper limit of 29. These are called the written limits. The real or mathematical limits are understood to extend half a unit above and below the written class limits. For convenience, researchers almost always use the written class limits in tables and charts.

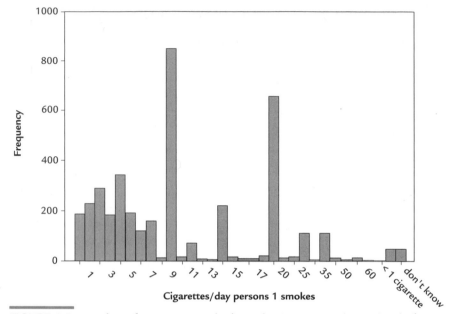

FIGURE 1-7. Number of cigarettes smoked per day in a national sample of 16,197 community-dwelling adults. (Data from US Department of Health and Human Services [DHHS]. [1996]. *Third National Health and Nutrition Examination Survey, 1988–1994,* NHANES III Laboratory Data File [CD-ROM]. US Department of Health and Human Services. National Center for Health Statistics. Public Use Data File Documentation Number 76200. Hyattsville, MD: Centers for Disease Control.)

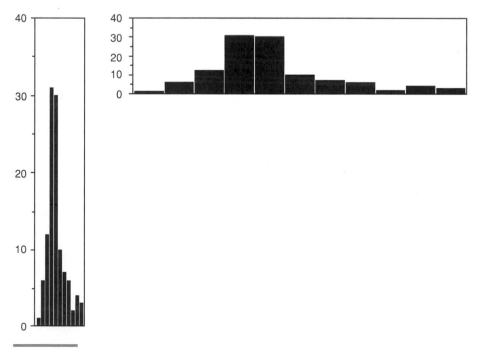

FIGURE 1-8. Illustration of the importance of the graph's height when designing a histogram for a set of data.

the same data by a tall, narrow chart and by a flat, wide chart. The tall, narrow chart seems to emphasize the clustering of the data in the middle, whereas the flat, wide chart appears to emphasize the scatter of the data to the right.

POLYGON

The polygon, a chart for interval or ratio variables, is equivalent to the histogram but appears smoother. For any set of data, the histogram and the polygon will have equivalent total areas of 100%. The polygon is constructed by joining the midpoints of the top of each bar of the histogram and then closing the polygon at both ends by extending lines to imaginary midpoints at the left and right of the histogram. Figure 1-9 illustrates a polygon superimposed on a histogram. In the process of construction, triangles of area are removed from the histogram, but congruent triangles are added to the polygon. Two such congruent triangles are shaded in Figure 1-9 to show why the areas of the two types of chart are equivalent.

Polygons are especially appropriate for comparing two univariate distributions by superimposing them (Fig. 1-10). The percentages were used on the vertical scale because the sizes of the two samples differed.

WHAT TO LOOK FOR IN A HISTOGRAM OR POLYGON

A chart can help us see quickly the shape of a distribution. Frequency distributions have many possible shapes. Often they have a bell-shaped appearance, as in the computer printout in Figure 1-11. In this case, older women rated themselves on the

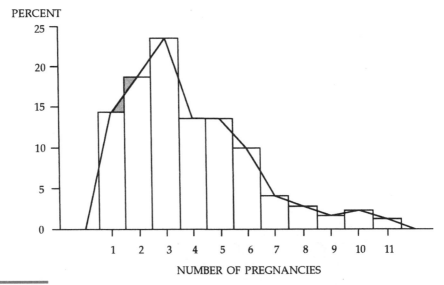

FIGURE 1-9. Polygon superimposed on histogram. The two shaded triangles are congruent. (Data collected with a grant funded by the National Institute of Nursing Research, NR-02867. P.I., Brooten, D. University of Pennsylvania School of Nursing, *Nurse Home Care for High Risk Pregnant Women: Outcome and Cost.*)

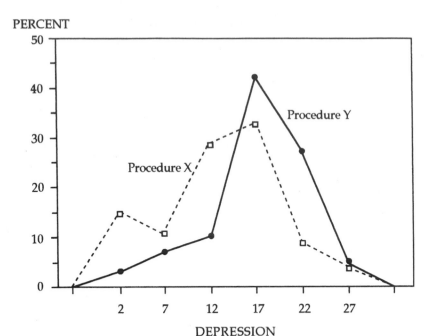

FIGURE 1-10. Comparison of depression scores for patients having surgical procedure X ($N = 104$) and patients having surgical procedure Y ($N = 61$).

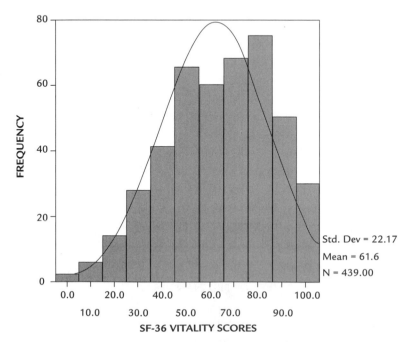

FIGURE 1-11. Example of a histogram produced by SPSS 12.0 for Windows: SF-36 Transformed Vitality Scores from a sample of 439 older women. (Data from Wood, R. Y. [1997]. The development and testing of video breast health kits for older women. National Cancer Institute Small Business Innovation Research (SBIR) Phase II R43 CA 63935-02.)

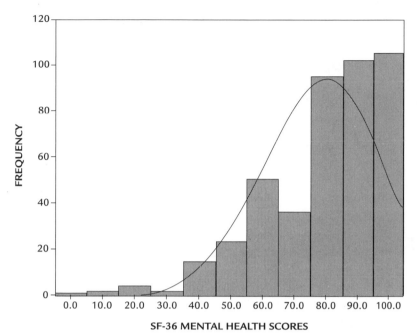

FIGURE 1-12. Relative frequency distribution of SF-36 transformed mental health scale scores from a sample of 439 older women. (Data from Wood, R. Y. [1997]. The development and testing of video breast health kits for older women. National Cancer Institute Small Business Innovation Research (SBIR) Phase II R43 CA 63935-02.)

Vitality subscale of the Short Form-36 Health Survey (SF-36), consisting of four items, with each item rated for evidence of vitality, energy, or fatigue on a 6-point scale, transformed so that scores ranged from 1 to 100 for comparison purposes. Technically, such a scale is ordinal, because there is no accepted physical unit of vitality, and the zero point is arbitrary. An ordinal scale with such a large range, however, is usually treated as interval in the research literature. In Figure 1-11, the frequency count is given at the left. The programmer chose an interval width of 10 and a starting point of 0. Thus, the first class is 0 to 10. In addition, the programmer instructed the computer program to plot the bell-shaped (normal) curve atop the histogram with a Line. The reader can then visually compare the distribution of transformed SF-36 vitality scores with the theoretical bell-shaped, or normal, curve.

Distributions also may be skewed, as in Figure 1-12. Occasionally, data may clump at several places, as in Figure 1-13.

Charts also can be helpful in spotting where the data cluster, how the data are scattered around the clustering points, whether there are far-out observations that may be outliers, and whether there are gaps in the data. These are the kinds of features that researchers need to know, and they become immediately evident with simple graphic representation (Cohen, 1990). With the assistance of a computer, researchers have no excuse for failing to know their data (Jacobsen, 1981). As with tables, all charts included in a research report should be cited in the text, and the important features of the distribution should be discussed.

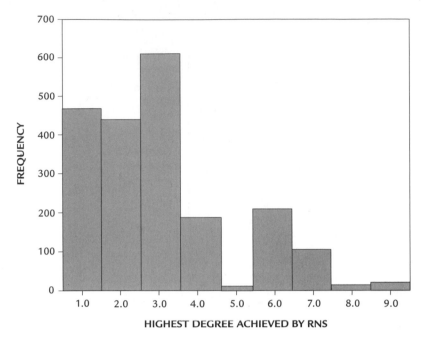

FIGURE 1-13. Relative frequency distribution of the highest degree achieved by registered nurses. (Data from Fry, S., & Duffy, M. [2000]. *Ethics and Human Rights in Nursing Practice: A Study of New England Registered Nurses.* Chestnut Hill, MA: Nursing Ethics Network & The Center for Nursing Research, Boston College.)

GENERAL SUGGESTIONS FOR CONSTRUCTING CHARTS

The purpose of a chart is to promote understanding without distorting the facts; therefore, the chart should make the desired point *honestly*. Because gross misuses of charts are not generally found in respected research journals, some researchers believe that they need not pay attention to the construction of their charts because editors and reviewers will tell them how to fix the charts. This is not true: Read some of the references cited on developing charts, and follow their advice to avoid having your research report rejected.

Wallgren et al. (1996) advise researchers to ask themselves the following questions after completing a chart:

- **Is the chart easy to read?** Simplicity is the hallmark of a good chart. What you want to display in a chart should be quickly and clearly evident. Keep in mind the target audience for whom you are constructing the chart. Keep grid lines and tick marks to a minimum. Avoid odd lettering and ornate patterns (Schmid, 1983).
- **Is the chart in the right place?** Locate the chart close to the place in the text where the topic is discussed. Make sure the chart is well positioned on the page.
- **Does the chart benefit from being in color (if color is used)?** Color should have a purpose; it should not be used solely for decorative reasons.
- **Have you tried the chart out on anybody?** Try the chart out on someone whom you consider to correspond to the target group before you make the

final diagram. Ask that person questions about the chart to gain information on how the person perceives the chart.

Wallgren et al. offer the caveat that "a poor chart is worse than no chart at all" (1996, p. 89).

SUMMARY

The first steps toward understanding data are univariate analyses. The researcher should study each variable separately by means of tables and charts. The type of table or chart varies according to the type of measurement scale. For nominal variables, the table should be a simple listing of categories with corresponding frequencies and percentages, and the bar chart is appropriate for graphic display. For interval or ratio variables, it may be necessary first to group the data into appropriate numeric intervals before constructing a frequency table, histogram, or polygon. For ordinal variables, the researcher must decide whether the values should be treated as nominal data or as continuous (interval or ratio) data. Once this decision has been made, the researcher can then apply the rules for either nominal or interval and ratio variables. The best tables and charts are self-explanatory and present data in a clear and straightforward manner.

Application Exercises and Results

General Introduction

Appendix G contains a survey instrument that was developed at Boston College's William F. Connell School of Nursing for doctoral students to gather data for use in a statistics class. Each student is responsible for getting 10 people to fill out the questionnaire. Students are asked to have variety in terms of the respondents' gender, age, and so forth. We also ask them to try to minimize missing data by checking questionnaires for completeness.

The students then enter the data from their 10 subjects into a data file, called a *dataset*. They examine a printout of file information, run frequencies, and examine the output carefully to be sure they have entered their data correctly. The students make corrections as necessary, and then their data files are merged and we provide them with a large dataset they can use for all their homework assignments.

The CD at the back of this book contains data collected by these students on 701 respondents. If the same survey is used for several years, a fairly substantial dataset can be developed. The reader may use our survey form, collect data, and add it to the dataset we have provided.

When the students collect and enter data and then clean the datasets, they achieve a much better understanding of data and how to manage it. Although our students use their dataset for all homework exercises, other large datasets that we get from researchers in the school are used for the midterm and final exams. Each student is provided with data from a randomly drawn subset of one of these large datasets. Thus, each student has a slightly different sample of respondents but the same variables so they can answer the same questions on the exam. Their answers will differ because they have different cases in their sample dataset.

The major dataset for the exercises throughout the book is named MUNRO04.SAV and was created in SPSS for Windows, version 12.0. For the purpose of this book, we have posed specific research questions for students to answer. In our courses, however, we often just ask the students to state a research question or hypothesis that can be answered using their dataset and the statistical technique being studied that week. They then run the analysis and write up the results. We have found that students need more guidance in how to write the results in a manner that would be acceptable for a research journal than in how to run the analysis. We have not provided step-by-step guidance in the use of statistical software for several reasons: so many statistical packages are available, students are more computer literate today, and statistics software is very user-friendly. When we first began teaching doctoral students how to use SPSS for Windows several years ago, it took a full-day workshop to accomplish this task. Now, it takes students about 1 hour to use later versions of SPSS for Windows.

Exercises

1. Access the dataset called MUNRO04.SAV, which contains data collected using the survey form contained in Appendix G. Either bring it into SPSS or convert it into a file for SAS or whatever software you are using. Print the dictionary, which contains a list of the variables, formats, and labels. In most versions of SPSS for Windows, this is done by clicking on Utilities, then on File Info. Once the file is in the output screen, it can be printed from the File menu.

2. Compare the file information with the survey form in Appendix G. Note that the variable names have been selected to reflect each variable, making it easy to recognize them when working with the file. Variable labels and value labels have been added to enhance the output. Look for any discrepancies between the survey form and the file information.

3. Produce charts/graphs. Many options are available for producing charts in statistical software programs. They may be produced within specific techniques and in separate graphics sections. We will confine ourselves to requesting graphics that are available with the specific techniques. The following can be requested as part of the output from frequencies in most software programs. Within the frequencies program, request a bar graph for GENDER, a histogram for SATCURWT, and a histogram with a polygon (normal curve) for SATCURWT.

Results

1. Exercise Figure 1-1 contains a portion of the dictionary.

2. If you look carefully, you should note the following:
   a. Compared to what is printed in the survey form in Appendix G, the value labels for the following items from the Inventory of Personal Attitudes (IPPA) have been reversed: 1, 2, 4, 6, 8, 13, 15, 20, 22, 24, 27, and 29. This had to be done to prepare these items for scoring the scale. For example, look at item 1. On the questionnaire, we see that a very high level of energy is scored 1 and a very low level is scored 7. Because the inventory measures positive attitudes, the originators (Kass et al., 1991) reversed this item before adding it to the scale. We have already done the reverse-scoring for you. We recoded all of these items so that 1 = 7, 2 = 6, 3 = 5, 4 = 4, 5 = 3, 6 = 2, and 7 = 1. Thus, with item 1, if someone checked a 1, it would now be scored a 7. We also reversed the value labels to reflect the new scoring.

      If you add your own data to our dataset, recode these items and be sure the value labels are correct **before** adding them to our dataset. If you add your data to the dataset first, then reverse-score the IPPA items, you will also change the previously reverse-scored items back to their original, unreversed-score values.

   b. Three "extra" variables are listed in the dictionary. These new variables follow the 30 IPPA items.

```
                     List of variables on the working file
Name                                                             Position

CODE          subject's identification number                        1
              Print Format: F3
              Write Format: F3

GENDER        gender                                                  2
              Print Format: F1
              Write Format: F1

              Value     Label
                 0      male
                 1      female

AGE           subject's age                                          3
              Print Format: F3
              Write Format: F3

MARITAL       marital status                                         4
              Print Format: F1
              Write Format: F1

              Value     Label
                 1      Never Married
                 2      Married
                 3      Living with Significant Other
                 4      Separated
                 5      Widowed
                 6      Divorced
```

```
DEPRESS       depressed state of mind                                9
              Print Format: F1
              Write Format: F1

              Value     Label
                 1      Rarely
                 2      Sometimes
                 3      Often
                 4      Routinely
```

```
IPA1          energy level                                          19
              Print Format: F8
              Write Format: F8

              Value     Label
                 1      very low
                 7      very high

IPA2          reaction to pressure                                  20

              Print Format: F1
              Write Format: F1

              Value     Label
                 1      I get tense
                 7      I remain calm
```

EXERCISE FIGURE 1-1. A portion of the SPSS dictionary.

FREQUENCIES
   VARIABLES=marital
   /BARCHART   FREQ
   /ORDER=   ANALYSIS

Frequencies

Statistics

MARITAL marital status

N	Valid	688
	Missing	13

MARITAL marital status

		Frequency	Percent	Valid Percent	Cumulative Percent
Valid	1 never married	230	32.8	33.4	33.4
	2 married	346	49.4	50.3	83.7
	3 living with significant other	44	6.3	6.4	90.1
	4 separated	13	1.9	1.9	92.0
	5 widowed	20	2.9	2.9	94.9
	6 divorced	35	5.0	5.1	100.0
	Total	688	98.3	100.0	
Missing System		13	1.7		
Total		701	100.0		

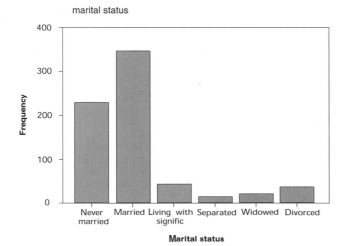

EXERCISE FIGURE 1-2. Frequencies for marital status (MARITAL) and bar graph.

FREQUENCIES
  VARIABLES=qolcur
  /HISTOGRAM
  /ORDER=   ANALYSIS

Frequencies

Statistics

QOLCUR quality of life in past month

N	Valid	699
	Missing	2

QOLCUR quality of life in past month

		Frequency	Percent	Valid Percent	Cumulative Percent
Valid	1 very dissatisfied, unhappy most of time	8	1.1	1.1	1.1
	2 generally dissatisfied, unhappy	27	3.9	3.9	5.0
	3 sometimes fairly satisfied, sometimes fairly unhappy	113	16.1	16.2	21.2
	4 generally satisfied, pleased	238	34.0	34.0	55.2
	5 very happy most of time	245	35.0	35.1	90.3
	6 extremely happy, could not be more pleased	68	9.7	9.7	100.0
	Total	699	99.7	100.0	
Missing System		2	.3		
Total		701	100.0		

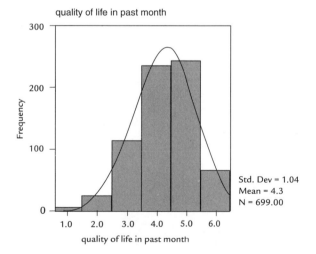

EXERCISE FIGURE 1-3. Frequencies for quality of life in the past month (QOLCUR) and two histograms.

CONFID is the sum of the following IPPA items: 2, 5, 7, 10, 14, 15, 16, 17, 18, 22, 24, 26, and 29. It is defined as self-confidence during stressful situations. Because it includes 13 items and each item is rated on a scale from 1 to 7, the potential range of scores for CONFID is 13 to 91.

LIFE is the sum of the following IPPA items: 1, 3, 4, 6, 8, 9, 11, 12, 13, 19, 20, 21, 23, 25, 27, 28, and 30. It is defined as life purpose and satisfaction and includes 17 items, with a potential range of scores of 17 to 119.

IPPATOT is the sum of all 30 items and is the total score on the IPPA. The potential range of scores is 30 to 210.

3. Exercise Figure 1-2 contains the frequencies for marital status (MARITAL) and its associated bar graph. Exercise Figure 1-3 contains the frequencies for quality of life in the past month (QOLCUR), and the histogram with the normal curve superimposed.

Univariate Descriptive Statistics

Mary E. Duffy and
Barbara S. Jacobsen

Objectives for Chapter 2

After reading this chapter, you should be able to do the following:

1. Define measures of central tendency and dispersion.
2. Select the appropriate measures to use for a particular dataset.
3. Discuss methods to identify and manage outliers.
4. Discuss methods to handle missing data.

Although charts may bring facts to life vividly, the information they present for our inspection is often inexact. Frequency distribution tables provide many details, but often a researcher will want to condense a distribution further. After the data have been organized, quantitative measures are frequently calculated to capture the essence of the four basic characteristics of a distribution: central tendency, variability, skewness, and kurtosis. These statistics may be used not only in a descriptive summary, but also in statistical inference.

Symbols and formulas for descriptive statistics vary depending on whether one is describing a sample or a population. As mentioned in Chapter 1, a population includes all members of a defined group; a sample is a subset of a population. Characteristics of populations are called *parameters*; characteristics of samples are called *statistics*. To distinguish between them, different sets of symbols are used. Usually, lowercase Greek letters are used to denote parameters, and Roman letters are used to denote statistics.

MEASURES OF CENTRAL TENDENCY

The typical value of a variable is summarized using measures of central tendency. These statistics, commonly called *averages,* describe where the values of a variable's distribution cluster. The most commonly reported measures of central tendency are the *mean*, the *median*, and the *mode*.

Mean

The *mean*, the best known and most widely used average, describes the center of a frequency distribution. The mean of a sample[1] is represented symbolically by $\overline{X}$, which is read "X bar." Many journals simply use "M" to represent the mean.

To compute the mean, add up all the values in the distribution and divide by the number of values. Expressed as a formula, the sample mean is defined as:

$$M = \Sigma X/N$$

The uppercase Greek letter sigma (Σ) means "the sum of." If the letter X represents a single quantitative value in a distribution, then ΣX means "sum up all the values."

For example, the following list of values for length of stay (in hours) in the hospital in the past year for a sample of older women has 10 entries: 8, 10, 10, 18, 24, 29, 36, 48, 60, 72. The mean is:

$$8 + 10 + 10 + 18 + 24 + 29 + 36 + 48 + 60 + 72 = 315/10$$
$$= 31.5 \text{ hours}$$

In this example, the mean is located near the middle of the 10 values. It is clear from the formula and the example that each value in the distribution contributes to the mean. Because the mean is influenced by all of the data points, it is not appropriate as a descriptive statistic for a variable when not all the data points are known. For instance, not everyone with cancer will have a recurrence of that disease; therefore, some of the values of the variable "time to recurrence" may be absent or "censored."

Any extreme values in the distribution also influence the mean. For example, in the previous distribution relating to length of stay in hours in the hospital for the group of older women, suppose the value of 72 hours was instead 224 hours. The new mean would be

$$8 + 10 + 10 + 18 + 24 + 29 + 36 + 48 + 60 + 224 = 467/10$$
$$= 46.7 \text{ hours}$$

This mean would not be located in the middle of the 10 values; only three women would have a length of hospital stay greater than the mean. Thus, the mean works best as an average for symmetrical frequency distributions that have a single peak, more commonly called a normal distribution.

---

[1]The mean of a population (N) is represented by the lowercase Greek letter mu (μ). The formula is the same as that for the sample mean.

TABLE 2-1 *Demonstration of Several Important Properties of the Mean*

X	X − M	(X − M)²
4	4 − 6 = −2	(−2)² = 4
4	4 − 6 = −2	(−2)² = 4
10	10 − 6 = +4	(+4)² = 16
5	5 − 6 = −1	(−1)² = 1
7	7 − 6 = +1	(+1)² = 1
ΣX = 30	Σ(X − M) = 0	Σ(X − M)² = 26
N = 5		sum of squares
M = 6		

The mean has several other interesting properties. First, for any distribution, the sum of the deviations of the values from the mean always equals zero. This helps to explain why the mean is the center of a distribution. Table 2-1 demonstrates this property. The mean (6) is subtracted from each value to form *deviations* (X − M). These deviations from the mean sum to zero. If any value other than the mean is subtracted from each value, the sum of the deviations will not be zero.

A second property of the mean relates to the sum of the squared deviations—that is, $\Sigma(X - M)^2$. In Table 2-1, each of the deviations from the mean has been squared, and the sum of these squared deviations equals 26. This sum, called the *sum of squares* in statistics, is at a minimum; that is, it is smaller than the sum of squares around any other value. If any value other than the mean (6) is subtracted from each value and squared, the total will exceed 26. This characteristic of the mean underlies the idea of *least squares*, which is important in later chapters.

Third, because the mean has a formula, it is algebraic and can be manipulated in equations. For example, if two or more means are available from samples of different sizes, a mean of the total group can be calculated. By transposing terms in the formula for the mean, the following shows that the sum of the values is equal to the mean multiplied by the size of the sample.

$$\Sigma X = Mn$$

Therefore, a formula for a combined mean for two samples (which can be easily extended to include more than two samples), weighted according to sample size, logically follows:

$$M_{total} = M_1 n_1 + M_2 n_2 / n_1 + n_2$$

Finally, when repeatedly drawing random samples from the same population, means will vary less among themselves and less from the true population mean than other measures of central tendency. Thus, the mean is the most reliable average when making inferences from a sample to a population.

The mean is intended for interval or ratio variables when values can be added, but many times it is also sensible for ordinal variables. Computer programs, however, will compute means for nominal level variables, reporting such uninterpretable results for a sample as "the mean gender = 0.75."

Median

The median, the middle value of a set of ordered numbers, is the point or value below which 50% of the distribution falls. Thus, 50% of the sample will be below the median regardless of the shape of the distribution. The median is sometimes called the 50th percentile and symbolized as P_{50}. It may also be conceived as the bisector of the total area of the histogram or polygon. There is no algebraic formula for the median, just a procedure:

1. Arrange the values in order.
2. If the total number of values is odd, count up (or down) to the middle value. If there are several identical values clustered at the middle, the median is that value.
3. If the total number of values is even, compute the mean of the middle values.

In the previous example relating to length of stay of older women in the hospital, the 10 values, arranged in order, were 8, 10, 10, 18, 24, 29, 36, 48, 60, 72. Counting to the center of these 10 entries (an even number), the two middle values are 24 and 29. Thus, the median is (24 + 29)/2 = 26.5. Note that the mean for these data was 31.5, slightly higher than the median.

From the procedure, it is clear that every value does not enter into the computation of the median; only the number of values and the values near the midpoint of the distribution enter the computation. If the value of 72 is changed to 224 in the previous example, the new distribution is 8, 10, 10, 18, 24, 29, 36, 48, 60, 224. The median of this distribution is still located midway between 24 and 29 and is still 26.5 hours. Thus, the median is not sensitive to extreme scores. It may be used with symmetrical or asymmetrical distributions, but is especially useful when the data are skewed. However, this property of not summarizing all values in a distribution is also the median's chief shortcoming: it means that the median cannot be algebraically derived. The median merely represents the point in a distribution below which 50% of the scores fall.

The median is appropriate for interval or ratio data and for ordinal data but not for nominal data. It can be used for open-end or censored data, such as "time to recurrence," if more than half of the sample has contributed a value to the distribution.

Mode

The mode, the most frequent value or category in a distribution, is not calculated but is simply spotted by inspecting the values in a distribution. In the previous example of length of hospital stay in hours, the 10 entries were 8, 10, 10, 18, 24, 29, 36, 48, 60, and 72. The mode for this distribution is 10 because that score occurs most frequently.

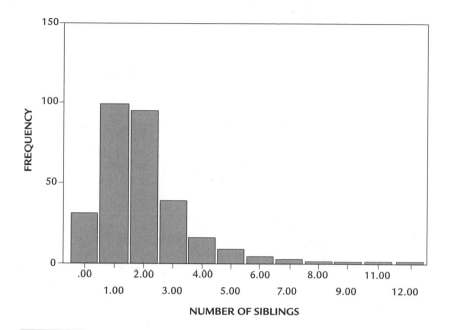

FIGURE 2-1. Relative frequency distribution of number of siblings a child has. (Data collected with a grant funded by the National Institute of Nursing Research, R01 NR04838-01A2. P.I., Vessey, J. (2000). *Development of the CATS: Child-Adolescent Teasing Scale.* The William F. Connell School of Nursing, Boston College.)

If all scores in a distribution are different, the mode does not exist. If several values occur with equal frequency, then there are several modes. If the values of a distribution cluster in several places but with unequal frequency, then there are primary and secondary modes. For example, when discussing the bar chart showing the frequency distribution of number of siblings a child has in Fig. 2-1, it is helpful to note that the primary mode was 1 (the midpoint of the second bar) with a secondary mode of 2 (the midpoint of the third bar). Alternatively, the primary mode for Fig. 2-1 could be reported as 1 sibling and the secondary mode 2 siblings.

For strictly nominal-level variables, the mode is the only appropriate measure of central tendency. It is reported as the modal category. For instance, in Fig. 2-2, the modal category for data collection site is "Albuquerque, NM."

The mode can also be used with interval, ratio, or ordinal variables as a rough estimate of central tendency. Obtaining the mode for numeric data consists of noting which value occurs most frequently. The modal value is the most frequently occurring actual value in the distribution, not the value that has the largest frequency of scores.

Comparison of Measures of Central Tendency

The mean is the most common measure of central tendency. It has a formula and is the most trustworthy estimate of a population average. Generally, researchers prefer

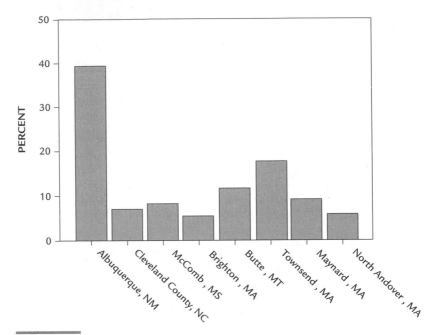

FIGURE 2-2. Data collection site, $N = 764$. (Data collected with a grant funded by the National Institute of Nursing Research, R01 NR04838. P.I., Vessey, J. (2000). *Development of the CATS: Child-Adolescent Teasing Scale.* The William F. Connell School of Nursing, Boston College.)

to use the mean, unless there is a good reason for not doing so. The most compelling reason for not using the mean is a distribution that is badly skewed. The effect of extreme values on the mean diminishes as the size of the sample increases; therefore, another good reason for not using the mean is a small sample with a few extreme values. The mean is best when used with distributions that are reasonably symmetrical and that have one mode.

The median is easy to understand as the 50th percentile of a distribution or the bisector of the area of a histogram. It has no formula but is calculated by a counting procedure, and is usually produced by statistical computer programs. The median may be used with distributions of any shape but is especially useful with very non-symmetrical distributions because it is not sensitive to skewness.

The main use of the mode is for calling attention to a distribution in which the values cluster at one or more places. It can also be used for making rough estimates. In addition, the mode is the only measure of central tendency available for nominal data.

When a distribution has only one mode and is symmetrical, the mean, median, and mode will have, or very nearly have, the same value. In a skewed, or nonsymmetrical, distribution like that in Fig. 2-3, the mode is the value under the high point of the polygon, the mean is pulled to the right by the extreme values in the tail of the distribution, and the median usually falls in between. Thus, if the mean is greater than the median, then the distribution is *positively skewed*, with the mean being

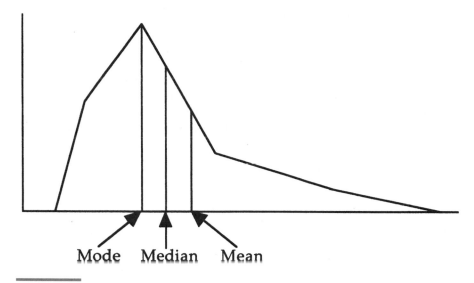

FIGURE 2-3. Sketch of frequency polygon for a distribution skewed to the right, indicating the relative positions of mean, median, and mode.

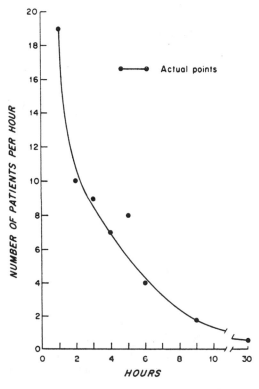

FIGURE 2-4. Graph illustrating a distribution (rate at which patients seek medical care for coronary symptoms as a function of time from onset of symptoms) in which mean, median, and mode are quite different. (From Hackett, T. P., & Cassem, N. H. [1969]. Factors contributing to delay in responding to the signs and symptoms of acute myocardial infarction. *American Journal of Cardiology, 24,* 653. With permission from Excerpta Medica Inc.) Mean, 10.6 hours; median, 4 hours; mode, 1 hour.

dragged to the right by a few high scores. If the mean is less than the median, then the distribution is *negatively skewed*, with the mean being pulled to the left by a small number of low scores.

Weisberg (1992) points out that it is not always necessary to select only a single measure of central tendency because these statistics provide different information. Sometimes it is useful to examine multiple aspects of a distribution. An example from a research journal is presented in Fig. 2-4. In this case, the mode for delay in seeking treatment was 1 hour, the median was 4 hours, and the mean was 10.6 hours. If the objective of reporting an average is to present a fair view of the data, consider which average (or averages) should be used here.

MEASURES OF VARIABILITY OR SCATTER

Reporting only an average without an accompanying measure of variability, or dispersion, is a good way to misrepresent a set of data. A common story in statistics classes tells of the woman who had her head in an oven and her feet in a bucket of ice water. When asked how she felt, the reply was, "On the average, I feel fine." Researchers tend to focus on measures of central tendency and neglect how the data are scattered, but variability is at least equally important (Tulman & Jacobsen, 1989). Two datasets can have the same average but very different variabilities (Fig. 2-5). If scores in a distribution are similar, they are *homogeneous* (having low variability); if scores are not similar, they are *heterogeneous* (having high variability).

The three measures of variability discussed in this text are the standard deviation (SD), range, and interpercentile measures. Unlike averages, which are points

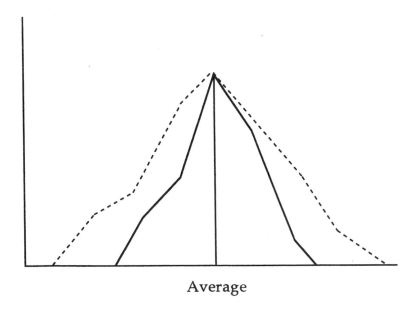

Average

FIGURE 2-5. Two frequency distributions with equal averages but different variabilities.

X	X − M	(X − M)²
8	8 − 31.5 = −23.5	(−23.5)² = 552.25
10	10 − 31.5 = −21.5	(−21.5)² = 462.25
10	10 − 31.5 = −21.5	(−21.5)² = 462.25
18	18 − 31.5 = −13.5	(−13.5)² = 182.25
24	24 − 31.5 = − 7.5	(− 7.5)² = 56.25
29	29 − 31.5 = − 2.5	(− 2.5)² = 6.25
36	36 − 31.5 = + 4.5	(+ 4.5)² = 20.25
48	48 − 31.5 = +16.5	(+16.5)² = 272.25
60	60 − 31.5 = +28.5	(+28.5)² = 812.25
72	72 − 31.5 = +40.5	(+40.5)² = 1640.25
ΣX = 315	Σ(X − M) = 0	Σ(X − M)² = 4466.50 = Sum of squares

TABLE 2-2 *Demonstration of the Calculation of the Sample Standard Deviation for Length of Stay (in Hours) in the Hospital for a Sample of Older Women*

M = 31.5

Variance = 4466.50/9 = 496.28 square hours

SD = Square root of 496.3 = 22.28 hours

representing a central value, measures of variability should be interpreted as distances on a scale of values.

Standard Deviation

This is the most widely used measure of variability. The sample[2] SD is defined as:

$$SD = \text{square Root of } \Sigma(X − M)^2/n − 1$$

The reason for dividing by the quantity (n − 1) involves a theoretical consideration called *degrees of freedom*. This concept is discussed later in this text. Briefly, it can be shown that using (n −1) produces, for a random sample, an unbiased estimate of a population variance. This consideration assumes more importance with small samples.

Table 2-2 illustrates the calculation of the SD for the list of 10 values for the variable "length of stay in the hospital" for a sample of older women. The first step is to calculate the mean and then subtract it from each value, making sure that the sum

[2]The SD of a population is represented symbolically by the lowercase Greek letter sigma (σ). The formula differs from the sample SD in that the denominator is simply N, not n − 1.

of the deviations is zero. Next, each deviation is squared. The sum of the squared deviations (or sum of squares) is then divided by (n − 1). This quantity is called the *variance*. Although it is a measure of variability, the variance is not used as a descriptive statistic because it is not in the same unit as the data. For example, the variance of the data in Table 2-2 is 496.28 square hours. Most people would have difficulty interpreting a "square hour." Therefore, the square root is taken to return the statistic to its original scale of measurement. The resulting statistic of 22.28 hours is the SD. Again, as with the mean, it is clear that every value in the distribution enters into the calculation of the SD. It is also clear from the formula that the SD is a measure of variability around the mean. The formula in Table 2-2 provides the basic understanding of the SD.

The SD, like the mean, is sensitive to extreme values. For example, in Table 2-2, if the value of 72 is changed to 224, the new SD is 35.15 hours, a large inflation from the original SD of 22.28 hours. Therefore, the SD serves best for distributions that are symmetrical and have a single peak. In general, if it is appropriate to calculate the mean, then it is appropriate to calculate the SD.

The SD has a straightforward interpretation if the distribution is bell-shaped or normal (the normal curve is discussed in detail in the next chapter). If the distribution is perfectly bell-shaped, 68% of the values are within 1 SD of the mean, 95% of the values are within 2 SD of the mean, and more than 99% of the data will be within 3 SD of the mean. For example, Table 2-3 displays the basic statistics for the approximately bell-shaped distribution of a set of denial scores from a sample of 152 heart attack patients. The mean for the denial scale is 46.5, and the SD is 16.4. To determine the range of patients falling ±1 SD from the mean, you subtract the SD from the mean to determine the lower limit (46.5 − 16.4 = 30.1) and add the SD to the mean to determine the upper limit (46.5 + 16.4 = 62.9). After rounding

TABLE 2-3 *Descriptive Statistics Produced by SPSS for a set of Denial Scores From a Sample of 152 Heart Attack Patients*

Program

FREQUENCIES VARIABLES = DENIAL/FORMAT. = NOTABLE/STATISTICS = ALL.

Output

Mean	46.533	Std err	1.328	Median	45.500
Mode	45.000	SD	16.374	Variance	286.092
Kurtosis	−.249	S E Kurt	.391	Skewness	.195
S E Skew	.197	Range	76.000	Minimum	11.000
Maximum	87.000	Sum	7073.000		
Valid cases	152	Missing cases	0		

Jacobsen, B. S., & Lowery, B. J. (1992). Further analysis of the psychometric properties of the Levine Denial of Illness Scale. *Psychosomatic Medicine, 54,* 372–381.

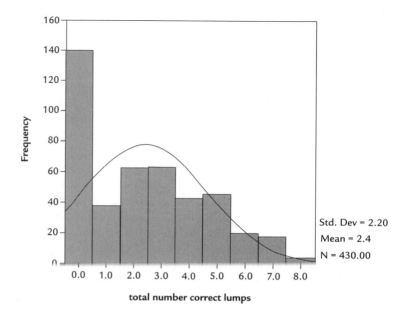

FIGURE 2-6. Number of correct breast lumps identified by a sample of 246 older Black women. (Data from Wood, R. Y. [1997]. The development and testing of video breast health kits for older women. National Cancer Institute Small Business Innovation Research (SBIR) Phase II R43 CA 63935-02.)

to whole numbers, 46 of the 152 heart attack patients, or 68% of the sample, had denial scores ranging from 30 to 63 and falling within 1 SD of the mean on the denial scale.

Even if the distribution is not perfectly symmetrical, however, this percentage holds fairly well. Chebyshev's theorem maintains that even in oddly shaped distributions, at least 75% of the data will fall within 2 SD of the mean (Freund, 1988). Figure 2-6 displays a positively skewed distribution, with a mean of 2.4 and an SD of 2.2. By actual count, about 87% of the values lie within the interval of mean ±1 SD. Because this distribution is decidedly not bell-shaped, the percentage in this interval is different from the expected 68%. Subtracting 2 SD from the mean of 2.4 leads to the absurd conclusion that some older women had a −2.0 correct identification of breast lumps score!

Because the SD, like the mean, is algebraic, formulas have been developed for combining SD from several distributions with different sample sizes to compare measures of variability across different samples from different studies. The *coefficient of variation* (CV) is a useful statistic for comparing SD between several investigations examining the same variable (Daniel, 1987). This statistic is defined as:

$$CV = 100 \ (SD/\overline{X}) \ \text{or} \ 100 \ (SD/m)$$

Because the CV expresses the SD as a percentage of the mean value, it lets the researcher compare the variability of different variables (Norusis, 2002). For example, Spielberger (1983) reported the following statistics on the State-Trait Anxiety Inventory for a sample of depressed patients: mean = 54.43 and SD = 13.02. For general medical or surgical patients without depression, the statistics were: mean = 42.68 and SD = 13.76. The CV for the depressed group was 24%; the

CV for the nondepressed group was 32%. Thus, the nondepressed group was more variable relative to their mean than the depressed group.

Range

The range, the simplest measure of variability, is the difference between the maximum value of the distribution and the minimum value. In Table 2-2, the range is $72 - 8 = 64$. If the range is reported in a research journal, it would ordinarily be given as a maximum and a minimum, without the subtracted value.

The range can be unstable because it is based on only two values in the distribution and because it tends to increase with sample size. It is sensitive to extreme values. For example, in Table 2-2, if the single value of 72 is changed to 224, the range would then be $224 - 8 = 216$, a tremendous increase.

The main use of the range is for making a quick estimate of variability, but it can be informative in certain situations. For example, a health researcher who is considering subgroup analyses may be interested in knowing the most extreme values in a particular variable's distribution. A researcher who intends to report the SD may also choose to report the range for the additional information it provides about the two endpoints of a distribution.

Interpercentile Measures

A *percentile* is a score value above which and below which a certain percentage of values in a distribution fall (Norusis, 2002). Percentiles are symbolized by the letter *P*, with a subscript indicating the percentage below the score value. Hence, P_{60} refers to the 60th percentile and stands for the score below which 60% of values fall. The statement "$P_{40} = 55$" means that 40% of the values in the distribution fall below the score 55.

Percentiles allow us to describe a score in relation to other scores in a distribution. The 25th percentile is called the *first quartile*; the 50th percentile, the *second quartile* or more commonly the *median*; and the 75th percentile, the *third quartile*. A score is not said to fall within a quartile, because the quartile is only one point. Therefore, the third quartile is not from 50 to 75; it is just the 75th percentile.

There are several interpercentile measures of variability, the most common being the *interquartile range* (IQR). The IQR is defined as the range of the values extending from the 25th percentile to the 75th percentile. To locate the first quartile, first locate the median of the distribution. The first quartile is the middle value of all the data points below the median; the third quartile is the middle value of all the data points above the median. In the previous example, the set of ordered values was 8, 10, 10, 18, 24, 29, 36, 48, 60, 72. The 50th percentile was noted to be 26.5; there are five values below 26.5. The median of those five values is 10, and the median of the five values above the 50th percentile is 48. Thus, the IQR is 48 to 10.

Other frequently used interpercentile ranges are (P_{10} to P_{90}) and (P_3 to P_{97}). The latter interpercentile range identifies the middle 94% of a distribution, a percentage similar to that identified in a bell-shaped distribution by the mean ± 2 SD. Table 2-4

TABLE 2-4 *Selected Percentiles Produced by SPSS 12.0 for the Data in FIGURE 2-6; Number of Correct Breast Lumps Identified by Older Black Women (N = 246).(Data from Wood, R. Y. [1997]. The development and testing of video breast health kits for older women. National Cancer Institute Small Business Innovation Research (SBIR) Phase II R43 CA 63935-02.)*

Frequencies

ACLUMPS

Statistics
Total Number of Correct Lumps

N	*Valid*	*430*
	Missing	*9*
Percentiles	10	.0000
	20	.0000
	30	.0000
	40	1.0000
	50	2.0000
	60	3.0000
	70	3.0000
	80	4.0000
	90	5.0000

contains a printout of selected computer percentiles for the variable, number of correct breast lumps identified by a sample of older Black women.

These interpercentile ranges, like the median, are not sensitive to extreme values. If a distribution is badly skewed and the researcher judges that the median (P_{50}) is the appropriate average, then the IQR (or other interpercentile measure) is also appropriate. One of the most common uses of interpercentile measures is for growth charts.

Comparison of Measures of Variability

The SD is the most widely reported measure of variability. It has a formula and is the most reliable estimate of population variability. Generally, researchers prefer to use the SD, unless there is a good reason for not doing so. Like the mean, the most compelling reason for not using the SD is a distribution that has extreme values. The SD is best with distributions that are reasonably symmetrical and have only one mode.

The main uses of the range are to call attention to the two extreme values of a distribution and for quick, rough estimates of variability. The range has a serious shortcoming as a measure of variability because it is greatly influenced by sample size. Because the range is determined by only the smallest and largest values in a distribution, other things being equal, the larger the sample, the larger the range (Glass & Hopkins, 1996).

Interpercentile measures are easy to understand. In a histogram, they mark off a certain percentage of area around the median. For example, the IQR, extending from P_{25} to P_{75}, delineates the middle 50% of a distribution. These measures have no formulas but are calculated by a counting procedure. They can be used with distributions of any shape but are especially useful with very skewed distributions.

To choose the appropriate measures of variability, the researcher must know how a set of scores on a variable is distributed. All of the above measures of variability are intended for use with interval or ratio variables, and often they are sensible for ordinal values. There are no measures of variability for nominal data in common use (Weisberg, 1992).

MEASURES OF SKEWNESS OR SYMMETRY

In addition to central tendency and variability, *symmetry* is an important characteristic of a distribution. A *normal distribution* is *symmetrical* and bell-shaped, having only one mode. When a variable's distribution is asymmetrical, it is skewed. A skewed variable is one whose mean is not in the center of the distribution. If there is positive skewness, there is a pileup of cases to the left and the right tail of the distribution is too long. Negative skewness results in a pileup of cases to the right and a too-long left tail (Tabachnick & Fidell, 2001).

Two sets of data can have the same mean and SD but different skewness (see Fig. 2-5). Two measures of symmetry are considered here: Pearson's measure and Fisher's measure. Although rarely mentioned in research reports, these statistics are very useful in determining the degree of symmetry of a variable's distribution. Researchers routinely compute them using statistics produced when running frequency distributions and descriptive statistics on study variables.

Pearson's Skewness Coefficient

This measure of skewness is nonalgebraic but is easily calculated and is useful for quick estimates of symmetry. It is defined as:

$$\text{Skewness} = (\text{mean} - \text{median})/\text{SD}$$

For a perfectly symmetrical distribution, the mean will equal the median, and the skewness coefficient will be 0. If the distribution is positively skewed, as in Fig. 2-1, the mean will be more than the median, and the coefficient will be positive. If the coefficient is negative, the distribution is negatively skewed, and the mean will be less than the median. In general, skewness values will fall between -1 and $+1$ SD units. Values falling outside this range indicate a substantially skewed distribution (Hair et al., 1998). Hildebrand (1986) states that skewness values above 0.2 or below -0.2 indicate severe skewness.

For the denial score data of Table 2-3, the skewness coefficient is $(46.53 - 45.50)/16.37$. The resulting value of 0.06 is close to zero. Using Hildebrand's guideline, the value of 0.06 indicates minor, not severe, skewness. The reader should verify this result visually by means of the chart of the denial score data in Fig. 2-7.

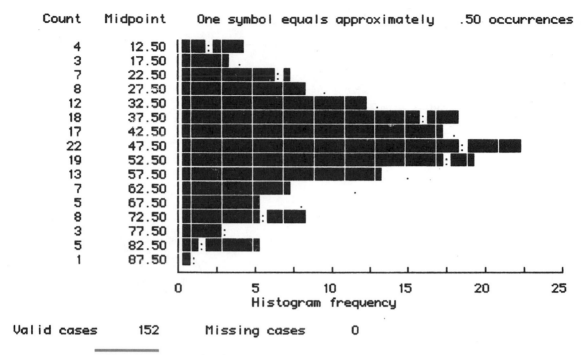

Count   Midpoint   One symbol equals approximately   .50 occurrences

FIGURE 2-7. Example of a histogram produced by SPSS: Denial scores from a sample of 152 heart attack patients. (Jacobsen, B., & Lowery, B. [1992]. Further analysis of the psychometric characteristics of the Levine Denial of Illness Scale. *Psychosomatic Medicine, 54,* 372–381.)

It is a different story for the negatively skewed data in Fig. 2-8. The SF-36 transformed mental health score mean for that distribution is 79.7, the median is 84.0, and the SD is 18.5. Therefore, Pearson's coefficient is (79.7 − 84.0)/18.5, producing a value of −0.23, indicating severe negative skewness.

Fisher's Measure of Skewness

The formula for Fisher's skewness statistic, found in Hildebrand (1986), is based on deviations from the mean to the third power. A symmetrical curve will result in a value of 0. If the skewness value is positive, then the curve is skewed to the right, and vice versa for a distribution skewed to the left. For the denial score data in Table 2-3, Fisher's skewness measure is 0.195. The measure of skewness can be interpreted in terms of the normal curve. (This concept is explained further in the next chapter.) A z-score is calculated by dividing the measure of skewness by the standard error for skewness (0.195/0.197 = 0.99). Values above +1.96 or below −1.96 are significant at the 0.05 level because 95% of the scores in a normal distribution fall between +1.96 and −1.96 SD from the mean. Our value of 0.99 indicates that this distribution is not significantly skewed. Because this statistic is based on deviations to the third power, it is very sensitive to extreme values.

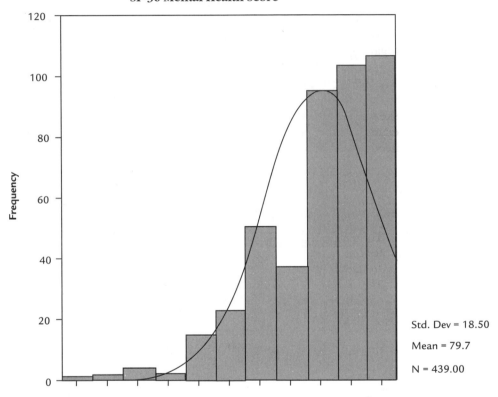

Statistics

TMH

N	Valid	439
	Missing	0
Mean		79.7267
Median		84.0000
Std. Deviation		18.50085

SF-36 Mental Health Score

Std. Dev = 18.50

Mean = 79.7

N = 439.00

FIGURE 2-8. Example of a histogram produced by SPSS 12.0 for Windows: SF-36 transformed mental health scores from a sample of 439 older women. (Data from Wood, R. Y. [1997]. The development and testing of video breast health kits for older women. National Cancer Institute Small Business Innovation Research (SBIR) Phase II R43 CA 63935-02.)

Types of Data Transformations

Markedly skewed data indicate that the mean is not a good measure of central tendency of scores in the distribution. It is often possible to transform the skewed data so that the new scores display normality and equality of variances. Because variables differ in the extent to which they deviate from normal, Tabachnick and Fidell (2001) recommend the following:

- For moderate skewness, use a square root transformation.
- For substantial skewness, use a log transformation.
- For severe skewness, use an inverse transformation.

Although these authors do not define "moderate," "substantial," and "severe," a practical approach is to start with a square root transformation and see if that results in a more normally distributed variable. If not, then proceed to use a log transformation on the original variable and so on, always checking to see if the transformation reduces the skewness problem. If it does, then use the transformed variable in subsequent statistical analyses.

The direction of the skewness is also considered. For example, when data have a positive skewness, one can proceed directly to undertake either a square root or logarithmic transformation, which often produces data that are more nearly normal. In some cases, the same transformation also achieves equality of variances (Maxwell & Delaney, 1990; Tabachnick & Fidell, 2001). With negative skewness, however, an additional step is required, that of "reflecting" the variable to make the negative skewness a positive skewness. This means that the variable is reverse-scored. For example, with moderate or severe negative skewness, the following procedure needs to be done:

1. "Reflect" the variable by finding the largest score in the distribution, and add one to it to form a constant that is larger than any other score in the distribution.
2. Form a new variable by subtracting each person's score from the constant. Thus, the negative skewness is converted to a positive skewness before transformation. At this stage, the resulting variable, because it was derived from a "reflected" variable, means just the opposite of what it meant before reflection. Thus, if high scores on a self-esteem total score mean high self-esteem, they now mean low self-esteem after reflection.
3. Then apply the appropriate transformation to the newly formed variable.
4. Check the skewness for the transformed variable; if close to zero, then use the transformed variable in subsequent analyses.

If you then use the transformed variable in subsequent analyses, remember that its meaning has been reversed so that a high score now means just the opposite of what it meant before reflecting the variable and transforming it. In order to change the transformed variable back to its original meaning, it is often useful to perform another reflection on the transformed variable. This can be accomplished by finding the largest score in the transformed variable's distribution, add one to it to form a constant that is larger than any other score in the distribution, and form a new variable by subtracting each person's score from the constant. The resulting variable now is interpreted exactly as it was interpreted prior to the first reflection (#s 1 and 2 in the earlier list). If high numbers meant more of that characteristic (ie, self-esteem) before the first reflection, then high numbers again mean more of that characteristic (ie, high self-esteem) after the second reflection.

As a rule, it is best to transform significantly skewed variables to normality unless the transformed scores make interpretation impractical (Tabachnick & Fidell,

2001). Once transformed, always check that the transformed variable is normally or nearly normally distributed. If one type of transformation does not work, try another until you achieve a transformation that produces variables with skewness close to zero and/or the fewest outliers. Finally, if transforming the variable does not work, the best thing might be to create a categorical variable.

There are potential disadvantages to transforming data. Chief among them is that transformed variables may be harder to interpret. Whether or not to transform depends on the scale that measures the variable. If the scale is widely known and used, transformations often hinder interpretation. If the scale is not well known, transformations often do not particularly increase the difficulty of interpretation (Tabachnick & Fidell, 2001). Most computer programs permit various types of transformations through the use of the Compute command.

Hair et al. (1998) recommend keeping several guidelines in mind when carrying out data transformations:

1. For a transformation to have a noticeable effect, the ratio of the variable's mean to its SD should be less than 4.0.
2. When the transformation can be done on either of two variables, transform the variable with the smallest ratio from guideline #1.
3. Transformations should be applied to the independent variable except when heteroscedasticity, or the failure of the assumption of homoscedasticity, is present. (Homoscedasticity is the assumption that the dependent variable displays equal levels of variance across the range of predictor variables.)
4. Heteroscedasticity can be corrected only by transforming the dependent variable in a dependence relationship. If a heteroscedastic relationship is also nonlinear, the dependent variables and possibly the independent variables must also be transformed.
5. Transformations may change how you interpret the variable's score. Thus, you should carefully explore the possible interpretations of the transformed variables.

MEASURES OF KURTOSIS OR PEAKEDNESS

Fisher's Measure of Kurtosis

This statistic, indicating whether a distribution has the right bell shape for a normal curve, measures whether the bell shape is too flat or too peaked. Fisher's measure, based on deviations from the mean to the fourth power, can also be found in Hildebrand (1986). However, the calculation is tedious and is ordinarily done by a computer program. A curve with the correct bell shape will result in a value of zero. If the kurtosis value is a large positive number, the distribution is too peaked to be normal (*leptokurtic*). If the kurtosis value is negative, the curve is too flat to be normal (*platykurtic*). For the denial score data in Table 2-3, the kurtosis statistic is given as -0.249, a value close to zero, indicating that the shape of the bell for this distribution can be called normal. Dividing this value by the standard error for kurtosis

$(-0.249/0.391 = -0.64)$, our distribution is not significantly kurtosed; that is, the value is not beyond ±1.96 SD. Because this statistic is based on deviations to the fourth power, it is very sensitive to extreme values. If a distribution is markedly skewed, there is no particular need to examine kurtosis because the distribution is not normal.

ROUNDING DESCRIPTIVE STATISTICS FOR TABLES

When reporting descriptive statistics in a table, too many digits are confusing. Even though a computer program has provided the statistic to the fourth decimal place, not all the digits need to be reported. If diastolic blood pressure is measured to the nearest whole number, why report descriptive statistics for blood pressure to the nearest 10,000th?

In rounding to the nearest 10th (or 100th), if the last digit to be dropped is less than 5, round to the lower number; if it is higher than 5, round to the higher number. If the last digit to be dropped is exactly 5, no change is made in the preceding digit if it is even, but if it is odd, it is increased by 1. Thus, 4.25 to the nearest 10th is 4.2, but 4.35 becomes 4.4.

CHARTS USING DESCRIPTIVE STATISTICS

Line Charts

In health care research, the line chart is frequently used to display longitudinal trends. Time points in equal intervals are placed on the horizontal axis and the scale for the statistic on the vertical axis. Dots representing the statistic (eg, means, medians, or percentages) at each time point are then connected. The line chart presents a smoother appearance than drawing bars over each time point. Frequently, vertical error bars are added to each time point to indicate the accuracy of the statistic as an estimate of a population parameter. These error bars represent standard errors, which are discussed in detail in Chapter 3. Examples of several types of line charts from research journals are given in Figs. 2-9 through 2-11. When several groups are being compared in the same line chart, Tufte (1983) recommends that labels be integrated into the chart rather than having a separate legend, so the eye is not required to go back and forth.

The issue of whether to place a zero on the vertical axis of a time series line chart is determined by the purpose of the chart and the target group for whom it was designed. Different authors of books on charting have differing views on this subject. Cleveland (1985) and Tufte (1983) both maintain that the vertical axis should start immediately below the lowest value in the dataset. It is best to choose the scale for the vertical axis so that the data fill up the chart. You may assume that the reader of a scientific journal will look at tick mark labels and breaks in the axes or line plot and understand them (Cleveland, 1985).

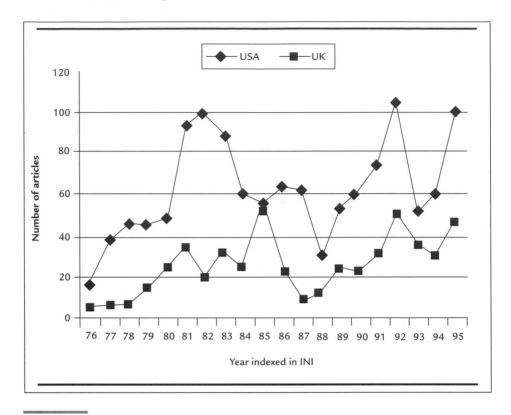

FIGURE 2-9. Comparison of numbers of articles published on patient advocacy in the USA and the UK (1876–1995). (From Mallik, M., & Rafferty, A. [2000]. Diffusion of the concept of patient advocacy. *Journal of Nursing Scholarship, 32*(4), 402.)

Box Plots

A *box plot,* also called a *box-and-whiskers plot,* is a graphic display that uses descriptive statistics based on percentiles (Tukey, 1977). It simultaneously displays the median, the IQR, and the smallest and largest values for a group (Norusis, 2002). Although more compact than a histogram, it does not provide as much detail.

The first step in constructing the box plot is to draw the box. Its length corresponds to the IQR; that is, the box begins with the 25th percentile and ends with the 75th percentile (Fig. 2-12). A line (or other symbol) within the box indicates the location of the median or 50th percentile. Thus, the box provides information about the central tendency and the variability of the middle 50% of the distribution.

The next step is to locate the wild values of the distribution, if any. Calculate the IQR ($P_{75} - P_{25}$), and then multiply this value by 3. Individual scores that are more than three times the IQR from the upper and lower edges of the box are extreme outlying values and are denoted on the plot by a symbol such as E. Next, multiply the IQR by 1.5. Individual scores between 1.5 times the IQR and 3 times the IQR

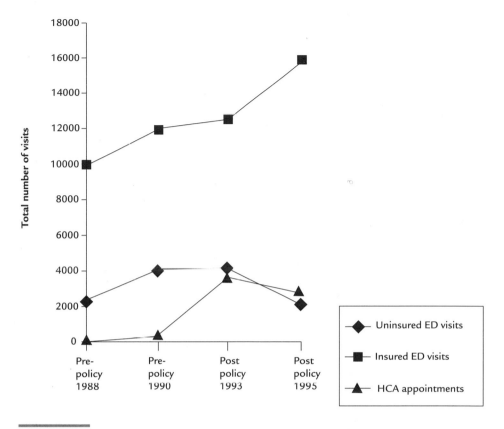

FIGURE 2-10. Total emergency department (ED) visits and HCA (health care access) appointments by year, before and after state funding. (From Smith-Campbell, B. [2000]. Access to health care: Effects of public funding on the uninsured. *Journal of Nursing Scholarship, 32*(3), 298.)

away from the edges of the box are minor outlying values. They are denoted on the box plot with a different symbol, such as O. Finally, draw the whiskers of the box. These lines should extend to the smallest and largest values that are not minor or extreme outlying values. Thus, the whiskers and designation of the outlying values provide more detail about how the lower 25% and upper 25% of the distribution are scattered.

The box plot is particularly well suited for comparisons among several groups. Examples of box plots are given in Fig. 2-13, comparing psychological adjustment to illness in a sample of breast cancer patients according to stage of cancer. As the stage of cancer became higher, adjustment worsened (ie, the average score increased). Also, it is clear that the variability of the adjustment scores was greater as the stage became higher. The subject identification numbers can be placed on the plot for convenient reference.

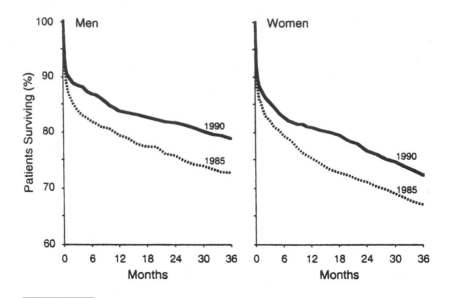

FIGURE 2-11. Trends in survival in the 3 years after hospitalization for definite acute myocardial infarction in 1985 and 1990 among residents of the Twin Cities area who were 30 to 74 years of age. (From McGovern, P. G., Pankow, J. S., Shahar, E., Doliszny, K. M., Folsom, A. R., Blackburn, H., & Leupker, R. V. [1996]. Recent trends in acute coronary heart disease. *New England Journal of Medicine, 34*(14), 887. © 1996, Massachusetts Medical Society. All rights reserved.)

OUTLIERS

Outliers are values that are extreme relative to the bulk of scores in the distribution. They appear to be inconsistent with the rest of the data. Outliers must be appraised by the types of information they provide. In some cases, outliers, despite being different from most of the sample, may be beneficial: They may indicate characteristics of the population that would not be known in the normal course of analysis. In other cases, outliers may be problematic because they do not represent the population, run counter to the objectives of the analysis, and can seriously distort statistical tests (Hair et al., 1998). Thus, it is important to detect outliers to ascertain their type of influence.

The source of an outlier may be any of the following:

1. An error in the recording of the data
2. A failure of data collection, such as not following sample criteria (eg, inadvertently admitting a disoriented patient into a study), a subject not following instructions on a questionnaire, or equipment failure
3. An actual extreme value from an unusual subject

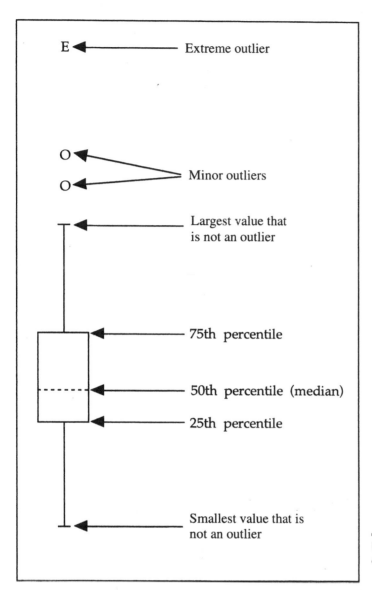

FIGURE 2-12. Schematic diagram of the construction of a box plot.

Outliers must first be identified by an objective method. A traditional way of labeling outliers has been to locate any values that are more than 3 SD from the mean. The problem with this method is that outliers inflate the SD, making it less likely that a value will be 3 SD away from the mean. Tukey's (1977) recommendation was described earlier in connection with the box plot. Values that are more than 3 IQRs from the upper or lower edges of the box are extreme outliers. Values between 1.5 and 3 IQRs from the upper and lower edges of the box are minor outliers. The reason for having an objective method is to prevent undue (perhaps

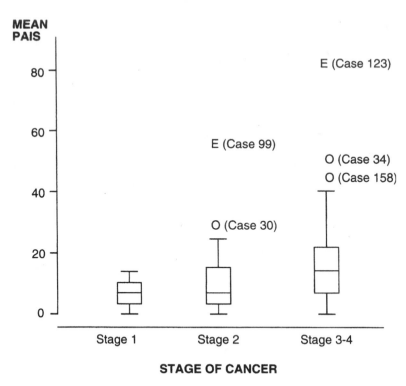

FIGURE 2-13. Box plots of psychological adjustment to illness (PAIS) in a sample of breast cancer patients by stage of cancer (hypothetical data). Higher scores indicate poorer adjustment.

unethical) data manipulation, such as pruning very high or very low values that are not really outliers.

Outliers in a dataset can be identified from univariate, bivariate, and multivariate perspectives. In data analysis, it is best to use as many of these perspectives as possible. Although in-depth discussion of the various approaches is beyond the scope of this chapter, Hair et al. (1998) and Tabachnick and Fidell (2001) provide excellent discussions on detecting and handling outliers in various circumstances.

Once outliers have been identified, the next step is to try to explain them. If they represent errors in coding or a failure in the data collection, then those observations are either discarded or corrected. If the outliers represent actual values or their occurrence in the distribution cannot be explained, the researcher must decide how to deal with them.

Handling Outliers

A frequent suggestion for handling outliers is to analyze the data two ways: with the outliers in the distribution and with the outliers removed. If the results are similar, as they are likely to be if the sample size is large, then the outliers may be ignored. If the results are not similar, then a statistical analysis that is resistant to outliers can be used (eg, median and IQR).

If the researcher wants to use a mean with outliers, then the *trimmed mean* is an option. This statistic is calculated with a certain percentage of the extreme values removed from both ends of the distribution. For example, if the sample size is 100, then the 5% trimmed mean is the mean of the middle 90% of the observations. Formulas for using the trimmed mean in statistical inference are given by Koopmans (1987).

Another alternative is a *winsorized mean*. In the simplest case, the highest and lowest extremes are replaced, respectively, by the next-to-highest value and by the next-to-lowest value. If the sample size is 100, the resulting 100 data points are then processed as if they were the original data. Winer (1971) outlines the techniques for handling statistics computed from winsorized samples.

For univariate outliers, Tabachnick and Fidell (2001) suggest changing the score(s) on the variable(s) for the outlying cases so they are deviant, but not as deviant as they originally were. For example, give the outlying case(s) a raw score on the specific variable that is one unit smaller (or larger) than the next most extreme score in the distribution. Thus, if the two largest scores in the distribution are 125 and 122, and the next largest score is 87, recode 122 as 88 and 125 as 89. This moves these outliers closer to the bulk of scores in the distribution. Sometimes, this conversion is all it takes to handle the problem of severe skewness in a distribution, discussed in Chapter 3.

The actual score a case has is somewhat arbitrary. What is important is that the case still retains its place in the distribution: If the case has the lowest score, it will still have the lowest score after being assigned a number closer to the bulk of scores in the distribution. Any changes in scores should be noted, along with the rationale, in the results section of the research report.

Further details on the treatment of outliers can be found in Mertler and Vannatta (2002), Tabachnick and Fidell (2001), and Hair et al. (1998). A researcher can also view these actual outliers as case material and adopt the advice of Skinner (1972), who advocates that when you encounter something interesting, study it.

MISSING DATA

One of the most pervasive problems in data analysis is what to do about missing data. Most studies have missing information for some variables for some cases. Missing data can occur at the subject and/or item level (Kneipp & McIntosh, 2001). Missing data at the subject level are usually found in longitudinal and repeated measures studies when one or more subjects are lost to follow-up or decide not to continue participation in the study. Missing data at the item level are quite common when one or more items on a survey or questionnaire are not answered by a respondent. Missing data are a problem because all standard statistical techniques presume that each case in a dataset has information on all the variables to be included in the particular analysis (Allison, 2001).

With missing data, the researcher faces three major tasks: to identify the pattern and amount of missing data, to assess why it is missing, and to determine what to do about it.

Pattern and Amount of Missing Data

There are two characteristic patterns of missing data: random and systematic. A *random pattern* consists of values missing in an unplanned or haphazard fashion throughout a dataset. A *systematic pattern* consists of values missing in a methodical, nonrandom way throughout the data. The pattern of missing data is more important than the amount of missing data (Tabachnick & Fidell, 2001). If only a few data values are absent in a random pattern from a large dataset, almost any procedure for handling missing values can be used. However, if many data are missing from a small or moderately sized dataset, serious problems can ensue unless the researcher takes steps to handle the problem. Missing data is such a serious problem in a dataset that all statistical packages have conventions for coding missing data for further study and for special treatment in statistical procedures. For example, SPSS has a "System Missing" category that shows up in the data spreadsheet and on the computer printout as a period.

Random missing data can be one of three categories (Allison, 2001; Little & Rubin, 1987): missing completely at random (MCAR), missing at random (MAR), and not missing at random (NMAR). MCAR data have the highest degree of randomness, displaying no underlying reason that would contribute to biased data (Musil et al., 2002). MCAR data are randomly distributed across all cases and are completely unrelated to other variables in the dataset (Hair et al., 1998). In contrast, MAR data display some randomness to the pattern of omission that can be traced or predicted from cases with no missing data. In other words, MAR occurs when the probability of a missing value is not dependent on the value itself but may rely on the values of other variables in the dataset (Allison, 2001). The third type of missing data, NMAR, occurs when the missing values are systematically different from those observed, even among respondents with other similar characteristics (Kneipp & McIntosh, 2001). Systematic missing data, even in a few cases, should always be treated seriously because they affect the generalizability of results.

If you are not sure whether the missing data are random or systematic, you can test for patterns with the following procedure. First, create a grouping variable with two levels (using the Recode, or comparable, command in your computer program), making 1 = cases with missing values on the variable and 0 = cases with no missing values on the variable. Then, perform a test of differences, such as the *t* test, between the two levels on the dependent variable(s). If there are no meaningful differences, how you handle the missing data is not so important. If serious differences are noted, then handling missing data is critical and care should be taken to preserve the missing cases for further analyses (Tabachnick & Fidell, 2001). A useful program for examining missing data is SPSS Missing Values Analysis, which permits you to analyze patterns of missing data and to replace them in the dataset using one of several methods.

Assessing Why Data Are Missing

It is important to understand what, if any, factors led up to missing data in a research study, because the researcher needs to grasp what may have happened to handle the problem. Hair et al. (1998) define a missing data process as "any systematic event external to the respondent (such as data entry errors or data collection problems) or action on the part of the respondent (such as refusal to answer) that leads to missing data" (p. 46). If the missing data process is under the researcher's control and can be explicitly defined, these missing data can be ignored and no specific remedies are needed because allowances have been made for missing data in the technique used (Allison, 2001; Little & Rubin, 1987).

An example of ignorable missing data inherent in the technique used is the application of probability sampling to select respondents for a study. This sampling method permits the researcher to stipulate that the missing data process leading to the missing data points is random and that the missing data are explained as sampling error in the statistical procedures (Hair et al., 1998).

More often than not, however, the researcher has no idea why specific data are missing. Thus, examining the pattern of missing data becomes important. Are the respondents with missing data on some variables different than the respondents who provided information on these variables? Only by understanding to the greatest extent possible why missing data occurred can the researcher take appropriate steps to handle the impact that it can have on the analyses, the results, and the subsequent interpretation of the data.

Handling Missing Data

Missing data can be handled in several ways: Using complete-case (listwise deletion) and available-case (pairwise deletion) analysis (Kneipp & McIntosh, 2001); deleting cases or variables (Tabachnick & Fidell, 2001); weighting techniques (Patrician, 2002); and estimating missing data through imputation (Tabachnick & Fidell, 2001).

USING OBSERVATIONS: COMPLETE-CASE AND AVAILABLE-CASE ANALYSIS

The easiest and most direct method for dealing with missing data values is to analyze only those cases with complete data. This procedure, called *listwise deletion*, is the default procedure in most major statistical programs such as SPSS, SAS, BMDP, and Systat. As such, numerous cases can be deleted without the researcher's knowledge, resulting in a substantial loss of subjects. Thus, it is important to check the number of cases when running statistical analyses to ensure that all desired cases are used. Hair et al. (1998) suggest using this method if the amount of missing data is small, the sample is sufficiently large to permit deletion of cases with missing data, and the relationships in the data are so strong that they will not be influenced by any missing data process. With MCAR data, listwise deletion produces unbiased parameter estimates but larger standard errors due to the decrease in sample size and can lead to misleading results and decreased analytic power especially if a large number of cases is removed (Patrician, 2002).

Available-case analysis using only those cases that have available data on the variables for a specific analysis is a common research practice. This can be accomplished using *pairwise deletion* of cases with missing data, commonly available as an option in most statistical packages. This method permits cases to be deleted only if the variables being used in the analysis have missing data. Both listwise and pairwise deletion procedures are ad hoc in nature, have no theoretical justification, and are designed solely to provide complete data for specific analyses. Pairwise deletion is often used for correlations, factor analysis, and linear regression (Allison, 2001).

DELETING CASES OR VARIABLES

Dropping the case or variable is another remedy for handling missing data. The researcher simply determines the extent of missing data on each case and variable in the dataset, then removes the cases or variables with excessive levels. Although there are no hard-and-fast rules for determining excessive levels of missing data, many researchers use a predetermined percentage of missing data as a cutoff for deciding whether to exclude a variable from analysis. It is not unusual to see a 5% or 10% cutoff being used. Usually, this planned cutoff level is based on theoretical and empirical reasons. In many situations, given a large enough sample, this is the most efficient solution. Once cases or variables with missing data are removed, the researcher may discover that the missing data were localized in a small set of cases or variables. Once excluded, the extent of missing data is considerably decreased (Hair et al., 1998).

WEIGHTING TECHNIQUES

Another, less common, way to handle missing data is to disregard missing values and assign a weight to cases with complete data. Little and Rubin (1987) believe that weighting those cases with no missing data higher than those with missing data decreases the bias from case-deletion methods as well as the sample variance, but makes calculating standard errors more difficult.

ESTIMATING MISSING DATA BY IMPUTATION

Imputation is the process of estimating missing data based on valid values of other variables or cases in the sample. The goal of imputation is to use known relationships that can be identified in the valid values of the sample to help estimate the missing data (Hair et al., 1998). Tabachnick and Fidell (2001) discuss five popular ways to estimate missing data: using prior knowledge, inserting mean values, using regression, expectation maximization (EM), and multiple imputation.

- **Prior knowledge** involves replacing a missing value with a value based on an educated guess. This is a reasonable method if the researcher has a good working knowledge of the research domain, the sample is large, and the number of missing values is small. In such circumstances, the researcher is confident that the missing value would have been near the median, or other, value.
- **Mean replacement** (or median replacement for skewed distributions) involves calculating mean values from available data on that variable and using them to replace missing values before analysis. This is a conservative

procedure because the distribution mean as a whole does not change and the researcher does not have to guess at missing values. Hair et al. (1998) cite three disadvantages to this approach: It invalidates the variance estimates derived from the standard variance formulas by understating the data's true variance; it distorts the actual distribution of values; and it depresses the observed correlation that this variable will have with other variables because all missing data have a single constant value, thus reducing variance.

Mean substitution, however, has the advantage of being easily implemented and provides all cases with complete data. A compromise procedure is to insert a group mean for the missing value. If, for example, the case with a missing value is a female patient with hypertension, the mean value for female patients with hypertension is computed and inserted in place of the missing value. This procedure is less conservative than inserting the overall mean value but not as liberal as using prior knowledge (Tabachnick & Fidell, 2001).

Using regression, a more sophisticated method for estimating missing values, involves using other variables in the dataset as independent variables to develop a regression equation for the variable with missing data serving as the dependent variable. Cases with complete data are used to generate the regression equation; the equation is then used to predict missing values for incomplete cases. More regressions are computed, using the predicted values from the previous regression to develop the next equation, until the predicted values from one step to the next are comparable. Predictions from the last regression are the ones used to replace missing values.

Hair et al. (1998) cite four disadvantages to using the regression approach: It reinforces the relationships already in the data, resulting in less generalizability; the variance of the distribution is reduced because the estimate is probably too close to the mean; it assumes that the variable with missing data is correlated substantially with the other variables in the dataset; and the regression procedure is not constrained in the estimates it makes. Thus, the predicted values may not fall in the valid ranges for variables—for instance, a value of 6 may be predicted for a 5-point scale. The main advantage of the regression approach is that it is more objective than the researcher's guess but not as blind as simply using the overall mean (Tabachnick & Fidell, 2001).

Expectation maximization (EM) method, available for randomly missing data, is an iterative process that proceeds in two discrete steps. First, in the Expectation (E) step, the conditional expected value of the complete data is computed and then given the observed values, such as correlations. Second, in the maximization (M) step, these expected values are then substituted for the missing data and maximum likelihood estimation is then computed as though there were no missing data. The procedure iterates until convergence is reached and the filled-in data are saved in the dataset. SPSS Missing Values

Analysis performs EM to produce imputed values and allows some specifications of other nonnormal distributions (Tabachnick & Fidell, 2001).

Multiple imputation (MI), similar to maximum likelihood estimation, produces several datasets and analyzes them separately. One set of parameters is then formed by averaging the resulting estimates and standard errors. The number of datasets to impute derives from the extent of missing data in the dataset, although most statisticians recommend 3 to 5 sets (Patrician, 2002). For an excellent discussion of the various types of multiple imputation, the reader is referred to Allison (2001) and Little and Rubin (2002).

Multiple imputation has a number of advantages:

- It makes no assumptions about whether data are randomly missing (Tabachnick & Fidell, 2001) but incorporates random error because it requires random variation in the imputation process (Patrician, 2002);
- It permits use of complete-data methods for data analysis and also includes the data collector's knowledge (Patrician, 2002);
- It permits estimates of nonlinear models (Allison, 2001);
- It simulates proper inference from data and increases efficiency of the estimates (Patrician, 2002) by minimizing standard errors (Rubin, 1987); and
- It is the method of choice for databases that are made available for analyses outside the agency that collected the data (Tabachnick & Fidell, 2001).

MI has the following major disadvantages:

- It requires computational intensiveness to carry out MI, including special software and model building (Kneipp & McIntosh, 2001), although this has become less so in recent years due to technological advances;
- It does not produce a unique answer because randomness is preserved in the MI process, making reproducibility of exact results problematic (Patrician, 2002); and
- It requires large amounts of data storage space that often exceeds space on personal computers' hard drives or the amounts allotted on university-shared drives, especially when national datasets with thousands of respondents are used (Kneipp & McIntosh, 2001).

When using imputation methods, Tabachnick and Fidell (2001) recommend repeating analyses with and without missing data to make sure that the results do not get distorted by imputed values. This can be particularly problematic if the dataset is small.

SUMMARY

Descriptive statistics based on the mean are best for distributions that are reasonably symmetrical and have a single peak. These measures include the mean, the SD, Pearson's skewness coefficient, and Fisher's measures of skewness and kurtosis. For skewed distributions, the median and the IQR are less influenced by extreme scores. The range, the mode, Pearson's coefficient of skewness, and Fisher's measure of skewness are quick estimates. In addition, the mode is informative when a distribution has several peaks. The range is useful for locating the most extreme values. Outliers are extreme values that meet objective criteria, and researchers must consider carefully how to handle them in data analysis. Two charts that make use of summary statistics are the line chart and the box plot. A line chart uses statistics such as means at various time points to portray longitudinal trends. Box plots emphasize extreme values in a distribution and are handy for displaying outliers. Missing data are a fact of life in data analysis. The researcher must determine the pattern and amount of missing data, why it occurred, and what method is best for handling it. No one technique can solve all problems with missing data.

Application Exercises and Results

Exercises

1. Access the dataset named SURVEY03.SAV. Run frequencies and include statistics for all variables. Examine the output for outliers, marked skewness, unequal groups, and missing data. Decide what to do about the problems you encounter.

2. Construct a table that includes some of the categorical variables in this dataset. Write a description of the table.

3. Construct a table that includes some of the continuous variables in this dataset. Write a description of the table.

4. Construct a box plot (sometimes called a box-and-whiskers plot) for the variable EDUC by GENDER.

Results

1. Generally, when you first look at output, you will find invalid numbers—that is, a number that is not valid for a particular variable. With SURVEY03.SAV, we tried to remove all invalid numbers, so unless we missed one, you should not have found any.

    For an example of an outlier, find the frequencies for the variable AGE in the printout and examine them. You should see one 78-year-old, one 79-year-old, two 82-year-olds, one 83-year-old, and one 95-year-old. The next largest age is 74 years. We questioned whether the 95-year-old was a data entry error but were assured by the student who collected the data that the individual was indeed 95 years old. These five data points could be viewed as outliers because they are several units away from the next highest age score of 74 years. If we follow Tabachnick and Fidell's (2001) suggestion for univariate outliers, we would change the scores of the five outliers in the AGE variable to bring them closer to the bulk of the distribution's scores. In all versions of SPSS for Windows, we accomplish this by clicking on the Transform, Recode, and Into Different Variables menus. In this last window, highlight the AGE variable in the variable column and paste it in the Numeric Variable box. Give the output variable a new name such as RECAGE, then click Change. This will move the new variable name into the Numeric Variable window following the arrow.

Click on Old and New Values and specify how to recode the values. Under Old Value, type the number 78 in the Value box. Under New Value, type the number 74 in the Value box. Click Add to paste the conversion into the Old → New window. Repeat this procedure for the additional four values (79, 82, 83, and 95, making them 75, 76, 77, and 78, respectively). Then, in the Old Value column, click on All Other Values at the bottom, then click on the Copy All Value(s) in the New Value column and hit the Add button. (If you do not Copy All Values, your resulting variable will have only six cases because all of the other values were not moved to the new variable, RECAGE.) When you have completed these operations, you should have five value statements in the Old S New window. To complete the Recode procedure, click Continue, then OK. The transformation will then take place and the new variable RECAGE will appear as the last variable in the data file window. Next, return to the spreadsheet and switch to the Variable View. Scroll down the variable list to the last variable, RECAGE. Now, move horizontally to the column named Value and type in the following: Recoded Age Variable Making 78, 79, 82, 83, 95 into 74, 75, 76, 77, and 78. Finally, to make sure you do not lose this newly created variable when you exit the program, save the data file at this time.

Exercise Fig. 2-1 contains the descriptive statistics for several variables in the dataset. The recoded AGE variable (RECAGE) resulted in small changes in the mean, standard error of the mean, SD, variance, range, and minimum and maximum values. Skewness was reduced from 0.753 to 0.643; kurtosis was greatly changed from 0.796 to 0.287.

Skewness is often a problem in data analysis and violates the assumptions underlying parametric tests. Look at the variable HEALTH (overall state of health). It was scored from 1 = Very Sick to 10 = Very Healthy. Only 12.9% of the distribution falls between the scores of 1 and 5. Only one respondent had a rating of 1; no respondents rated themselves as 2. This is understandable because students are not likely to request data from people who are very ill. You can tell by looking at the distribution that it is negatively skewed (ie, the values tail off at the lower end). The value for skewness (-0.961) divided by the standard error of skewness (0.092) yields -10.44, indicating significant skewness beyond the 0.01 level (critical value = 2.58 SD from the mean). You might try to transform this variable and see if you can create a normally distributed variable. Remember, it is negatively skewed and would require "reflecting" before being transformed.

There are a number of examples of *unequal groups* in the dataset, SURVEY03.SAV. Males make up only 36.6% of the sample. Only 11.3% of the sample still smokes, and only 1.6% are routinely depressed. What other examples of unequal groups can you find?

Although there are quite a lot of *missing data* across the dataset, no variable has more than 5% missing data. This indicates a random rather than a systematic pattern of missing data. If you examine the frequency distributions, you will note that EDUC has 28 (4.0%) missing data points and SMOKE (Smoking History) has 4 (0.6%) missing data points. Are there any other variables with similar amounts of missing data?

We now need to determine what method we should use to handle the missing data problem. If we choose the most conservative method and use only the cases with no missing data, we might end up with just a few cases in our dataset. This is because there are missing data in 44 (86.3%) of the 51 variables in our dataset. So, we now consider the next most conservative approach for handling missing data: dropping the case or the variable with excessive levels of missing data. If we examine the frequencies for the variables in the dataset, we see that TOTAL, the total score for the IPPA scale, has missing data for 40 (5.7%) of cases. Why is this so high when the items that were summed to compute the total

(text continues on page 69)

Statistics

		AGE subject's age	RECAGE Recorded Age (78,79,82 83,95 into 75,76,77, 78,79)
N	Valid	684	684
	Missing	17	17
Mean		38.06	38.0073
Std. Error of Mean		.496	.48884
Median		37.00	37.0000
Mode		28	28.00
Std. Deviation		12.972	12.78479
Variance		168.266	163.45090
Skewness		.753	.643
Std. Error of Skewness		.093	.093
Kurtosis		.796	.287
Std. Error of Kurtosis		.796	.287
Range		80	64.00
Minimum		15	15.00
Maximum		95	79.00

Statistics

HEALTH overall state of health

N	Valid	700
	Missing	1
Mean		7.85
Std. Error of Mean		.066
Median		8.00
Mode		9
Std. Deviation		1.740
Variance		3.027
Skewness		−.961
Std. Error of Skewness		.092
Kurtosis		.555
Std. Error of Kurtosis		.185
Range		9
Minimum		1
Maximum		10

EXERCISE FIGURE 2–1. Descriptive statistics for study variables.

HEALTH overall state of health

		Frequency	Percent	Valid Percent	Cumulative Percent
Valid	1 Very Sick	1	.1	.1	.1
	3	17	2.4	2.4	2.6
	4	21	3.0	3.0	5.6
	5	51	7.3	7.3	12.9
	6	31	4.4	4.4	17.3
	7	117	16.7	16.7	34.0
	8	170	24.3	24.3	58.3
	9	182	26.0	26.0	84.3
	10 Very Healthy	110	15.7	15.7	100.0
	Total	700	99.9	100.0	
Missing	System	1	.1		
Total		701	100.0		

Frequency Table

GENDER gender

		Frequency	Percent	Valid Percent	Cumulative Percent
Valid	0 male	255	36.4	36.6	36.6
	1 female	441	62.9	63.4	100.0
	Total	696	99.3	100.0	
Missing	System	5	.7		
Total		701	100.0		

SMOKE Smoking History

		Frequency	Percent	Valid Percent	Cumulative Percent
Valid	0 Never Smoked	433	61.8	62.1	62.1
	1 Quit Smoking	185	26.4	26.5	88.7
	2 Still Smoking	79	11.3	11.3	100.0
	Total	697	99.4	100.0	
Missing	System	4	.6		
Total		701	100.0		

EXERCISE FIGURE 2–1. (*Continued*).

DEPRESS depressed state of mind

		Frequency	Percent	Valid Percent	Cumulative Percent
Valid	1 Rarely	361	51.5	51.6	51.6
	2 Sometimes	280	39.9	40.0	91.6
	3 Often	48	6.8	6.9	98.4
	4. Routinely	11	1.6	1.6	100.0
	Total	700	99.9	100.0	
Missing	System	1	.1		
Total		701	100.0		

Frequency Table

EDUC education in years

		Frequency	Percent	Valid Percent	Cumulative Percent
Valid	7	1	.1	.1	.1
	8	12	1.7	1.8	1.9
	9	2	.3	.3	2.2
	10	6	.9	.9	3.1
	11	5	.7	.7	3.9
	12	70	10.0	10.4	14.3
	13	25	3.6	3.7	18.0
	14	3	.4	.4	18.4
	14	63	9.0	9.4	27.8
	15	28	4.0	4.2	31.9
	16	147	21.0	21.8	53.8
	17	40	5.7	5.9	59.7
	18	1	.1	.1	59.9
	18	84	12.0	12.5	72.4
	19	46	6.6	6.8	79.2
	20	1	.1	.1	79.3
	20	65	9.3	9.7	89.0
	21	27	3.9	4.0	93.0
	22	21	3.0	3.1	96.1
	23	7	1.0	1.0	97.2
	24	1	.1	.1	97.3
	24	7	1.0	1.0	98.4
	25	5	.7	.7	99.1
	26	2	.3	.3	99.4
	28	3	.4	.4	99.9
	30	1	.1	.1	100.0
	Total	673	96.0	100.0	
Missing	System	28	4.0		
Total		701	100.0		

EXERCISE FIGURE 2–1. (*Continued*).

SMOKE Smoking History

		Frequency	Percent	Valid Percent	Cumulative Percent
Valid	0 Never Smoked	433	61.8	62.1	62.1
	1 Quit Smoking	185	26.4	26.5	88.7
	2 Still Smoking	79	11.3	11.3	100.0
	Total	697	99.4	100.0	
Missing	System	4	.6		
Total		701	100.0		

Statistics

		TOTAL	CONFID	LIFE	IPA1 energy level	IPA2 reaction to pressure	IPA3 characterization of life as a whole
N	Valid	661	681	676	700	695	693
	Missing	40	20	25	1	6	8
Mean		152.7035	62.6975	89.7544	5.01	4.05	5.20
Median		155.0000	64.0000	92.0000	5.00	4.00	5.00
Std. Deviation		28.07608	12.92818	17.08832	1.351	1.705	1.270

AUTHOR COMMENTS
TOTAL = IPPA TOTAL SCORE; PERCENT MISSING: 40/661 = 6.1%
CONFID = IPPA CONFIDENCE SCALE; PERCENT MISSING: 20/681 = 2.9%
LIFE = IPPA LIFE SCALE; PERCENT MISSING: 25/676 = 3.7%

MARITAL marital status

		Frequency	Percent	Valid Percent	Cumulative Percent
Valid	1 Never Married	230	32.8	33.4	33.4
	2 Married	346	49.4	50.3	83.7
	3 Living with Significant Other	44	6.3	6.4	90.1
	4 Separated	13	1.9	1.9	92.0
	5 Widowed	20	2.9	2.9	94.9
	6 Divorced	35	5.0	5.1	100.0
	Total	688	98.1	100.0	
Missing	System	13	1.9		
Total		701	100.0		

EXERCISE FIGURE 2–1. (*Continued*).

score had only one or two missing data points each? The large amount of missing data in the TOTAL IPPA scale score is due to the default option in the Compute command in SPSS for Windows. Only cases that have scores for each variable in the Compute statement will be used in the procedure. Any case that is missing a data point for a variable in the equation will be dropped, resulting in missing data in the computed scale score. Thus, if the missing data problem is not addressed **before** forming subscale and total scores, the resulting scores will have a fair amount of missing data. That is what happened to TOTAL (IPPA total score) as well as to the CONFID and LIFE IPPA subscale scores.

Although we are getting ahead of ourselves a bit, we can correct this problem in one of two ways. We can replace the missing data in each of the IPA1 through IPA30 items by substituting the mean or median (if the data are markedly skewed) on that variable for the missing data point using the Recode command. Once completed, we recompute the total score for TOTAL and for the CONFID and LIFE subscales. Then, we rerun the frequencies for these variables and compare them to the original frequencies. You should find that these recomputed variables have no missing data.

What we have just described is another way to handle missing data through substituting the mean or median of the distribution for missing data points. Given the relatively small amount of missing data throughout the SURVEY03.SAV dataset, this choice is most likely the best, and the easiest, way to handle the missing data problem. However, you must decide, based on the amount of skewness in the continuous variables, whether to use the mean or the median as the replacement value. For example, what value would you use for the AGE variable, or for the HEALTH variable?

For nominal level variables such as MARITAL (Marital Status) and POLAFF (Political Affiliation), it is usually best to use the modal value if there is only one mode and not a great deal of missing data. If there is more than one mode or lots of missing data, it might be best to consider using another method or methods. If all else fails, you may have to live with the fact that some cases will have some missing data and, in some analyses, you will use only those cases with complete data on the variables of interest.

2. Exercise Figure 2-2 contains a sample table of two categorical variables. Often, variables are combined into one table, but because SPSS for Windows 12.0 presents separate tables that can be copied into a manuscript, we have kept them as they appear in the SPSS output. Tables are used to present data clearly and succinctly. Not all the information is repeated in the text; generally just the highlights are presented. In our text description, we could describe these three variables by stating that over 62% of the sample is employed full time, and almost half list their political affiliation as independent. When choosing a winter vacation, the most popular choice was a beachfront condo in Hawaii, followed by a Caribbean cruise and a chalet in the Swiss Alps: about 86% of the respondents selected one of those choices. A trip to Disney World was the least popular choice.

3. Exercise Figure 2-3 contains a sample table of continuous variables for respondents' age, education, and total scores on the IPPA scale. We created the table using the descriptives program in SPSS. We could describe the table in the text by stating that respondents ranged in age from 15 to 95 years, with a mean age of 38.1 ± 13 years. They were a well-educated group, with an average of 16.6 ± 3.5 years of education. On the IPPA scale, in which scores can range from 30 to 210, respondents' actual scores ranged from 51 to 210.

4. Exercise Figure 2-4 contains the box plot that we ran in SPSS for Windows 12.0 by clicking on Graphics, then Box plot. The box encloses the data from the 25th to the 75th percentile (50% of the data) for the IPPA total score (TOTAL) by gender. The median is represented by the horizontal line within the box. In SPSS, extreme outlying values are defined as those that

WORK current work status

		Frequency	Percent	Valid Percent	Cumulative Percent
Valid	0 Unemployed	105	15.0	15.0	15.0
	1 Part Time	159	22.7	22.7	37.8
	2 Full Time	435	62.1	62.2	100.0
	Total	699	99.7	100.0	
Missing	System	2	.3		
Total		701	100.0		

POLAFF political affiliation

		Frequency	Percent	Valid Percent	Cumulative Percent
Valid	1 Republican	137	19.5	19.8	19.8
	2 Democrat	225	32.1	32.5	52.3
	3 Independent	330	47.1	47.7	100.0
	Total	692	98.7	100.0	
Missing	System	9	1.3		
Total		701	100.0		

WINTER choosing a winter vacation

		Frequency	Percent	Valid Percent	Cumulative Percent
Valid	1 beachfront condo in Hawaii	294	41.9	42.2	42.2
	2 chalet in Swiss Alps	145	20.7	20.8	63.0
	3 luxury hotel at Disney World in Florida	97	13.8	13.9	76.9
	4 ocean cruise through Caribbean Islands	161	23.0	23.1	100.0
	Total	697	99.4	100.0	
Missing	System	4	.6		
Total		701	100.0		

EXERCISE FIGURE 2-2. Tables of categorical variables.

Statistics

		AGE subject's age	EDUC education in years	TOTAL
N	Valid	684	673	661
	Missing	17	28	40
Mean		38.06	16.60	152.7035
Std. Error of Mean		.496	.133	1.09203
Median		37.00	16.00	155.0000
Mode		28	16	162.00
Std. Deviation		12.972	3.460	28.07608
Variance		168.266	11.973	788.26649
Skewness		.753	.153	−.612
Std. Error of Skewness		.093	.094	.095
Kurtosis		.796	.474	.472
Std. Error of Kurtosis		.187	.188	.190
Range		80	23	159.00
Minimum		15	7	51.00
Maximum		95	30	210.00
Sum		26034	11171	100937.00

EXERCISE FIGURE 2–3. A table describing continuous variables.

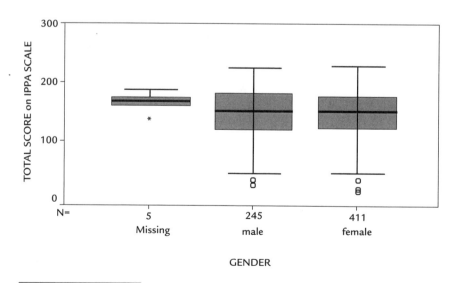

EXERCISE FIGURE 2-4. A box plot of the variable IPPA total score by gender.

are more than three box lengths from the upper or lower edge of the box and are designated by asterisks. In this figure, there are no extreme outlying scores. Cases with values between 1.5 and 3 box lengths from the edges of the box are called outliers and are designated by a circle. Although not seen on the box plot, SPSS will print next to the circle the code number(s) of the case(s) with the outlier value. We can then find that specific outlying cases on the variable of interest. The plot helps us determine quickly which subjects are associated with the outlying values.

Key Principles of Statistical Inference

Mary E. Duffy, Barbara Hazard Munro, and
Barbara S. Jacobsen

Objectives for Chapter 3

After reading this chapter, you should be able to do the following:

1. Describe the principles of statistical inference.
2. Describe the characteristics of a normal distribution.
3. Discuss the types of hypothesis testing.
4. Discuss type I and type II statistical errors.
5. Define sensitivity, specificity, predictive value, and efficiency.
6. Discuss tests of significance.
7. Interpret a confidence interval.
8. Examine the components of sample size estimation for study populations.

*S*tatistical inference involves obtaining information from a sample of data about the population from which the sample is drawn and setting up a model to describe this population. For example, the average birth weight of all newborns in a hospital in 2002 (population) can be estimated using observations from a sample of those newborns. Suppose 810 infants were born in the hospital in 2002, and the birth weights of the first 81 newborns (starting January 1) were recorded and averaged. Would the average (mean) birth weight in that sample of 81 be a good estimate of the mean birth weight in the 810 (the population of interest)? It would not be if birth weight depends on time of year or if an effective prenatal nutrition program to improve birth weight had begun in the surrounding community near that time. How can a sample that is representative of that population of 810 be selected? One way is by random selection.

When a *random sample* is drawn from the population of interest, every member of the population has the same probability (chance) of being selected in the sample. If the population is a finite one in which every person in the population can be listed, a table of random numbers can then be used to select a random sample of any size. Prior to using the World Wide Web (WWW), most people would use a table of random numbers to draw the sample. Now, using the WWW, it is very easy to generate a table of random numbers for many different purposes. Two websites that researchers have used extensively to generate random number tables are *Research Randomizer* (http://www.randomizer.org) and *Random.org* (http://www.random.org). Both sites also permit downloading of randomly generated numbers in a variety of formats, including Microsoft Excel. It is very worthwhile to use one of these sites to accomplish random number generation for research purposes.

Random samples have a high likelihood of being representative of the population from which they were drawn. In contrast, nonprobability samples, or samples nonrandomly selected, are very likely not to represent the populations from which they were selected. Suppose a 10% random sample was selected from the population of 810 newborns. It is very unlikely that the resulting random sample would be the first 81 infants born in 2002.

Random samples are likely to represent the target population because they are based on the principle that each unit in the population has an equal chance of being chosen for the sample. Thus, random samples are considered unbiased in that the process of random sampling produces samples that theoretically represent the population. Most important, the statistical theory on which this book is based assumes random sampling.

Statistical inference is of two types: parameter estimation and hypothesis testing. *Parameter estimation* takes two forms: point estimation and interval estimation. When an estimate of the population parameter is given as a single number, it is called a *point estimate*. The sample mean, median, variance, and standard deviation would all be considered point estimates. Thus, the average birth weight for the random sample of 81 newborns would be a point estimate. In contrast, *interval estimation* of a parameter involves more than one point; it consists of a range of values within which the population parameter is thought to be. A common type of interval estimation is the construction of a confidence interval (CI) and the upper and lower limits of the range of values, called confidence limits. Both point and CI estimates are types of statistical estimates that let us *infer* the true value of an unknown population parameter using information from a *random sample* of that population.

Hypothesis testing, the second and more common type of parameter estimation, will be discussed later in this chapter.

NORMAL CURVE

The *normal curve*, also called the Gaussian curve, is a theoretically perfect frequency polygon in which the mean, median, and mode all coincide in the center, and it takes the form of a symmetrical bell-shaped curve (Fig. 3-1). De Moivre, a French mathematician, developed the notion of the normal curve based on his observations of games of chance. Many human traits, such as intelligence, attitudes,

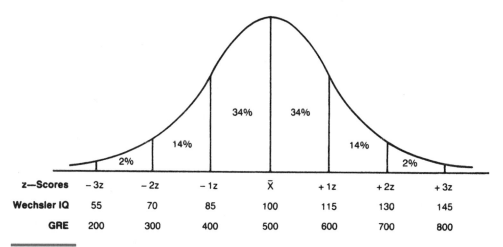

z—Scores	– 3z	– 2z	– 1z	x̄	+ 1z	+ 2z	+ 3z
Wechsler IQ	55	70	85	100	115	130	145
GRE	200	300	400	500	600	700	800

FIGURE 3-1. The normal curve.

and personality, are distributed among the population in a fairly normal way; that is, if you measure something, such as an intelligence test, in a representative sample of sufficient size, the resulting scores will assume a distribution that is similar to the normal curve. Most scores will fall around the mean (an IQ of 100), and there will be relatively few extreme scores, such as an IQ below 55 or above 145.

The normal curve is the most important distribution in statistics for three reasons (Vaughan, 1998). First, although most distributions are not exactly normal, most variables tend to have approximately normal distributions. Second, many inferential statistics assume that the populations are distributed normally. Third, the normal curve is a probability distribution and is used to answer questions about the likelihood of getting various particular outcomes when sampling from a population. For example, when we discuss hypothesis testing, we will talk about the probability (or the likelihood) that a given difference or relationship could have occurred by chance alone. Understanding the normal curve prepares you for understanding the concepts underlying hypothesis testing.

The baseline of the normal curve is measured off in standard deviation (SD) units. These are indicated by the lowercase letter z in Fig. 3-1. A score that is 1 SD above the mean is symbolized by $+1z$, and $-1z$ indicates a score that is 1 SD below the mean. For example, the Wechsler IQ test has a mean of 100 and an SD of 15. Thus, 1 SD above the mean ($+1z$) is determined by adding the SD to the mean ($15 + 100 = 115$), and 1 SD below the mean ($-1z$) is found by subtracting the SD from the mean ($100 - 15 = 85$). A score 2 SD above the mean is $15 + 15 + 100 = 130$; a score 2 SD below the mean is $100 - (15 + 15) = 70$.

When a variable's mean and SD are known, any set of scores can be transformed into z-scores, which have a mean of 0 and an SD of 1. Thus, the z-score tells how many SD a given score is above or below the mean of the distribution. The general formula for converting a score into a z-score is:

$$z = (\text{Score} - M)/SD$$

However, do not assume that converting variable raw scores to z-scores will result in a normal distribution: A distribution of z-scores has exactly the same distribution as the original distribution. Thus, if the original distribution was positively skewed, the resulting z-score distribution will be positively skewed.

In a normal distribution, approximately 34% of the scores fall between the mean and 1 SD above the mean. Because the curve is symmetrical, 34% also fall between the mean and 1 SD below the mean. Therefore, 68% of scores fall between $-1z$ and $+1z$. With the Wechsler IQ test, this means that 68%, or approximately two thirds of the scores, will fall between 85 and 115. Of the one third of the scores remaining, one sixth will fall below 85, and one sixth will be above 115.

Of the total distribution, 28% fall between 1 and 2 SD from the mean, 14% fall between 1 and 2 SDs above the mean, and 14% fall between 1 and 2 SD below the mean. Thus, 96% of the scores $(14 + 34 + 34 + 14)$ fall between ±2 SD from the mean. For the Wechsler IQ test, this means that 96% of the population receive scores between 70 and 130. Most of the last 4% fall between 2 and 3 SD from the mean, 2% on each side. Thus, 99.7% of those taking the Wechsler IQ test score between 55 and 145.

Two other z-scores are important because we use them when constructing confidence intervals. They are $z = \pm1.96$ and $z = \pm2.58$. Of the scores in a distribution, 95% fall between $\pm1.96z$, and 99% fall between $\pm2.58z$. For additional practice with the normal curve, look at the Graduate Record Examination (GRE) scores in Fig. 3-1. Each section of the GRE was scaled to have a mean of 500 and an SD of 100. A person who scored 600 on this test would be 1 SD above the mean, or at the 84th percentile. (The 50th percentile is the mean, and 34% above the mean equals the 84th percentile.)

PERCENTILES

In Chapter 2, we pointed out that percentiles allow us to describe a given score in relation to other scores in a distribution. A *percentile* tells us the relative position of a given score and allows us to compare scores on tests that have different means and SDs. A percentile is calculated as

$$\frac{\text{number of scores less than a given score}}{\text{total number of scores}} \times 100$$

Suppose you received a score of 90 on a test given to a class of 50 people. Of your classmates, 40 had scores lower than 90. Your percentile rank would be:

$$(40/50) \times 100 = 80$$

You achieved a higher score than 80% of the people who took the test, which also means that almost 20% who took the test did better than you.

As mentioned in Chapter 2, the 25th percentile is called the *first quartile*; the 50th percentile, the *second quartile* or more commonly the *median*; and the 75th percentile, the *third quartile*. The quartiles are points, not ranges like the interquartile range (IQR). Therefore, the third quartile is not from 50 to 75; it is just the 75th percentile. A score is not said to fall within a quartile, because the quartile is only one point.

As demonstrated with the GRE score of 600, we also can determine percentile rank by using the normal curve. For another example, in Fig. 3-1, the IQ score of 85 exceeds the score of 16% of the population, so a score of 85 is equal to a percentile rank of 16. To test your understanding, determine the percentile rank of a GRE score of 700. Remember that a percentile rank is not a percentile. The *percentile rank* is the *percentage of observations* below a certain score value; a *percentile* is a *score value* below which a certain number of observations in a distribution falls.

Tables make it possible to determine the proportion of the normal curve found between various points along the baseline. They are set up as in Appendix A. To understand how to read the table, go down the first column until you come to 1.0. Note that the percentage of area under the normal curve between the mean and a standard score (z-score) of 1.00 is 34.13. This is how the 34% was determined in Fig. 3-1. Moving down the row to the right, note that the area under the curve between the mean and 1.01 is 34.38, between the mean and 1.02 is 34.61, and so forth.

Suppose you have a standard score of $+1.39$ (the next section discusses how to calculate the z-scores). Finding this score in the table, we see that the percentage of the curve between the mean and 1.39 is 41.77. A plus z-score is above the mean, so 50% of the curve is on the minus z side, and another 41.77% is between the mean and $+1.39$; the percentile rank is 91.77 (50 + 41.77). If the z-score were -1.39, the score would fall below the mean, and the percentile rank would be 8.23 (50 − 41.77).

In summary, to calculate a percentile when you have the standard score, you first look up the score in the table (Appendix A) to determine the percentage of the normal curve that falls between the mean and the given score. Then, if the sign is positive, you add the percentage to 50. If the sign is negative, you subtract the percentage from 50.

When using percentiles to determine relative position, it is important to remember the following points:

1. Because so many scores are located near the mean and so few at the ends, the distance along the baseline in terms of percentiles varies a great deal.
2. The distance between the 50th percentile and the 55th percentile is much smaller than the distance between the 90th and the 95th.

What this means in practical terms is that if you raise your score on a test, there will be more impact on your percentile rank if you are near the mean than if you are near the ends of the distribution. For example, suppose three people again took the GRE quantitative examination in hopes of raising their scores and thus their percentile ranks (Table 3-1). All three subjects raised their score by 10 points. For subject 1, who was right at the mean, that meant an increase of 4 points in percentile rank, whereas for subject 3, who was originally 2 SD above the mean, the percentile rank went up only half a point.

Subject	Scores	GRE-Q	Percentile
1	1st score	500	50
	2nd score	510	54
2	1st score	600	84
	2nd score	610	86
3	1st score	700	97.7
	2nd score	710	98.2

TABLE 3-1 *Relationship of Scores to Percentiles at Varying Distances from the Mean*

STANDARD SCORES

Standard scores are a way of expressing a score in terms of its relative distance from the mean. A z-score is one such standard score. The meaning of an ordinary score varies depending on the mean and the SD of the distribution from which it was drawn. In research, standard scores are used more often than percentiles. Thus far, we have used examples when the z-score was easy to calculate. The GRE score of 600 is 1 SD above the mean, so the z-score is +1. The formula used to calculate z-scores is:

$$z = \frac{X - M}{SD}$$

The numerator is a measure of the deviation of the score from the mean of the distribution. The following calculation is for the GRE example:

$$z = (600 - 500)/100 = 100/100 = 1$$

As another example, suppose a person obtained a score of 50 on a test in which the mean was 36 and the SD was 4.

$$z = (50 - 36)/4 = 14/4 = 3.5$$

Using the table in Appendix A, we find that 49.98% of the curve is contained between the mean and 3.5 SD above the mean, so the percentile rank for this score would be 99.98 (50 + 49.98).

Suppose the national mean weight for a particular group is 130 pounds, and the SD is 8 pounds. An individual from the group, Jane, weighs 110 pounds. What is Jane's z-score and percentile rank?

$$z = (110 - 130)/8 = -20/8 = -2.5$$

Jane's percentile rank is 50 − 49.38, or 0.62.

If all the raw scores in a distribution are converted to z-scores, the resulting distribution will have a mean of zero and an SD of 1. If several distributions are converted to z-scores, the z-scores for the various measures can be compared directly. Although each new distribution has a new SD and mean (1 and 0), the shape of the distribution is not altered.

Transformed Standard Scores

Because calculating z-scores results in decimals and negative numbers, some people prefer to transform them into other distributions. A widely used distribution is one with a mean of 50 and an SD of 10. Such *transformed standard scores* are generally called *T-scores*, although some authors call them *Z-scores*. Some standardized test results are given in *T*-scores. To convert a z-score to a *T* score, use the following formula:

$$T = 10z + 50$$

For example, with a z-score of 2.5, the *T*-score would be:

$$T = (10)(2.5) + 50$$
$$T = 25 + 50$$
$$T = 75$$

In the new distribution, the mean is 50 and the SD is 10, so a score of 75 is still 2.5 SD above the mean.

In the same way, other distributions can be established. This is the technique used to transform z-scores into GRE scores with a mean of 500 and an SD of 100. The basic formula for transforming z-scores is to multiply the z-scores by the desired SD and add the desired mean:

$$\text{transformed } z\text{-scores} = (\text{new SD})(z\text{-score}) + (\text{new mean})$$

Suppose you wanted to transform your z-scores into a scale with a mean of 70 and an SD of 10. Then your formula would be $10z + 70$. Transforming scores in this way does not change the original distribution of the scores. In some circumstances, however, a researcher may want to change the distribution of a set of data. This might occur when you have a set of data that is not normally distributed.

CORRECTING FAILURES IN NORMALITY THROUGH DATA TRANSFORMATIONS

Many statistical techniques assume that data are normally distributed in the population being studied. Even though many methods will work just as well when this assumption is violated (Glass & Hopkins, 1996), data transformation is often recommended to convert original scores to another metric that approximates normality. Such transformations, however, should be approached with caution because they make interpretation of the results more difficult. The transformed scales are not in the same metric as the original; thus, measures of central tendency and dispersion are not clear in relation to the original measure.

As discussed in Chapter 2, Tabachnick and Fidell (2001) recommend procedures for handling skewness problems. Because the impact of skewness on data analysis, results, and interpretation is often overlooked, this information bears repeating.

First, determine the direction of the deviation. Positive skewness, with the long tail to the right, can be handled in a straightforward manner. However, if a variable has negative skewness, with the long tail to the left, it is best to make it positive by "reflecting" it before transformation. (Reflecting a variable is the same as reverse-coding of all scores in the distribution using a RECODE command so that what was once the lowest score becomes the highest score and so on for all values in the distribution.) This is done as follows:

1. Find the largest value in the distribution and add one to it to form a constant that is larger than any score in the distribution. For example, if the largest score in a distribution is 24, adding one forms a constant of 25 ($24 + 1 = 25$).
2. Create a new variable by subtracting each score in the distribution from this constant. The new variable, which originally was negatively skewed, now has a positive skewness.

The reflected variable's interpretation changes in the opposite direction as well. If high scores on a variable before it was reflected indicated a large amount of a characteristic, these scores, after reflection, signify a small amount of that characteristic.

Once the direction of the skew has been addressed, use

- A square root transformation for moderate skewness,
- A log transformation for severe skewness,
- An inverse transformation for very severe, or J-shaped, skewness (Tabachnick & Fidell, 2001).

After each attempt at correcting the skew, recalculate the measure of skewness to determine whether the variable is normally, or nearly normally, distributed after transformation. If the transformed variable has a more normal distribution, then use it in subsequent data analyses. Report your use of the transformed variable in subsequent tables and in the narrative of the research report. If transformations are not successful, consider creating a categorical (nominal) variable in place of the continuous variable.

CENTRAL LIMIT THEOREM

If you draw a sample from a population and calculate its mean, how close have you come to knowing the mean of the population? Statisticians have provided us with formulas that allow us to determine just how close the mean of our sample is to the mean of the population.

When many samples are drawn from a population, the means of these samples tend to be normally distributed; that is, when they are charted along a baseline, they tend to form the normal curve. The larger the number of samples, the more the distribution approximates the normal curve. Also, if the average of the means of the samples is calculated (the mean of the means), this average (or mean) is very close to the actual mean of the population. Again, the larger the number of samples, the closer this overall mean is to the population mean.

If the means form a normal distribution, we can then use the percentages under the normal curve to determine the probability statements about individual means. For example, we would know that the probability of a given mean falling between $+1$ and -1 SD from the mean of the population is 68%.

To calculate the standard scores necessary to determine position under the normal curve, we need to know the SD of the distribution. You could calculate the SD of the distribution of means by treating each mean as a raw score and applying the regular formula. This new SD of the means is called the *standard error of the mean*. The term *error* is used to indicate the fact that due to sampling error, each sample mean is likely to deviate somewhat from the true population mean.

Fortunately, statisticians have used these techniques on samples drawn from known populations and have demonstrated relationships that allow us to estimate the mean and SD of a population given the data from only one sample. They have established that there is a constant relationship between the SD of a distribution of sample means (the standard error of the mean), the SD of the population from which the samples were drawn, and the size of the samples. We do not usually know the SD of the population. If we had measured the whole population, we would have no need to infer its parameters from measures taken from samples. The formula for the standard error of the mean can be written as:

$$\frac{\text{standard deviation}}{\text{square root of } n}$$

The formula indicates that we are estimating the standard error given the SD of a sample of n size. A sample of 30 (Vaughan, 1998) is enough to estimate the population mean with reasonable accuracy. Given the SD of a sample and the size of the sample, we can estimate the standard error of the mean. For example, given a sample of 100 and an SD of 40, we would estimate the standard error of the mean to be:

$$40/\sqrt{100} = 40/10 = 4$$

Two factors influence the standard error of the mean: the SD of the sample and the sample size. The sample size has a large impact on the size of the error because the square root of n is used in the denominator. As the size of n increases, the size of the error decreases. Suppose we had the same SD as just demonstrated, but a sample size of 1,000 instead of 100. Now we have $40/\sqrt{1,000} = 40/31.62 = 1.26$ a much smaller standard error. This shows that the larger the sample, the less the error. If there is less error, we can estimate more precisely the parameters of the population.

If there is more variability in the sample, the standard error increases. If there is much variability, it is harder to draw a sample that is representative of the population. Given wide variability, we need larger samples. Note the effect of variability (SD) on the standard error of the mean.

$$20/\sqrt{100} = 20/10 = 2$$
$$40/\sqrt{100} = 40/10 = 4$$

As is shown later in this chapter, the standard error of the mean underlies the calculation of the confidence interval.

PROBABILITY

Ideas about probability are of primary importance to health care researchers. The use of data in making decisions is a hallmark of our information world, and probability provides a means for translating observed data into decisions about the nature of our world (Kotz & Stroup, 1983). For example, probability helps us to evaluate the accuracy of a statistic and to test a hypothesis. Thus, research findings in journals often are stated in terms of probabilities and are often communicated to patients using this language. The approach to probability in this chapter is practical, with special attention given to concepts that are important later in this text. Probability also underlies the use of logistic regression, presented in Chapter 13.

In the life of a health care professional, questions about probability frequently occur in connection with a patient's future. For example, suppose patient X's mammogram revealed a cluster of five calcifications with no other signs of breast abnormality. The patient is told she should have a breast biopsy based solely on these X-ray findings. If the patient asks about the probability that the biopsy will reveal a malignancy, health care professionals refer to the literature. Powell, McSweeney, and Wilson (1983) studied 251 patients who underwent a breast biopsy with mammographic calcifications as the only reason for the biopsy. Everyone in the sample had at least five microcalcifications in a well-defined cluster. Cancer was found in 45 of these patients (17.9%). Consequently, the patient might be told that the probability of cancer was 17.9%.

What has really been stated? The health care practitioner has presumably imagined that the names of the 251 patients in the study were placed in a hat, and one name was drawn by chance. The odds of drawing the name of one of the 45 patients with cancer are 45 in 251, or 17.9%. Patient X, of course, is not one of the 251 names in the hat, but the practitioner is thinking along the lines of, "What if she were?" This way of thinking, although hypothetical, is reasonable if patient X is similar to the group of 251 patients in the study. Powell et al. (1983) described the sample of 251 patients as consecutively chosen over a period of 18 years from the practice of one surgeon at one hospital. Although this information implies a fairly broad sample, it does not provide any breakdown by prognostic variables.

An outcome may vary according to membership in a certain subset of a total group. For example, in 1982, a male patient was diagnosed with a rare form of abdominal cancer (Gould, 1985). The patient read that the median mortality was 8 months after diagnosis; therefore, he reasoned that his chances of living longer than 8 months were 50%. On reading further, he decided that his chances of being in that 50% who lived longer were good: He was young, the disease was discovered early, and he was receiving the best treatment. He also realized that the survival distribution was undoubtedly skewed to the right, indicating that some patients lived for years with the disease. Therefore, if he was in the upper 50%, his chances of living a lot longer than 8 months were very good.

Self-Evident Truths (Axioms) about Probabilities

All probabilities are between 0% and 100%, as illustrated in Fig. 3-2. There are no negative probabilities. If the probability of something happening is 0%, then it is

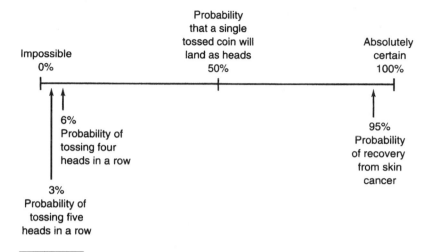

FIGURE 3 2. Diagram of the scale of probabilities.

impossible. Although one must be careful about assigning a probability of 0% to an event, it is highly likely that the probability is 0% that a 98-year-old woman would give birth to a newborn. If the probability of an event is 100%, then we are certain that it will occur. The eventual death of a person has a probability of 100%.

The probability of an event is 100% minus the probability of the opposite event. Perhaps a different health care worker would have preferred to tell patient X there was an 82.1% chance that the breast microcalcifications would *not* be malignant. This would be accurate because 100% − 17.9% = 82.1%.

Table 3-2 lists the four possibilities for the sample of 45 women who were diagnosed with cancer after a biopsy based on a suspicious mammogram, as given by Powell et al. (1983). The sum of all the possibilities for an event is 100%. The sum

TABLE 3-2 *Malignant Pathology of X-Ray Calcifications*	
Pathology	**N**
Duct cancer, in situ	25
Lobular cancer, in situ	9
Duct, invasive	9
Lobular, invasive	2
	45
	(*100%*)

Data from Powell, R. W., McSweeney, M. B., & Wilson, C. E. (1983). X-ray calcifications as the only basis for breast biopsy. *Annals of Surgery, 197*, 555–559. Modified slightly to represent individual patients rather than 47 breasts from 45 patients.

of the four outcomes in Table 3-2 is 100%, indicating that it is certain that one of these possibilities will occur.

Definitions of Probability

FREQUENCY PROBABILITY

Most health care professionals, however, think of probability in the sense of a frequency or statistical probability—that is, they think of probability as a percentage based on empirical observation, which allows them to make an intelligent guess about the future. Their definition for such a probability, based on observations from a sample, is:

$$\text{sample probability} = \frac{\text{number of times the event occurred}}{\text{total number of people in the sample}} \times 100$$

For patient X with the suspicious mammogram findings, the health care worker would substitute as follows:

$$\text{probability of cancer} = (45/251) \times 100 = 17.9\%$$

Patient X was not a member of the group of 251 patients, but the hypothetical type of thinking, "What if patient X were from that group?" is at least reasonable as a practical type of probability. It helps to be able to argue logically that patient X might have been a member of the total group of 251 patients.

In mathematical theory, however, probabilities are meaningful only in the context of chance. We also have to imagine that patient X was chosen "by chance" from the total sample, which implies a random choice. There are two criteria for a random process. First, every item must have an equal chance of being chosen. In the case of drawing from a hat, this means that attention must be given to details, such as whether each name was written on the same-size slip of paper, whether the slips were well mixed, whether the person who drew from the hat was blindfolded, and so forth.[1] Second, each choice must be independent of every other choice. This means that we must not be able to predict whose name will be drawn after patient X.

These criteria for a random process also are important when we consider the larger question of whether the 17.9% probability of cancer would still be the same if more patients were followed. The mathematical definition for a frequency probability invokes the law of averages; that is, we must think of drawing more patients at random. As the sample becomes larger and larger, the percentage will converge to the true or population value.

$$\text{population probability} = \frac{\text{total number of times the event occurred}}{\text{total number of people in the population}} \times 100$$

Thus, the sample probability is an estimate of the population probability. A random sample provides, in theory, a better estimate of the population probability.

---

[1]Health care researchers who wish to draw a random sample avoid having to deal with such details by using a random number table or Research Randomizer.

In a brief discussion section following the article by Powell et al. (1983), Letton reported on a second sample of 269 patients collected for 10 years. A mammogram indicated calcium deposits, and subsequent biopsies revealed that 46 patients (17.1%) had cancer. Thus, a second study, again with a nonrandom sample, produced remarkably similar results to those of Powell et al.

Random sampling is infrequently used in health care research (Burns & Grove, 2001; Jacobsen & Meininger, 1985; McLaughlin & Marascuilo, 1990). Patients who arrive for care become the sample, and health care researchers take all they can get rather than drawing random samples. These sample probabilities, although not based on a chance process, remain as our only estimates of the true or population probabilities.

Frequency probabilities are based on empirical observations and can thus be termed objective. However, not all probabilities that can be considered objective are determined empirically. For example, when tossing a fair coin, the probabilities of heads or tails can be deduced logically without ever actually tossing the coin. These are called a priori (before the fact), or prior, probabilities. Derdiarian and Lewis (1986) provided an illustration of how a priori probabilities could be used in health care research. Each of three raters was asked to code an item from an interview transcript as belonging to category 1 or category 2. There are eight possible outcomes, as listed in Table 3-3. All three raters could agree that the item belonged in category 1 (1-1-1), or they could disagree, for example, with the first rater coding the item as category 1 and the other two coding the item as category 2 (1-2-2). If all of these outcomes are equally probable by chance, then each will have a probability of 1 in 8. Derdiarian and Lewis (1986) showed how comparing actual results to the tabled probabilities can provide a measure of inter-rater agreement.

TABLE 3-3 *Probability of Eight Possible Outcomes for Three Raters Coding an Item Into Dichotomous Categories (1 or 2) by Chance*

	Outcome		
Rater #1	Rater #2	Rater #3	Probability
1	1	1	$\frac{1}{8}$
1	1	2	$\frac{1}{8}$
1	2	1	$\frac{1}{8}$
2	1	1	$\frac{1}{8}$
1	2	2	$\frac{1}{8}$
2	1	2	$\frac{1}{8}$
2	2	1	$\frac{1}{8}$
2	2	2	$\frac{1}{8}$

Derdiarian, A. K., & Lewis, S. (1986). The D-L test of agreement: A stronger measure of interrater reliability. *Nursing Research, 35*, 375–378.

SUBJECTIVE PROBABILITY

Another definition for probability is a percentage that expresses our personal, subjective belief that an event will occur. Fisher and van Belle (1993) emphasize that these judgments are not whimsical or irrational; they are based on empiric evidence chosen for some personal reason. In the example of patient X with the suspicious mammogram findings, what is the health care professional's opinion about the probability of 17.9% that the calcifications are cancer? If the patient was told that the probability was close to zero that the biopsy findings would be malignant, then we would be surprised if it turned out to be cancer. On the other hand, most health care professionals would not view a probability of 17.9% as "close to zero." A practitioner would not be very surprised if the calcifications turned out to be cancer, and that is why patient X with five or more calcifications in a cluster was recommended for biopsy.

When testing hypotheses, which is discussed later in this text, researchers focus on probabilities (often called *p* values) that fall at the lower end of the continuum in Fig. 3-2. Generally, probabilities that are 5% or less are considered unusual in research. The reasons for this are partly intuitive and partly historic. For example, as part of a statistics class, the professor would toss a coin and arrange for it to turn up heads all the time. Intuitively, students begin to laugh and become skeptical after seeing four or five heads in a row. The probability of four heads in a row by chance is approximately 6%, and the probability of five heads in a row is approximately 3%. Note that 5% falls between the two.

The historic reasons for the 5% cutoff are partly based on the preference of Sir Ronald Fisher. Moore (1991) quotes Fisher as writing in 1926 that he preferred the 5% point for marking off the probable from the improbable. Because Fisher was an extremely influential statistician, others adopted this rule too. Moreover, the past inconveniences of calculating have influenced the choice of the 5% mark. Before the computer age, the tables for probabilities for various distributions in textbooks were constructed with handy columns such as 20%, 10%, 5%, and 1%—presumably because we have five fingers and our number system is based on 10. Today, these tables and the use of the 5% level are "almost obsolete" (Freedman et al., 1991, p. 494) because the computer can produce an exact probability based on a mathematical equation. Many researchers and editors of journals, however, persist in using the 5% mark as a cutoff for "unusual" simply because it is convenient to have some general standard that is easy to grasp.

Instead of using the 5% criterion, however, researchers often adopt probability cutoffs that are more generous (eg, 10%) or more strict (eg, 1%) based on their own intuition or the purposes and design of their research. Oftentimes when the researcher is interested in exploring relationships among variables and not hypothesis-testing, a less-stringent cutoff, such as 10% or 20%, might be used. In contrast, a researcher might set the cutoff level at 1% because of testing several hypotheses using one dataset.

At the higher end of the probability continuum, researchers consider probabilities of 95% or more as evidence for reporting potential events that they are confident will occur. The oft-quoted probability of 95% for recovery from skin cancer is empirically derived, and most health care workers would be surprised if recovery did not occur. Likewise, probabilities near the upper end of the probability scale frequently are used to express confidence in a statistic. For example, a poll reported that 38% of a pre-election random sample favored candidate A. The margin of error was given as 3%, with 95% confidence.

HYPOTHESIS TESTING

Given an underlying theoretical structure, a representative sample, and an appropriate research design, the researcher can test hypotheses. We test to see whether the data support our hypothesis. We do not claim to prove that our hypothesis is true, because one study can never prove anything; it is always possible that some error has distorted the findings.

Null Hypothesis and Alternative Hypothesis

Hypothesis testing is a predominant feature of quantitative health care research. Hypotheses originate from the theory that underpins the research. When a hypothesis relates to the characteristics of a population, such as population parameters, statistical methods can be used with sample data to test its soundness.

There are two types of hypotheses: null and alternative. The *null hypothesis* proposes no difference or relationship between the variables of interest. Often written as H_o, the null hypothesis is the foundation of the statistical test. When you statistically test a hypothesis, you assume that H_o correctly describes the state of affairs between the two variables of interest. If a significant difference or relationship is found, the null hypothesis is rejected; if no difference or relationship is found, H_o is accepted.

The *alternative hypothesis*, represented by H_a, is a hypothesis that contradicts H_o. The alternative hypothesis can indicate the direction of the difference or relationship that you expect. Thus, the alternative hypothesis is often called the *research hypothesis*, represented by H_r (Agresti & Finlay, 1997).

Types of Error

When we sample, we select cases from a predetermined population. Due to chance variations in choosing the sample's few cases from the population's many possible cases, the sample will deviate from the defined population's true nature by a certain amount. This deviation is called *sampling error*. Thus, inferences from samples to populations are always *probabilistic*, meaning we can never be 100% certain that our inference was correct.

Drawing the wrong conclusion is called an *error of inference*. There are two types of errors of inference, defined in terms of the null hypothesis: *type I* and *type II*.

Before describing these errors, the possibilities related to decisions about the null hypothesis are presented using the following diagram:

	Null Hypothesis	
Decision	*True*	*False*
Accept H_o	OK	Type II
Reject H_o	Type I	OK

If H_o is true and we accept that hypothesis, we have responded correctly. The incorrect response would be to reject a true null hypothesis (type I error). If H_o is false and we reject it, we have responded correctly. The wrong response would be to accept a false null hypothesis (type II error).

Suppose you compared two groups of patients with diabetes taught by different methods (A and B) on how to care for themselves at home, and the data indicated that group A scored significantly higher than group B. You would then reject H_o. Suppose, however, that group A had more diabetics with knowledge about caring for themselves at home and that the method actually did not matter at all. Rejecting the null hypothesis is a type I error.

The probability of making a type I error is called alpha (a) and can be *decreased* by altering the significance level. In other words, you could set the *p* at 0.01 instead of 0.05; then there is only 1 chance in 100 (1%) that the result termed significant could occur by chance alone. If you do that, however, you will make it more difficult to find a significant result; that is, you will decrease the *power* of the test and increase the risk of a type II error.

A *type II error* is accepting a *false* null hypothesis. If the data showed no significant results, the researcher would accept the null hypothesis. If there were significant differences, a type II error would have been made. To avoid a type II error, you could make the level of significance less extreme. There is a greater chance of finding significant results if you are willing to risk 10 chances in 100 that you are wrong ($p = 0.10$) than there is if you are willing to risk only 5 chances in 100 ($p = 0.05$). Other ways to decrease the likelihood of a type II error are to increase the sample size, decrease sources of extraneous variation, and increase the effect size. The *effect size* is the impact made by the independent variable. For example, if group A scored 10 points higher on the diabetic self-care knowledge scale than group B, the effect size would be 10 divided by the SD of the measure (Cohen, 1988).

There is a trade-off, however, because there is an inverse relationship between type I and type II error. Decreasing the likelihood of a type II error increases the chance of a type I error. If decreasing the probability of one type of error increases the probability of the other type, the question arises: Which type of error are you willing to risk? As you might expect, that depends on the study. An example would be a test for a particular genetic defect. If the defect exists and is diagnosed early, it can be successfully treated; however, if it is not diagnosed and treated, the child will become severely retarded. On the other hand, if a child is erroneously diagnosed as having the defect and treated, no physical damage is done.

In terms of the types of errors, a type I error would be diagnosing the defect when it does not exist. In that case, the child would be treated but not harmed by the treatment. In contrast, a type II error would be declaring the child to be normal when he or she is not. In that case, irreversible damage would be done. In such a situation, it is obvious that you would make every attempt to avoid the type II error.

Suppose a national study was conducted to determine whether a particular approach to preschool preparation of underprivileged children leads to increased success in school. This approach would cost a great deal of money to implement nationwide. Those responsible for deciding whether to implement this approach would certainly want to be sure that a type I error had not been made. They would not want to institute a costly new program if it did not really have any effect on success in school.

Type I and II errors are hard for some people to grasp, so here are a few examples to help you understand the concept. Let's hypothesize that the two diabetic groups are equal in their knowledge of taking care of themselves. Has an error been made, and if so, what type of error, if the researcher does the following?

1. Accepts the null hypothesis when the groups are really equal in diabetic self-care knowledge.
2. Rejects the null hypothesis when the groups are really equal in diabetic self-care knowledge.
3. Rejects the null hypothesis when the groups are really different in their diabetic self-care knowledge.
4. Accepts the null hypothesis when one group has much more diabetic self-care knowledge than the other.

These four examples summarize the possibilities surrounding these errors. First, if we are given a situation in which H_0 is true—that is, there is no difference—we can either accept it and make the correct decision (#1), or reject it and make an incorrect decision, or a type I error (#2). Second, if H_0 is false, we can reject it, making a correct decision (#3), or accept it and make an incorrect decision, or a type II error (#4).

Sensitivity, Specificity, Predictive Value, and Efficiency

When thinking about types of errors, there is an analogy that can be drawn to diagnostic testing for specific diseases. Clinicians routinely order tests to screen patients for the presence or absence of disease. There are four possible outcomes to diagnosing and testing a particular patient: True Positive (TP), where both diagnosis and test are positive for the disease; True Negative (TN), where both diagnosis and test are negative; False Positive (FP), where the diagnosis is positive and the test is negative for the disease; and False Negative (FN) where the diagnosis is negative for the disease and the test is positive for it (Kraemer, 1992). Essex-Sorlie (1995) notes that a type I error resembles a *false positive outcome,* occurring when a clinical test result incorrectly indicates disease presence. A type II error is comparable to a *false negative* (FN) *outcome,* indicating a test result incorrectly points to disease absence. The following 2 × 2 table is often used as a way to depict the relationship between the various outcomes.

	Condition Present	**Condition Absent**
Test Positive	True Positive (TP)	False Positive (FP)
Test Negative	False Negative (FN)	True Negative (TN)

The terms used to define the clinical performance of a screening test are sensitivity, specificity, positive predictive value, negative predictive value, and efficiency. Test *sensitivity* (Sn) is defined as the probability that the test is positive when given to a group of patients who have the disease. It is determined by the formula Sn = (TP/(TP + FN)) × 100. In other words, sensitivity can be viewed as, **1 − the false negative rate**, expressed as a percent.

For example, Harvey and colleagues (1992) undertook a study to assess the use of plasma D-dimer levels for diagnosing deep venous thrombosis (DVT) in 105 patients hospitalized for stroke rehabilitation. Plasma samples were drawn from patients within 24 hours of a venous ultrasound screening for DVT. Of the 105 patients in the study, 14 had DVTs identified by ultrasound. The optimal cutoff for predicting DVT was a D-dimer > 1,591 ng/ml. Test results showed the following:

	Positive Ultrasound	**Negative Ultrasound**
d-Dimer > 1,591 ng/ml.	13 (TP)	19 (FP)
d-Dimer ≤ 1,591 ng/ml.	1 (FN)	72 (TN)
	14 (TP + FN)	91 (FP + TN)

Using the above formula, Sn = (TP/(TP + FN)) × 100 = 13/14 × 100 = 93, the sensitivity for the D-dimer test for diagnosing DVTs is 93%. The larger the sensitivity, the more likely the test is to confirm the disease. The D-dimer's test for diagnosing the presence of DVT is accurate 93% of the time.

The *specificity* (Sp) of a screening test is defined as the probability that the test will be negative among patients who do not have the disease. Its formula is Sp = (TN/(TN + FP)) × 100 and can be understood as **1 − the false positive rate**, expressed as a percent.

In the same example, the specificity for the D-dimer test was 79% (Sp = (72/(72 + 19)) × 100 = 72/91 × 100 = 79%). A large Sp means that a positive test can rule out the disease. The D-dimer's specificity of 79% indicates that that test is fairly good in ruling out the presence of DVTs in rehabilitation stroke patients.

The *positive predictive value* (PPV) of a test is the probability that a patient who tested positive for the disease actually has the disease. The formula for PPV is PPV = (TP/(TP + FP)) × 100. Again using the D-dimer test for predicting DVT, its PPV is calculated as PPV = (13/(13 + 19)) × 100 = 13/32 × 100 = 40.6 or 41%. This means that only 41 out of every 100 screened patients is likely to be a correctly diagnosed and 59 out of 100 are likely to be false positives.

The *negative predictive value* (NPV) of a test is the probability that a patient who tested negative for a disease will not have the disease. It is calculated as NPV = (TN/(TN + FN)) × 100. Using this formula in the above D-dimer test example, NPV = (72/(72 + 1)) × 100 = 72/73 × 100 = 98.6 or 99%. This value indicates that 99 out of 100 patients screened are likely to be true negatives. Thus, the D-dimer test is outstanding at ruling out DVTs in rehabilitation stroke patients who test negative for their presence.

The *efficiency* (EFF) of a test is the probability that the test result and the diagnosis agree (Kraemer, 1992) and is calculated as EFF = ((TP + TN)/(TP + TN + FP + FN)) × 100. In the D-dimer test example, EFF = ((13 + 72)/(13 + 72 + 19 + 1)) × 100 = 85/105 × 100 = 80.9%. Thus, the efficiency of this test in diagnosing rehabilitation stroke patients with DVTs is almost 81%.

SUMMARY

Sensitivity, specificity, predictive values, and efficiency of outcome measures are often reported in health care research studies. Sensitivity depends solely on how positive and negative test results are distributed within a diseased population whereas specificity depends only on how results are distributed in a nondiseased population. Positive predictive values are related to sensitivity and negative predictive values are associated with specificity. Efficiency is the overall accuracy of the test in measuring true findings divided by all of the test results.

In addition to the above calculations, clinical researchers may compute likelihood ratios and relative risks (discussed in later chapters in this book) and receiver operator characteristic (ROC) curve analysis, which graphically portrays a series of sensitivities and specificities for a given test. Kraemer (1992) provides a full treatment of ROC curve analysis. An excellent example of the use of ROC curve analysis in instrument validation can be found in Curley et al. (2003).

Significance Level (*p* Value)

In significance testing, we evaluate differences between what we expect on the basis of our hypothesis and what we observe, but only in relation to one criterion, the probability (*p*) that these differences could have happened by chance (Elwood, 1998; Henkel, 1986). Chance, or random, factors are those associated with the manner in which the observations used to test the hypothesis were chosen.

In significance testing, we have these two assumptions: H_0 is true and only chance factors could produce results different from what was hypothesized. We then obtain a distribution of possible outcomes, their relative frequency of occurrence, and the likelihood (or probability) that any particular observation would occur. The *p value* is the chief reported result of a significance test and enables us to judge the extent of the evidence against H_0. The *p* value, which ranges from 0.00 to 1.0, summarizes the evidence in the data about H_0. A large *p* value, such as 0.53 or 0.78, indicates that the observed data would not be unusual if H_0 were true. A small *p* value, such as 0.001, denotes that these data would be very doubtful if H_0 were true. This provides strong evidence against H_o. In such instances, results are said to be *significant at the 0.001 level*, indicating that getting a result of this size might occur only 1 out of 1,000 times.

The alpha level for a statistical test, usually chosen before analyzing data, reflects how careful the researcher wishes to be. The smaller the alpha level, the stronger the evidence must be to reject H_o.

In older studies, hypotheses were usually stated in null form; however, this is not done as often today. When you hypothesize, you state that you believe there is a difference or a relationship between the variables of interest (nondirectional relationship). It is stronger if you state what differences or relationships you expect (directional relationship), rather than write a string of null hypotheses.

It is important to understand the null hypothesis, however, because without it, there is no significance test. Suppose you stated that there is no significant difference between breast-fed and bottle-fed babies in terms of weight gain. If you really had no idea about this issue, it is more common not to state a hypothesis but simply to ask the research question: Is there a difference in weight gain between breast-fed and bottle-fed babies? Even though there is no explicit hypothesis, the null hypothesis (of no difference in weight gain between breast-fed and bottle-fed babies) is implied. If you had rationale for a hypothesis, you might state a directional research hypothesis (H_r) such as: Breast-fed babies gain more weight in the first week of life than bottle-fed babies.

Testing a Statistical Hypothesis

Statistical hypotheses are assumed to be true or false. When we use inferential statistics, we make a decision within a certain margin of error about whether to accept (H_o is true) or reject (H_o is false) the statistical hypothesis. By using the sampling distribution of the test statistic, we compute the probability, labeled p, that the values of the statistic like the one observed would occur if H_o were true.

Testing a statistical hypothesis involves several sequential steps (Glass & Hopkins, 1996; Henkel, 1986):

Step 1. State the statistical hypothesis to be tested; for example, H_o: population mean = 50.

Step 2. Choose the appropriate statistic to test H_o.

Step 3. Define the degree of risk of incorrectly concluding that H_o is false when it is true (type I error). This risk, commonly called alpha, is stated as the probability of a type I error (discussed in the next section). Unless otherwise indicated, alpha ≤ 0.05.

Step 4. Calculate the statistic from a set of randomly sampled observations.

Step 5. Decide whether to reject H_o on the basis of the sample statistic. For example, if p from Step 3 ≤ 0.05, H_o is rejected and we conclude the population mean is not 50. If $p > 0.05$, H_o is not rejected and we conclude the population mean = 50.

Power of a Test

The *power* of a test is the probability of detecting a difference or relationship if such a difference or relationship really exists. Anything that decreases the probability of a type II error increases power, and vice versa (Vaughan, 1998). A more powerful test is one that is more likely to reject H_o; that is, it is more likely to indicate a statistically significant result when such a difference or relationship exists in the population. The level of significance (probability level) and the power of the test are important factors to consider.

One-Tailed and Two-Tailed Tests

The "tails" refer to the ends of the normal curve. When we test for statistical significance, we want to know whether the difference or relationship is so extreme, so far out in the tail of the distribution, that it is unlikely to have occurred by chance alone. When we hypothesize the direction of the difference or relationship, we state in which tail of the distribution we expect to find the difference or relationship.

Although there is controversy about this, the practice among many researchers is to use a *one-tailed* test of significance when a directional hypothesis is stated and a *two-tailed* test in all other situations. The advantage of using the one-tailed test is that it is more powerful, because the value yielded by the statistical test does not have to be so large to be significant at a given p level. To gain this advantage, however, you must have a sound theoretical basis for the directional hypothesis; you cannot base it on a hunch.

The normal curve is used to demonstrate the difference between one-tailed and two-tailed tests (Fig. 3-3). Recall from our discussion of the normal curve that 95% of the distribution falls between ±1.96 SD from the mean. Thus, only 5% falls beyond these two points: 2.5% of the distribution falls below a z-score of -1.96, and

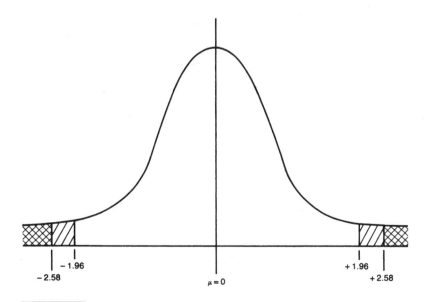

FIGURE 3-3. Two-tailed test of significance using the normal curve.

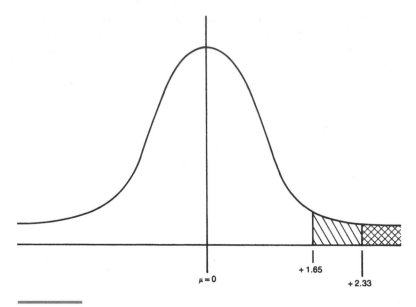

FIGURE 3-4. One-tailed test of significance using the normal curve.

2.5% falls above $+1.96z$. To be so "rare" as to occur only 5% of the time, a z-score would have to be $-1.96z$ or less or $+1.96z$ or greater. Note that we are using both tails of the distribution. Because 99% of the distribution falls between ± 2.58 SD from the mean of the normal curve, a score would have to be -2.58 or less or $+2.58$ or more to be declared significant at the 0.01 level.

Figure 3-4 shows what occurs when a directional hypothesis is stated. We examine only one tail of the distribution. In this example, we look at the positive side of the distribution. Fifty percent of the distribution falls below the mean and 45% falls between the mean and a z-score of $+1.65$ (see Appendix A). Thus, 95% (50 + 45) of the distribution falls below $+1.65z$. To score in the upper 5% would require a score of $+1.65$ or greater. Given a one-tailed test of significance, you would need a score of $+1.65z$ to be significant at the 0.05 level, whereas with a two-tailed test, you needed a score of $\pm 1.96z$. This is an example of the concept of power. With an a priori directional hypothesis, a lower z-score would be considered significant.

For the 0.01 level of significance and a one-tailed test, a z-score of $+2.33$ or greater is needed for significance. This is because 49% of the distribution falls between the mean and $+2.33$, and another 50% falls below the mean.

Degrees of Freedom

The effects of degrees of freedom (*df*) were included in the discussion of the denominator in the computation of the SD. In the sample formula, the denominator is $n - 1$, thus correcting for the possible underestimation of the population parameter. When describing the calculation of various statistics, we discuss dividing by the *df* and looking up levels of significance in tables using *df*s. Because this is sometimes a confusing concept, a simple example follows.

Degrees of freedom are related to the number of scores, items, or other units in a dataset and to the idea of freedom to vary. Given three scores (1, 5, 6), we have three degrees of freedom, one for each independent item. Each score is free to vary; that is, before collecting the data, we do not know what any of these scores will be. Once we calculate the mean, however, we lose one *df*. The mean of these three scores is four. Once you know the mean and two of the three scores, you can figure out what the third score is; it is no longer free to vary. In calculating the variance or SD, you are calculating how much the scores vary around the sample mean. Because the sample mean is known, one *df* is lost, and the *df*s become $n - 1$, the number of items in the set less one.

Confidence Intervals

When the means (point estimates) are normally distributed, we can use the standard error of the mean to calculate interval estimates. Typically, the 95% and 99% intervals are used. Recall that 95% of the curve is contained between ± 1.96 SD from the mean, and that 99% of the curve is contained between ± 2.58 SD from the mean. The term *confidence interval* (CI) refers to the degree of confidence, expressed as a percent, that the interval contains the population mean (or proportion), and for which we have an estimate calculated from our sample data (Newton & Rudestam, 1999).

The following formulas are used to calculate the CIs for the population means when the sample size is adequate (generally greater than 30). (For small samples, the *t* distribution may be used to calculate CIs.)

$$95\% = M \pm 1.96 \text{ (standard error)}$$
$$99\% = M \pm 2.58 \text{ (standard error)}$$

The following hypothetical examples are designed to illustrate point estimates and CI estimates derived from a random sample. Suppose that a random sample of 81 newborn infants from a hospital in a poor neighborhood during the last year had a mean birth weight of 100 oz, with an SD of 27 oz.

1. What is the point estimate for the unknown true value of the average (mean) birth weight of all infants born in that hospital in the last year (called the population parameter)?

   Answer: The mean value of 100 oz (computed from the 81 observations) is the best single number estimate (the point estimate) of the unknown value (parameter) for the population of interest. Another random sample of 81 would have given a sample mean different from 100 oz, so the mean value depends on the particular sample that was taken. The difference between the sample mean of 100 oz and the unknown population mean (which it estimates) is the sampling error.

Because the point estimate, 100 oz, is a single number, it gives no indication of its sampling error. CIs computed from random samples enable us to measure sampling error in numeric terms.

2. What is the value of the 95% CI estimate for mean birth weight?

Answer. First, we must calculate the standard error using the following formula:

$$SD/\sqrt{n}$$

For our example, this is:

$$27/\sqrt{81} = 27/9 = 3$$

Next, we calculate the 95% CI:

$$\bar{X} \pm 1.96 \text{ (standard error)}$$
$$100 \pm (1.96)(3)$$
$$100 \pm 5.88$$
$$94.12 \text{ and } 105.88$$

The 95% CI ranges from 94.12 to 105.88. It is a range or interval of estimates for the unknown true value. Thus, a CI consists of an entire interval of estimates for the population parameter.

3. How do we interpret the 95% CI?

Answer. First, another sample of 81 would almost surely yield a different point estimate. The width of the 95% CI reflects the sampling error resulting from using an estimate based on a random sample of 81 rather than the entire population. In other words, the width of the 95% CI indicates the range of variation for point estimates that may be expected by chance differences from one random sample of the hospital population to another. It is a 95% CI because about 95% of such CIs (obtained from different random samples of that size) will include the true mean value of hospital birth weights. Because that parameter value is usually unknown, we use statistical estimates, the point estimate and the CI estimate, to approximate it. However, if the parameter value (the true mean birth weight for all newborn infants born in that hospital during the last year) were known, approximately 95% of the 95% CIs computed from different random samples of 81 would include that true value.

The value of the point estimate and the CI estimate depends on the birth weights in the particular sample that was taken, and the estimates will vary from sample to sample. Therefore, we may *not* conclude that the probability is 95% that the mean hospital birth weight is between 94 and 106 oz.

Either the parameter (the mean of all birth weights in the hospital during 2002) is between 94 and 106 oz or it is not; we do not know which. The 95% denotes the typical accuracy in computing the varying CIs, and not the one CI calculated (Hahn & Meeker, 1991). However, the width of the CI provides useful information about the sampling error or uncertainty of the point estimate unavailable from the point estimate itself. To interpret the specific CI we computed from our sample (here, 95% CI, 94.12 to 105.88), it is necessary to understand the relationship between CIs and significance tests.

Relationship between Confidence Intervals and Significance Tests

To help explain the relationship between CIs and the levels of significance (p values) derived from statistical tests, the following four questions might be asked in relation to our sample mean:

1. Is the mean birth weight in this hospital sample (100 oz) statistically significantly different from 88 oz (5.5 lb, the definition of low birth weight)?
2. Is the mean birth weight in this sample statistically significantly different from 106 oz (6.6 lb, the mean birth weight in that city)?
3. Is the mean birth weight in this sample statistically significantly different from a birth weight of 103 oz?
4. Is the mean birth weight in this sample statistically significantly different from 100 oz, the sample estimate itself?

To test the null hypothesis that there is no statistically significant difference between the mean of 100 oz and each of the other values, we apply the t test. The results follow:

Question	Null Hypothesis	Difference between Values	p Value
1	88	12 oz	0.0006
2	106	6 oz	0.0456
3	103	3 oz	0.3174
4	100	0 oz	1.0000

For the first question, H_o is rejected. The observed mean of 100 oz is statistically significantly higher than the hypothesized value of 88 oz; that is, the 12-oz difference is a significant difference. The p value indicates that a difference that large would occur by chance alone only 6 times in 10,000. H_o is also rejected for question 2; that is, the hospital mean of 100 oz is statistically significantly lower than the city mean of 106 oz. A difference that large would occur by chance alone only 4.6 times in 100 random samples of equal size. For questions 3 and 4, H_o is not rejected; that is, the observed mean of 100 oz is not statistically significantly different from the values of 103 or 100 oz. In the case of the 3-oz difference (question 3), if there really was no difference between the population means, a difference at least that large could be expected to occur by chance in 32% of the random samples. In question 4, the point estimate and H_o are numerically indistinguishable (both 100 oz) and also statistically indistinguishable ($p = 1.0$), because the difference between the two values being compared is zero.

From the chart of the p values, you can see that the further a particular H_o is from the point estimate (100 oz), the lower the p value. In other words, hypotheses become less compatible with the mean of the observed values (here, 100 oz), the larger the difference between the point estimate and the hypothesized or comparison score becomes.

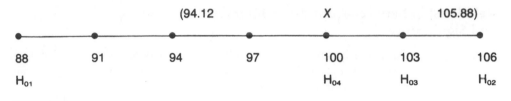

FIGURE 3-5. Relationship of confidence intervals to hypothesis testing.

Figure 3-5 summarizes our results. The null hypotheses are numbered and indicated by H_o. For example, our first H_o compared our mean of 100 with a value of 88. The CI of 94.12 to 105.88 is included in the figure.

What can be said about the p values for the null hypotheses that fall outside the 95% CI? The two that fall outside of the CI are 88 and 106 from questions 1 and 2, and in both cases the p was less than 0.05. Notice that the second null hypothesis of 106 is just outside the 95% CI, and its p value is barely below 0.05. If H_o falls at either end of a 95% CI, $p = 0.05$.

Because all numbers outside of the CI have p values less than 0.05, we would expect that all numbers within the CI would have p values greater than 0.05. This leads to a characterization of a 95% CI in terms of p values. A 95% CI contains all the (H_o) values for which $p \geq 0.05$. In other words, a 95% CI contains values (hypotheses) that are statistically compatible (will not be rejected at the 0.05 level) with the point estimate (observed value).

Consistency Checks for Evaluating Research Reports

The relationships between point estimates, CI estimates, and significance tests make it possible to uncover inconsistencies in research reports. The point estimate cannot be outside of the CI. A value for H_o within the 95% CI should have a p value greater than 0.05, and one outside of the 95% CI should have a p value less than 0.05.

Value of Confidence Intervals

Levels of significance (p values) determine whether a particular hypothesis is statistically compatible with the observed sample value, whereas 95% CIs specify all the population values that are statistically indistinguishable from the observed sample value. Smithson (2003) states that confidence intervals seem clearly superior to the traditional significance testing approach because they display the entire range of hypothetical values of a parameter that cannot be rejected compared to the significance test that focuses solely on one null hypothesis value. In addition, confidence intervals help researchers move toward cumulative knowledge because they enhance comparisons between research replications.

A Word of Caution

Statistical tests and statistical estimates assume random sampling. When using either significance tests or CIs, clear-cut conclusions regarding the entire population apply only when the study sample is a random sample of that population. Because study patients are rarely random samples from a population, we should be wary about making statistical inferences. If the sample appears to represent some population (but not a random sample), the width of the CI is often viewed as a lower bound (minimum) for the uncertainty in the point estimate. However, clinical judgment must supplement statistical analysis whenever nonrandom samples are used to generalize to individuals not studied (Riegelman, 1981).

When reading a research report, it is essential to determine whether there is an explicitly defined population of interest and whether and how the study sample was selected. Although a representative (nonrandom) sample from an explicitly defined population falls short of a random sample, it is superior to a nonrepresentative sample or to a situation in which the population or the study sample is not clearly defined. When inferences about the population are drawn using statistical tests or CIs in such situations, the reader should beware. Descriptions of the study sample (eg, using point estimates) provide useful information in all situations. When the population is ill defined, the study sample is unrepresentative, or the relation of the study sample to the population is unclear, point estimates and other statistics describing the sample may provide the only reliable information.

Statistical Significance Versus Meaningful Significance

A common mistake in research is to confuse statistical significance with substantive meaningfulness (Ingelfinger et al., 1994; Pedhazur & Schmelkin, 1991). A statistically significant result simply means that if H_o were true, the observed results would be very unusual. Given a sufficiently large sample (eg, $n \geq 100$), even the tiniest relationship can be statistically significant (Knapp, 1998; Piantadosi, 1997). Statistically significant results tell you nothing about the clinical importance or meaningful significance of the results.

The major task facing the health care researcher is not determining how statistically significant results are, but how meaningful, or substantively important, they are. Because statistical programs are widespread, readily accessible, and easy to use, it is simple to perform tests of statistical significance for various hypotheses. In contrast, it requires a good deal of knowledge and critical thinking skills to determine whether a finding is substantively meaningful. Perhaps this is why researchers still do not refrain from statistical "sanctification" of data (Pedhazur & Schmelkin, 1991; Tukey, 1969), despite numerous writings to this effect.

SAMPLE SIZE DETERMINATION

When planning research, the question always arises as to how large a sample is needed. Determining sample size involves ethical and statistical considerations. If the sample size is too small to detect significant differences or relationships or includes far more subjects than necessary, the cost to subjects and researchers cannot be justified.

In this section, the basic elements of sample size are addressed as they relate to the specific statistics covered in the rest of this book. Jacob Cohen (1988) made a major contribution to sample size determination. His book provides tables that help us determine the appropriate sample size for a particular statistical test.

Determining the right sample size for a specific study depends on several factors: power, effect size, and significance level. *Power* is defined as the likelihood of rejecting H_o (ie, avoiding a type II error). An 80% level is generally viewed as an adequate level. *Effect size* is the degree to which H_o is false; that is, the magnitude of the effect of an independent variable on the dependent variable. This magnitude must be known or estimated in order to determine the minimum sample size needed to achieve a statistical analysis with a power $\geq.80$. For example, in the absence of actual knowledge, for the *t* test, which compares the means of two groups, Cohen (1988) defines a small effect as 0.2 of an SD, a moderate effect as 0.5 SD, and a large effect as 0.8 SD. In relation to GRE scores with an SD of 100, a small effect would be 20 points (100 $\times$ 0.2), a moderate effect 50 points, and a large effect 80 points. The *significance level* is the probability of rejecting a true H_o (making a type I error); it is called *alpha* and is often set at 0.05.

Given three of these parameters, the fourth can be determined. Cohen's book has both power and sample size tables for most statistical procedures. If we know the sample size, effect size, and significance level, we can determine the power of the analysis. This can be particularly helpful when critiquing research because nonsignificant results may be related to an inadequate sample size, and significant results may be related to a very large sample rather than to a meaningful result.

When planning a study, the desired power, acceptable significance level, and expected effect size are determined, and these three parameters are used to determine the necessary sample size. In addition to Cohen's book, there are many other resources to help you determine appropriate sample sizes for different types of studies and related statistical techniques. These include books by Kraemer and Thiemann (1987), Maxwell and Delaney (1990), and Murphy and Myers (1998). There are also several stand-alone software programs that can be purchased. These include: Power and Precision, developed by Borenstein, Rothstein, and Cohen (1997) and also marketed as SamplePower, 2.0 (SPSS, 2002), and PASS (NCSS, 2002).

There are also many Web-based applications available to assist you with determining sample size. An excellent source of these websites is found at http://members.aol.com/johnp71/javastat.html. Another quick way to locate these websites is to use your favorite search engine, such as Google (http://www.google.com) and type in the terms "power analysis websites." Then, visit the found websites until you find the one calculator that will be most useful in calculating power or sample size. You will find discussions about power and sample size issues relevant to specific statistical tests in subsequent chapters.

SUMMARY

Topics covered in this chapter are basic to understanding the use of the specific statistical techniques contained in subsequent chapters of this book. Please be sure you understand these topics before proceeding.

Application Exercises and Results

Exercises

1. Scores on a particular test are normally distributed with a mean of 70 and an SD of 15. Between what two scores would you expect

   a. 68% of the scores to fall between: _____ and _____?

   b. 96% of the scores to fall between: _____ and _____?

2. In a positively skewed distribution, the "tail" extends toward the _____ (right/left) or toward _____ (higher/lower) scores of the distribution.

3. When raw scores are converted to standard scores, the resulting distribution has a mean equal to _____ and an SD equal to _____

4. A distribution of scores has a mean of 70 and an SD of 5. The following four scores were drawn from that distribution: 58, 65, 73, and 82.

   a. Transform the raw scores to standard scores and *T*-scores.

   b. Calculate the percentile for each score.

   c. Use the standard scores that you have calculated for the four scores, and transform them into scores from a distribution with a mean of 100 and an SD of 25.

5. Look at your frequencies for the variables AGE and EDUC. Determine whether the variables are significantly skewed. If they are skewed, perform the appropriate transformations and then run descriptives on the new variables to determine whether the transformations were successful.

6. At your hospital, there were 1,500 deliveries last year; 364 of the women had cesarean sections. What is the probability of having a cesarean section at your hospital?

7. You are testing for significant differences between the mean scores of two groups. You set the level of significance at 0.05. If the mean difference is so large that it would occur by chance 1% of the time, would you accept or reject the null hypothesis?

8. When you make a prediction about the direction of mean differences between an experimental and a control group, would you use a one-tailed or a two-tailed test of significance?

9. Which is the more powerful test, one tailed or two tailed?

10. You hypothesize that there is no significant difference in weight between infants in newborn nursery A and those in newborn nursery B. In each of the following, determine whether an error has been made and, if so, what type of error.

    a. Infants in newborn nursery A really weigh significantly more than infants in newborn nursery B, and you accept the null hypothesis.

    b. Infants in newborn nursery B really weigh more than infants in newborn nursery A, and you reject the null hypothesis.

    c. Infants in both newborn nurseries really do weigh the same, and you accept the null hypothesis.

    d. Infants in both newborn nurseries really do weigh the same, and you reject the null hypothesis.

11. You have measured 120 subjects on a particular scale. The mean is 75 and the SD is 6.

    a. What is the standard error of the mean?

b. Set up the 95% confidence interval for the mean.

c. Set up the 99% confidence interval for the mean.

12. You are reading a review paper discussing the use of serum ferritin as a diagnostic test for iron deficiency anemia, with the results summarized as follows:

		Anemia Present	Anemia Absent	Total
Serum Ferritin	+ (Positive)	731	270	1001
Test Result	− (Negative)	78	1500	1578
	Total	809	1770	2579

a. Calculate the sensitivity (Sn), specificity (Sp), positive predictive value (PPV), negative predictive value (NPV), and efficiency (EFF).

b. Describe the clinical performance of the serum ferritin test as a diagnostic tool.

Results

1. With a mean of 70 and an SD of 15:

   a. 68% of scores = ±1 SD; therefore, 68% fall between 55 and 85.

   b. 96% of scores = ±2 SD; therefore, 96% fall between 40 and 100.

2. In a positively skewed distribution, the tail is to the **right** or **higher** scores of the distribution.

3. A standard score distribution has a **mean of 0** and an **SD of 1**.

4. a. Standard scores and *T*-scores

Raw Score	Standard Score	T-Score
	$z = (X - X/SD)$	$T = 10z + 50$
58	$z = (58 - 70)/5 = -2.4$	$T = (10)(-2.4) + 50 = 26$
65	$z = (65 - 70)/5 = -1.0$	$T = (10)(-1.0) + 50 = 40$
73	$z = (73 - 70)/5 = 0.6$	$T = (10)(0.6) + 50 = 56$
82	$z = (82 - 70)/5 = 2.4$	$T = (10)(2.4) + 50 = 74$

b. Percentiles: Areas between mean and *z*-score (Appendix A)

Raw Score		z-Score	Tabled Values Percentiles
58	−2.4	49.18	50 − 49.18 = 0.82
65	−1.0	34.13	50 − 34.13 = 15.87
73	0.6	22.57	50 + 22.57 = 72.57
82	2.4	49.18	50 + 49.18 = 99.18

c. New distribution: Transformed z-scores = (new SD)(z) + (new X)
$$= 25z + 100$$

z-Scores	Transformed Scores
-2.4	$25(-2.4) + 100 = 40$
-1.0	$25(-1.0) + 100 = 75$
0.6	$25(0.6) \ + 100 = 115$
2.4	$25(2.4) \ + 100 = 160$

5. Here are the relevant values for the variables AGE and EDUC. To determine the degree of skewness using Fisher's measure of skewness formula, we divide the measure of skewness by its standard error. Values greater than 1.96 are significant at the 0.05 level and values greater than 2.58 are significant at the 0.01 level.

$$AGE = 0.753/0.093 = 8.096 = 8.10$$
$$EDUC = 0.153/0.094 = 1.627 = 1.62$$

The AGE variable is significantly skewed ($p < 0.01$), but the EDUC variable is not. Therefore, we can leave the EDUC variable alone, but we need to consider what method might be best to transform the AGE variable. We will use three methods for handling skewness that are recommended by Tabachnick and Fidell (2001). Each method requires us to create a new variable from the AGE variable. In the first method, we create the new variable, RECAGE, by using the Recode into a Different Variable approach, where we recode the outlier scores of 78, 79, 82, 83, and 95 to 75, 76, 77, 78, and 79, respectively, to make them closer to the bulk of scores in the distribution. In the second method, we use the Compute command to create a new variable, called SQRTAGE, which consists of the square root of every subject's age. In the third method, we again use the Compute command and create a new variable, called LG10AGE, which is a log transformation of the AGE variable. Here are the commands that were used to create these three new variables:

```
RECODE AGE (78=75)(79=76)(82=77)(83=78)(95=79)(ELSE=Copy)* INTO RECAGE.
COMPUTE SQRTAGE = SQRT(AGE).
COMPUTE LG10AGE = LG10(AGE).
EXECUTE.
```

(*If you don't use the ELSE command to bring over the rest of the scores in this type of Recode, the resulting variable will have only those scores that were created, in this case, an n = 6.)

After creating the three new variables, we check to see what, if any, transformation had corrected the skewness. We do this by computing descriptive statistics for the new variables and then calculating Fisher's measure of skewness.

$$RECAGE = 0.643/0.093 = 6.91$$
$$SQRTAGE = 0.268/0.093 = 2.89$$
$$LG10AGE = -0.190/0.093 = -2.04$$

Despite transformation, both RECAGE and SQRTAGE remained markedly skewed ($p < 0.01$). The log transformation, however, reduced the skewness level considerably but not less than the desired 1.96 SD unit level, indicating that the variable LG10AGE was almost normally transformed. Even though normal transformation was not achieved completely, we could use the log-transformed age variable LG10AGE in subsequent analyses as long as the sample size is not too small. Skewness tends to be more influential in small samples.

6. $100 \times 364/1{,}500 = 24.3\%$.

7. The researcher would reject H_o.

8. Use a one-tailed test of significance.

9. A one-tailed test is more powerful.

10. a. Type II error

    b. No error made

    c. No error made

    d. Type I error

11. a. S_x = SD/square root of n
    = 6/square root of 120
    = 6/10.95 = 0.547 = 0.55

    b. $95\% = \times \pm 1.96\, s_x$
    = 75 ± (1.96)(0.55)
    = 75 ± 1.08
    = 73.92 to 76.08

    c. $99\% = \times \pm 2.58\, s_x$
    = 75 ± (2.58)(0.55)
    = 75 ± 1.42
    = 73.58 to 76.42

12. a. The sensitivity is calculated as follows:

$$Sn = (TP/(TP + FN)) \times 100$$
$$= (731/(731 + 78)) \times 100$$
$$= 731/809 \times 100$$
$$= 90.4\% \text{ or } 90\%$$

The specificity is calculated as follows:

$$Sp = (TN/(TN + FP)) \times 100$$
$$= (1500/(1500 + 270)) \times 100$$
$$= 1500/1770 \times 100$$
$$= 84.7\% \text{ or } 85\%$$

Positive predictive value is calculated as follows:

$$PPV = (TP/(TP + FP)) \times 100$$
$$= (731/(731 + 270)) \times 100$$
$$= 731/1001 \times 100$$
$$= 73.0\%$$

Negative predictive value is calculated as follows:

$$NPV = (TN/(TN + FN)) \times 100$$
$$= (1500/(1500 + 78)) \times 100$$
$$= 1500/1578 \times 100$$
$$= 95.1\% \text{ or } 95\%$$

Efficiency is calculated as follows:

$$Eff = ((TP + TN)/(TP + TN + FP + FN)) \times 100$$
$$= ((731 + 1500)/(731 + 1500 + 270 + 78)) \times 100$$
$$= 2231/2579 \times 100$$
$$= 86.5\% \text{ or } 86\%$$

b. These results indicate that 90% of patients with iron deficiency anemia have a positive serum ferritin level test result (Sn), and 85% of patients who do not have the disorder test negative (Sp). Only 27 out of every 100 patients tested will be incorrectly diagnosed with the disorder (PPV) and only 5 out of every 100 patients will be incorrectly classified as not having the disorder when they in fact do have iron deficiency anemia (NPV). The serum ferritin level test is 86% accurate (EFF) in diagnosing patients with iron deficiency anemia.

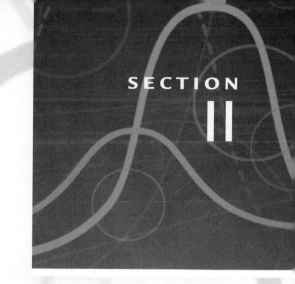

SECTION

II

Specific Statistical Techniques

Selected Nonparametric Techniques

Barbara Hazard Munro

Objectives for Chapter 4

After reading this chapter, you should be able to do the following:

1. Identify situations in which the use of nonparametric techniques is appropriate.
2. Interpret computer printouts containing specified nonparametric analyses.
3. Relate the results of the analysis to the research question posed.

RESEARCH QUESTION

Nonparametric tests can be used to answer research questions ranging from whether a relationship exists between two variables to whether groups differ on an outcome measure. The focus of this chapter is on comparing groups of subjects on outcome measures. The nonparametric techniques to be covered in this chapter are listed in Table 4-1. This chapter is intended to discuss only the commonly used nonparametrics. The parametric analogs covered in later chapters also are included.

TYPE OF DATA REQUIRED

Parametric Versus Nonparametric Tests

When we use *parametric* tests of significance, we are estimating at least one population parameter from our sample statistics. To be able to make such an estimation, we must make certain assumptions; the most important one is that the variable we have measured in the sample is normally distributed in the population to which we plan to generalize our findings. With *nonparametric* tests, there is no assumption

TABLE 4-1 *Nonparametric Tests and Corresponding Parametric Analogs*			
	Nonparametric Tests		
	Nominal Data	*Ordinal Data*	**Parametric Analog**
One-group case	Chi-square goodness of fit	—	—
Two-group case	Chi-square	Mann-Whitney U	*t* test
k-group case	Chi-square	Kruskal-Wallis H	One-way ANOVA
Dependent groups (repeated measures)	McNemar test for significance of change	Wilcoxon matched-pairs signed rank test Friedman matched samples	Paired *t* tests Repeated measures ANOVA

about the distribution of the variable in the population. For that reason, nonparametric tests often are called *distribution free*.

At one time, level of measurement was considered a critical element in deciding whether to use parametric or nonparametric tests. It was believed that parametric tests should be reserved for use with interval- and ratio-level data. However, it has been shown that the use of parametric techniques with ordinal data rarely distorts the results.

Parametric techniques have several advantages. Other things being equal, they are more powerful and more flexible than nonparametric techniques. They not only allow the researcher to study the effect of many independent variables on the dependent variable, but they also make possible the study of their interaction. Nonparametric techniques are much easier to calculate by hand than parametric techniques, but that advantage has been eliminated by the use of computers. Small samples and serious distortions of the data should lead one to explore nonparametric techniques. As discussed in Chapter 2, when the data are significantly skewed, thus failing the assumption of normal distribution, one might transform them to achieve a normal distribution. Rather than transform such variables, nonparametric techniques might be used. There are no clear rules for when one approach is preferred. An advantage of the nonparametric approach is that the data retain their original values, thus making interpretation easier. A disadvantage of nonparametrics is their inability to handle multivariate questions.

CHI-SQUARE

Research Question

Chi-square is the most commonly reported nonparametric statistic. It can be used with one or more groups. It compares the actual number (or frequency) in each group with the expected number. The expected number can be based on theory, experience, or comparison groups. The question is whether the expected number differs significantly from the actual number.

Type of Data Required

Chi-square is used when the data are nominal (categorical). In later chapters we discuss how the chi-square is used to test the fit of models in techniques such as logistic regression and path analysis.

Youngblut and colleagues (2001) compared family characteristics for their two groups of subjects, preterm and full-term deliveries. They used *t* tests to compare the groups on continuous variables and chi-square to compare them on categorical variables. Table 4-2 describes their results. They used an asterisk to indicate significant results. As you can see, none of the chi-square (χ^2) results are significant. The two groups (preterm and full term) did not differ on mother's race, mother's education, family income, mother's employment status, or child's sex. There were differences between the two groups. For example, 98% of the full-term group had family incomes of less than $20,000, whereas only 85% of the preterm group was in that category. This difference, however, was not greater than could occur by chance alone.

Assumptions Underlying Chi-Square

There are four assumptions underlying the chi-square:

1. Frequency data
2. Adequate sample size
3. Measures independent of each other
4. Theoretical basis for the categorization of the variables

The **first assumption** is that the data are frequency data, that is, a count of the number of subjects in each condition under analysis. The chi-square cannot be used to analyze the difference between scores or their means. If data are not categorical, they must be categorized before being used. Whether to categorize depends on the data and the question to be answered.

If the data are not normally distributed and violate the assumptions underlying the appropriate parametric technique, then categorization might be appropriate. The categories developed must adequately represent the data and must be based on sound rationale. If you had the ages of subjects, you could categorize them as 20 to 29, 30 to 39, and 40 to 49. However, you have treated all people within one of your three categories as being equal in age. Does a 29-year-old belong in the same group as a 20-year-old, or is he or she more like a 30-year-old? Specificity and variability are decreased through this categorization, and as a result the analysis will be less powerful.

The question addressed affects the categorization of subjects. Suppose the researcher was interested in whether being in school affects some categorical outcome measure. Then grouping the children as preschool and in school would make

TABLE 4-2 *Comparison of Families with Preterm and Full-Term Preschoolers*

Characteristic	Preterm M (SD)		Full-Term M (SD)		Statistic
Mother's age	29.90	(6.86)	29.20	(6.17)	$t = .58$
Proportion child's life employed	.27	(.37)	.22	(.32)	$t = .78$
Discrepancy	20.80	(12.94)	21.00	(14.59)	$t = .08$
Number of children	2.50	(1.55)	2.50	(1.34)	$t = .13$
Child's age (months)	48.70	(9.92)	48.40	(9.96)	$t = .18$
Birth weight (grams)	1444.10	(527.21)	3331.30	(514.18)	$t = 19.93^*$
Gestational age at birth (weeks)	30.50	(3.17)	39.60	(1.60)	$t = 19.98^*$
Proportion child's life single	.89	(.26)	.88	(.24)	$t = .23$
Mother's race	N (%)		N (%)		
White	16 (13%)		23 (19%)		$\chi^2 = 4.05$
Black	44 (36%)		36 (30%)		
Hispanic	0 (0%)		2 (2%)		
Mother's education					
<High school	12 (10%)		16 (13%)		$\chi^2 = 1.15$
High school grad	20 (16%)		22 (18%)		
>High school	28 (23%)		23 (19%)		
Family income					
<$20,000	51 (85%)		60 (98%)		$\chi^2 = 5.23$
$20,000–39,999	6 (10%)		1 (2%)		
≥$40,000	3 (5%)		0 (0%)		
Mother's employment status					
Employed	17 (14%)		17 (14%)		$\chi^2 = .003$
Nonemployed	43 (35%)		44 (36%)		
Child's sex					
Female	32 (26%)		25 (21%)		$\chi^2 = 1.85$
Male	28 (23%)		36 (30%)		

$^*p < .01$.
From Youngblut, J. M., Brooten, D., Singer, L. T., Standing, T., Lee, H., and Rodgers, W. L. (2001). Effects of maternal employment and prematurity on child outcomes in single parent families. *Nursing Research, 50*(6), 349.

sense, rather than using their actual ages. When categories have clinical relevance, statistical analyses that preserve these categories are more likely to provide useful interpretations. They are less likely to provide "differences that do not make a difference."

The **second assumption** is that the sample size is adequate. In cross-tabulation procedures, cells are formed by the combination of measures. None of the cells should be empty. Expected frequencies of less than five in 2 × 2 tables present problems. In larger tables, many researchers use the rule of thumb that not more than 20% of the cells should have frequencies of less than five (SPSS, 1999b, p. 67). If the cells do not contain adequate numbers, then the variables should be restructured to have fewer categories. It is very important to look at the frequencies of variables before running analyses to ascertain whether adequate numbers of subjects exist. Even with that, however, low numbers in particular cells may not be obvious until the cross-tabulation is run. Most statistical programs print a warning when cell sizes are inadequate. If the cell sizes are problematic, then the researcher should consider restructuring the variable to have less categories.

The **third assumption** is that the measures are independent of each other. This means that the categories created are mutually exclusive; that is, no subject can be in more than one cell in the design, and no subject can be used more than once. It also means that the response of one subject cannot influence the response of another. This seems relatively straightforward, but difficulties arise in clinical research situations when data are collected for a period of time. If you are testing subjects in a hospital or clinic, you must be sure that a person who is readmitted is not enrolled in the study for a second time. You also must be sure that subjects in one condition are not communicating with subjects in their own or different conditions in such a way that responses are contaminated.

The **fourth assumption** is that there is some theoretical reason for the categories. This ensures that the analysis will be meaningful and prevents "fishing expeditions." The latter would occur if the researcher kept recategorizing subjects, hoping to find some relationship between the variables. Research questions and methods for analysis are established before data collection. Although these may be modified to suit the data actually obtained, the basic theoretical structure remains.

Power

Power must be considered when planning sample size. If you have 40 subjects (10 in each of the four cells in a 2 × 2 design), set your probability level at 0.05 and expect a moderate effect, your power is only 0.47 (Cohen, 1987, p. 235). You have less than a 50% chance of finding a significant relationship between the two variables. Under the same conditions, a sample of 80 results in a power of .76, and a sample of 90 in a power of .81. After the description of the computer printout, an example of power is given.

Example for Computer Analysis

The research question is whether socioeconomic status (SES) is related to the abuse of women. The data were gathered in an AREA grant funded by NINR (Hawkins et al., 1996). Another way to state the question is whether women with low SES differ from women with high SES in their reports of abuse. The researchers used insurance as one way of measuring SES. They categorized the subjects into those who had private insurance against those who did not. They asked the women whether they had ever been emotionally or physically abused. Using the Hawkins et al. (1996) data

ever emotionally or physically abused * SES as risk factor Cross-tabulation

Count

		SES as risk factor		
		Has private insurance	Medicaid mass health or none	Total
Ever emotionally or physically abused	no	1,011	954	1,965
	yes	104	294	398
Total		1,115	1,248	2,363

FIGURE 4-1. Data for chi-square analysis.

and the SPSS program Crosstabs, we produced Fig. 4-1. All figures associated with this analysis were produced by SPSS for Windows version 12.0. Some have been edited slightly. Author comments have been added and appear in shaded boxes.

First, look at the totals for the columns (SES) and rows (abuse). Overall, there are 2,363 subjects, 1,115 with private insurance and 1,248 without private insurance. Fortunately, the group that reports being abused (n = 398) is much smaller than the group that reports no abuse (n = 1,965). Look closely at the figure. Do you think that SES as measured by insurance is related to abuse? The null hypothesis is that there is no difference between the two abuse groups in frequency of abuse.

Because the subjects are not divided equally between those with or without insurance or between those who have been abused and those who have not, adding percentages to the table is helpful in clarifying the results (Fig. 4-2). This was done by requesting row, column, and total percents. Requesting all of the possible percents results in a "busy" table, so take a moment to get comfortable with the figure. Generally, for publication, one uses the independent variable as the column variable and the dependent variable (outcome measure) as the row variable. Then, just the column percents are enough to interpret the results.

In each cell (box) the top number is the count, the second number is the row percent, the third is the column percent, and the bottom number is the total percent. Look at the top box on the left. The count is 1,011; that is 1,011 subjects had private insurance and said they had not ever been emotionally or physically abused. Abuse is the row variable. Here 51.5% (1,011/1,965) of those who had not been emotionally or physically abused had private insurance. SES is the column variable. In this box we see that 90.7% of those who had private insurance said they had not been abused (1,011/1,115). The bottom number in the box indicates that of all the subjects 42.8% had private insurance and had not been abused (1,011/2,363).

Looking at the totals for the row variable, abuse (right-hand column), we see that 1,965 or 83.2% of the women said they were never abused and 398 or 16.8%

ever emotionally or physically abused * SES as risk factor Cross-tabulation

			SES as risk factor		
			Has private insurance	Medicaid mass health or none	Total
Ever emotionally or physically abused	no	Count	1011	954	1965
		% within ever emotionally or physically abused	51.5%	48.5%	100.0%
		% within SES as risk factor	90.7%	76.4%	83.2%
		% of Total	42.8%	40.4%	83.2%
	yes	Count	104	294	398
		% within ever emotionally or physically abused	26.1%	73.9%	100.0%
		% within SES as risk factor	9.3%	23.6%	16.8%
		% of Total	4.4%	12.4%	16.8%
Total		Count	1115	1248	2363
		% within ever emotionally or physically abused	47.2%	52.8%	100.0%
		% within SES as risk factor	100.0%	100.0%	100.0%
		% of Total	47.2%	52.8%	100.0%

AUTHOR COMMENTS
Within a given cell, the percents are as follows:
Frequency (count)
Row %
Column %
Total %

FIGURE 4-2. Frequencies and all percents.

ever emotionally or physically abused *SES as risk factor Cross-tabulation

| | | | SES as risk factor | | Total |
			Has private insurance	Medicaid mass health or none	
Ever emotionally or	no	Count Expected Count	1,011 927.2	954 1037.8	1,965 1965.0
physically abused	yes	Count Expected Count	104 187.8	294 210.2	398 398.0
Total		Count Expected Count	1,115 1115.0	1,248 1248.0	2,363 2363.0

FIGURE 4-3. Actual and expected frequencies.

said they had been abused. The totals for the column variable, SES, show that 1,115 women or 47.2% had private insurance and 1,248 or 52.8% did not. If abuse were not related to SES, then we would expect that for each level of SES, the rate of abuse would be the same. For the entire sample the rate of abuse is 16.8%. Thus, if there were no differences between the groups, we would expect that within each insurance group, 16.8% would have been abused and 83.2% would not.

These expectations become the *expected frequencies* in the calculation of the chi-square. For those with private insurance (n = 1,115), the expected frequencies would equal 187.32 for the abused group (1,115 × .168 = 187.32). For those without private insurance, the expected frequencies for abuse would equal 209.664 (1248 × .168 = 209.664). Figure 4-3 contains the actual (observed) and expected frequencies. The slight discrepancies come from rounding errors. Actually the percent of those who were abused is 16.84304. If that number is used instead of 16.8, you will get the same expected counts as in Fig. 4-3.

Compare the observed and expected frequencies. Given a rate of 16.8%, we "expect" that 188 (187.8) of those with private insurance would report abuse, but only 104 actually reported abuse. For those without private insurance, more women reported abuse (294) than expected (210). There is a difference in reported abuse between the two groups. In the insurance group, 9.3% report abuse, whereas in the no private insurance group, 23.6% report abuse (see Fig. 4-4). The statistical test tells us whether or not such a difference could have happened by chance alone.

Computer Output for Chi-Square Analysis

Figure 4-4 contains the computer printout of this analysis. Under chi-square tests, we see four different values, with their degrees of freedom (*df*) and significance

ever emotionally or physically abused * SES as risk factor Cross-tabulation

			SES as risk factor		Total
			Has private insurance	Medicaid mass health or none	
Ever emotionally or physically abused	no	Count	1,011	954	1,965
		% within SES as risk factor	90.7%	76.4%	83.2%
	yes	Count	104	294	398
		% within SES as risk factor	9.3%	23.6%	16.8%
Total		Count	1,115	1,248	2,363
		% within SES as risk factor	100.0%	100.0%	100.0%

AUTHOR COMMENTS
The percents are column percents.

Chi-Square Tests

	Value	df	Asymp. sig. (2 sided)	Exact sig. (2 sided)	Exact sig. (2 sided)
Pearson chi-square	85.141(b)	1	.000		
Continuity correction (a)	84.128	1	.000		
Likelihood ratio	88.671	1	.000		
Fisher's exact test				.000	.000
Linear-by-linear association	85.105	1	.000		
N of valid cases	2363				

a Computed only for a 2 × 2 table
b 0 cells (.0%) have expected count less than 5. The minimum expected count is 187.80.

AUTHOR COMMENTS
The Pearson value is the usual chi-square value. The other values are described in the text.

FIGURE 4-4. Computer output of chi-square analysis.

Symmetric Measures

		Value	Approx. sig.
Nominal by nominal	Phi	.190	.000
	Cramer's V	.190	.000
	Contingency Coefficient	.186	.000
N of valid cases		2,363	

Not assuming the null hypothesis.
Using the asymptotic standard error assuming the null hypothesis.

AUTHOR COMMENTS

Symmetric measures are only reported when chi-square is significant.
Phi is a shortcut method of calculating a correlation coefficient that can be used when both variables are dichotomous (have only two levels).
Cramer's V is a modified version of Phi that can be used with larger tables.

FIGURE 4-4. (*Continued*)

levels. The *Pearson value* is what you would get if you did this by hand using the usual formula. It is based on the differences between the observed and expected frequencies. For example, the actual (or observed) number of abused women with private insurance is 104, but the expected number (based on an overall rate of 16.8%) is 187.8. The difference between these two values is 83.8. The chi-square value based on the differences between observed and expected frequencies in each of the four cells in our design is 85.141. There is one *df*, and the significance level is .000 (which is at least less than .001). Therefore, since the significance level is less than .05, we would say that the null hypothesis of no difference in abuse between the two insurance groups has not been supported. There is a significant difference between insured and uninsured women in their reported levels of abuse, with uninsured women reporting significantly more abuse.

Since the differences were quite large, this is probably what you expected.

In Chapter 3, the concept of degrees of freedom is defined as the extent to which values are free to vary given a specific number of subjects and a total score. In chi-square analysis, however, frequencies are used rather than scores. The number of cells that are free to vary depends on the number of cells found in the table. How many cell frequencies would we need to know to derive the others? The answer to that question will be equal to the *df*. Given the row and column totals, we only need to know one cell value in a 2 × 2 table to be able to calculate the rest by simple subtraction. Therefore, only one cell is free to vary; the others are dependent on that value. The *df* for a 2 × 2 chi-square analysis is always 1, regardless of sample size. The formula for calculating the *df* for any size table in a chi-square analysis is:

$$df = (r - 1)(c - 1)$$

For our 2 × 2 table, this becomes $df = (2 - 1)(2 - 1) = 1$.

The *continuity correction* is often referred to as the Yates' correction. Although nominal data are used to calculate a chi-square, chi-square values have a distribution (see Appendix B). The distribution is continuous, but when the expected frequency in any of the cells in a 2 × 2 table is less than 5, the sampling distribution of chi-square for that analysis may depart substantially from normal (Hinkle, Wiersma, & Jurs, 1998, p. 590). In those cases, the continuity correction is recommended. The correction consists of subtracting .5 from the difference between each pair of observed and expected frequencies. In our example, the difference of 83.8 would be reduced to 83.3 by subtracting .5, which results in an overall lower chi-square value. On the output we see that the Pearson value is 85.141, but with the continuity correction, this drops to 84.128. Thus, applying the correction reduces the power of the analysis.

In our example, the *minimum expected count* is 187.80; therefore, we would report the Pearson result. If the minimum expected count (or frequency) had been less than 5, the continuity correction value or Fisher's exact test should have been reported.

The *likelihood ratio* chi-square is an alternative to the Pearson chi-square used for log-linear models. When the sample is large, the likelihood ratio is very similar to the Pearson (SPSS, 1999b).

Fisher's exact test is an alternative to Pearson's chi-square for the 2 × 2 table. It assumes that the marginal counts remain fixed at the observed values and calculates exact probabilities of obtaining the observed results if the two variables are independent (SPSS, 1999b). It is most useful when sample sizes and expected frequencies are small. If the minimum expected value is less than 5, in a 2 × 2 table, Fisher's exact is more appropriate than Pearson's chi-square.

The *linear-by-linear association chi-square*, although printed when chi-square is requested, is not always appropriate because it is based on the relationship between the two variables as measured by the Pearson correlation coefficient. The Pearson correlation coefficient assumes normally distributed data, and this is not usually the case with nominal data, especially with two dichotomous variables, as in a 2 × 2 table (SPSS, 1999b).

Two measures are listed in the table in Figure 4-4 titled Symmetric Measures. They are Phi and Cramer's V.

Phi is a shortcut used for calculating a correlation coefficient. It can be used when both variables are dichotomous (have only two levels). It is appropriate only when the chi-square value is significant. It is interpreted as a measure of association; that is, in this example, the correlation between these two variables is .190. It allows us to interpret the strength of the relationship. It is most useful with 2 × 2 tables in

	Insured	Uninsured	Difference between Groups
TABLE 4-3 *Examples of Power*			
Null hypothesis	16.8%	16.8%	0%
Actual effect	9.3%	23.6%	14.3%
Small effect	10.0%	20.0%	10.0%
Moderate effect	8.0%	38.0%	30.0%
Large effect	5.0%	55.0%	50.0%

which the values of phi range from 0 to 1. In tables with more cells, the value can be greater than 1, decreasing its usefulness. It is complementary to chi-square because it is less sensitive to sample size. It could be used to compare the strength of the relationship across studies.

Cramer's V is a slightly modified version that can be used with larger tables. Phi is adjusted for the number of rows and columns. Thus, given a significant chi-square, report Phi for 2 × 2 tables and Cramer's V for larger tables.

Example of Power Analysis

Cohen (1987) defines the effect sizes related to the chi-square as small = 0.1, moderate = 0.3, and large = 0.5. Using our example, what do these mean? Table 4-3 demonstrates these effect sizes for our example. The null hypothesis in our example is based on the fact that overall, 16.8% of the women reported abuse. Thus, if the null hypothesis is true, 16.8% of the insured and 16.8% of the uninsured will report abuse. Our actual effect was a 14.3% difference between the groups. By Cohen's definition, a small effect would be a 10% difference between the two groups, such as 10% of the insured women being abused versus 20% of the noninsured. A moderate effect would be a 30% difference between the two groups, and a large effect would be a 50% difference. Look at the table to see examples of what those effects could look like.

Example from the Literature

Champion and colleagues (2001) compared genitourinary symptoms between abused and nonabused women. Table 4-4 contains the results. All of the comparisons are significant. Abused women reported significantly more vaginal discharge, abdominal pain, abnormal menses, and dyspareunia than did nonabused women. Look at the percentages, as well as the *p* values to see what the effects are. By Cohen's definition, the effects would be considered "small," since most are close to 10%.

TABLE 4-4 *Comparisons of Genitourinary Symptomatology of Abused and Nonabused Women*

Variable	Abused n = 194	Nonabused n = 418	p^a
Vaginal discharge	71.6%	60.0%	<.01
Abdominal pain	46.9%	38.0%	<.05
Abnormal menses	48.2%	36.4%	<.01
Dyspareunia	21.1%	12.0%	<.01

[a]p values from comparisons of abused and nonabused groups using chi-square analysis.
From Champion, J. D., Piper, J., Shain, R. N., Perdue, S. T., & Newton, E. R. (2001). Minority women with sexually transmitted diseases: Sexual abuse and risk for pelvic inflammatory disease. *Research in Nursing & Health, 24*(1), p. 27.

Calculation of Chi-Square

When calculating chi-square, the expected and observed frequencies in each cell are compared. Using the expected and observed frequencies in Fig. 4-3, we demonstrate the use of the chi-square formula. In each cell the expected frequency is subtracted from the observed frequency, and that result is squared and then divided through by the expected frequency. The sum of these calculations is the chi-square.

Chi-Square Formula

$$\sum \frac{(1011 - 927.2)^2}{927.2} + \frac{(954 - 1037.8)^2}{1037.8}$$

$$+ \frac{(104 - 187.8)^2}{187.8} + \frac{(294 - 210.2)^2}{210.2} = 85.141$$

Summary for Chi-Square

Chi-square is the appropriate technique when variables are measured at the nominal level. It may be used with one or more groups. In the *one-group* case comparison, data may be provided from a theoretical perspective, norms, or past experience. Suppose a hospital had a cesarean section rate of 30%. This percentage could be compared with reported rates (locally, regionally, or nationally) through the use of chi-square.

Although only a 2 × 2 design has been used as an example, this *two-group* case with two levels in each group can be extended to larger designs. The groups in a chi-square analysis must be mutually exclusive. However, an adaptation of chi-square is the *McNemar test* for use with repeated measures at the nominal level.

McNemar Test

lumps pretest & lumps posttest

Lumps pretest	Lumps posttest	
	0	1
0	199	100
1	15	112

Test Statistics (b)

	Lumps pretest & lumps posttest
N	426
Chi-square (a)	61.357
Asymp. Sig.	.000

a Continuity Corrected
b McNemar Test

AUTHOR COMMENTS
Row Totals—lumps found on pretest
  299 women (199 + 100) found 0 to 3 lumps (0)
  127 women (15 + 112) found 4 to 8 lumps (1)
Column Totals—lumps found on posttest
  214 women (199 + 15) found 0 to 3 lumps (0)
  212 women (100 + 112) found 4 to 8 lumps (1)
Cells
  Reflecting no change
    199 women found 0 to 3 lumps both times (0)
    112 women found 4 to 8 lumps both times (1)
  Reflecting change
    100 women who found 0 to 3 lumps at pretest, found 4 to 8 at posttest
    15 women who found 4 to 8 lumps at pretest, found 0 to 3 at posttest

---

FIGURE 4-5. Computer output of McNemar test.

NOMINAL-LEVEL DATA, DEPENDENT MEASURES

The McNemar test can be used with two dichotomous measures on the same subjects. It is used to measure change. Figure 4-5 contains an example of a computer printout produced by SPSS for Windows, using data collected by Wood (1997). In this example, we are interested in subjects' ability to identify lumps in models of breasts before and after training. There were 8 lumps in the model. Those who detected 0–3 lumps were scored 0, and those who detected 4–8 lumps were scored 1. Looking at the cells, we see that 311 people did not change in their ability to detect the lumps, 199 scored low both times (0), and 112 scored high (1) both times.

Among those who changed, 100 who scored low on the pretest, scored high on the posttest, whereas only 15 people who scored high on the pretest, scored low on the posttest. Thus, for those who changed their scores, more moved from low to high (100) than from high to low (15). This change is statistically significant at the .000 level. This indicates that the training provided to these women improved their ability to detect lumps in a model of a breast.

Summary for McNemar

The McNemar test uses an adaptation of the chi-square formula to test the direction of change. Only the two cells that include changes are included in the analysis; therefore, $df = 1$.

ORDINAL DATA, INDEPENDENT GROUPS

Two commonly used techniques are the *Mann-Whitney U*, which is used to compare two groups and is thus analogous to the *t* test, and the *Kruskal-Wallis H*, which is used to compare two or more groups and is thus analogous to the parametric technique *analysis of variance*. In these techniques, scores for subjects are converted into ranks, and the analyses compare the mean ranks in each group. Using data collected by Wood (1997), we seek to answer the question, Is type of living quarters related to knowledge about breast self-examination? The three types of living quarters are private home, apartment, and elder housing. The knowledge score was significantly skewed, thus making the nonparametric test appropriate. Figures 4-6 and 4-7 contain the computer printouts.

Kruskal-Wallis Test

Ranks

	Type of living quarters	N	Mean Rank
Knowledge score, time 2	Private home	199	245.35
	Apartment	87	206.43
	Elder housing	141	174.43
	Total	427	

Test Statistics (a, b)

	Knowledge score, time 2
Chi-square	28.240
df	2
Asymp. sig.	.000

a Kruskal Wallis Test
b Grouping variable: Type of living quarters

FIGURE 4-6. Computer output, Kruskal-Wallis.

Mann-Whitney Test

Ranks

	What type of living quarters?	N	Mean rank	Sum of ranks
Knowledge score, time 2	Private home	199	151.66	30180.00
	Apartrment	87	124.84	10861.00
	Total	286		

Test Statistics (a)

	Knowledge score, time 2
Mann-Whitney U	7033.000
Wilcoxon W	10861.000
Z	−2.557
Asymp. Sig. (2 tailed)	.011

a Grouping Variable: What type of living quarters?

Mann-Whitney Test

Ranks

	What type of living quarters?	N	Mean rank	Sum of ranks
Knowledge score, time 2	Private home	199	168.74	33579.00
	Elder housing	103	118.19	12174.00
	Total	302		

Test Statistics (a)

	Knowledge score, time 2
Mann-Whitney U	6818.000
Wilcoxon W	12174.000
Z	−4.825
Asymp. Sig. (2 tailed)	.000

a Grouping Variable: What type of living quarters?

FIGURE 4-7. Computer output, Mann-Whitney U.

Mann-Whitney Test

Ranks

	What type of living quarters?	N	Mean rank	Sum of ranks
Knowledge score, time 2	Apartment	87	103.79	9029.50
	Elder housing	103	88.50	9115.50
	Total	190		

Test Statistics (a)

	Knowledge score, time 2
Mann-Whitney U	3759.500
Wilcoxon W	9115.500
Z	−1.926
Asymp. Sig. (2 tailed)	.054

a Grouping Variable: What type of living quarters?

FIGURE 4-7. (*Continued*)

The Kruskal-Wallis test (see Fig. 4-6), with a significance level of .000, indicates that the three groups differ significantly on their knowledge of breast self-examination. Looking at the mean ranks, we can see that the group living in private homes scored highest (245.35), followed by those living in apartments (206.43). Those living in elder housing scored lowest (174.43). While we know that there is an overall difference across the three groups, we do not know if each pairwise comparison is significant.

For pairwise comparisons, we use the Mann-Whitney test (see Fig. 4-7), and make all the possible pairwise comparisons. Because we will be making three pairwise comparisons, we need to consider the chance of a type I error. To protect against that error, we can use a *Bonferroni correction*. This involves dividing the desired level of significance by the number of comparisons we are making (.05/3 = .0167). For a comparison to be considered significant, it must have a significance level of .0167, not 0.05. The first test compares those living in private homes with those living in apartments. The significance level of .011 indicates that these two groups are significantly different from each other. Specifically, those in private homes scored significantly higher on the knowledge test than did those living in apartments. The comparison of those living in private homes with those living in elder housing is also significant at the .000 level; that is, those living in private homes scored significantly higher than those living in elder housing. The third comparison between those in apartments and those in elder housing (p = .044) is not significant when we use the Bonferroni correction. Thus, these data indicate that women living in private homes score significantly higher on a test of knowledge of breast self-examination than those living in apartments or elder housing. There is no significant difference between those living in apartments and those living in elder housing.

TABLE 4-5 *Variables Contributing to Significant Differences between Frequent and Infrequent TSE Performers (N = 191)*

Variable	Mann-Whitney U	Z	p
Ethnic background	3082.50	−3.851	.000*
Education	3371.00	−2.449	.014*
Family problems	3570.50	−1.874	.050*
Social support	3390.50	−1.756	.035*

*$p < .05$ (two-tailed test)
From Wynd, C. A. (2002). Testicular self-examination in young adult men. *Journal of Nursing Scholarship, 34*(3), p. 254.

Example from the Literature

The Mann-Whitney test was used by Wynd (2002) to study factors related to the practice of testicular self-examination (TSE) among young adult men. Table 4-5 contains a table from her study. She compared frequent and infrequent TSE performers. Those two groups differed significantly in ethnic background, education, family problems, and social support. Additional analyses indicated that African American and Hispanic men practiced TSE less frequently than men from other ethnic groups. Men without a high school education were less likely to practice TSE. Those who reported more family problems and those who had less social support were less likely to practice TSE.

Summary of Kruskal-Wallis and Mann-Whitney U

The Kruskal-Wallis test is the nonparametric analog of the one-way analysis of variance and the Mann-Whitney U test is the nonparametric analog of the *t* test. They may be used when the data violate the assumptions underlying the parametric tests, especially when the data are not normally distributed.

ORDINAL DATA, DEPENDENT GROUPS

The last two nonparametric techniques to be presented are the *Wilcoxon matched-pairs signed rank test* and the *Friedman matched samples*. The Wilcoxon matched-pairs test is analogous to the parametric paired *t* test, and the Friedman matched samples is analogous to a repeated measures analysis of variance. They are used in within-subjects designs when subjects serve as their own controls or the outcome variables are measured more than once.

We will start with the Friedman to demonstrate once more how initial analysis and posthoc tests might be done using nonparametric techniques. Dr. Robin Wood (1997) tested her subjects on their ability to find lumps in models of breasts. She

Friedman Test

Ranks

	Mean rank
Lumps correct, time 1	2.93
Lumps incorrect, time 1	1.77
Lumps correct, time 2	3.47
Lumps incorrect, time 2	1.83

Test Statistics (a)

N	407
Chi-Square	749.367
df	3
Asymp. Sig.	.000

a Friedman Test

FIGURE 4-8. Computer output, Friedman.

counted the number of correct and the number of incorrect lumps they found at two points in time. These variables were not normally distributed, thus the use of non-parametrics is appropriate.

Each subject has a score on each of these variables. The question is whether the subjects differed significantly in their ability to find correct, versus incorrect lumps, and whether this ability changed over time. Figures 4-8 and 4-9 contain the results. The mean ranks for the three variables are given first. The ranks vary from a high of 3.47 for their ability to find correct lumps at time 2 to a low of 1.77 for the number of incorrect lumps they found at time 1. The chi-square has a significance level of .000. Because the initial analysis is significant, we will conduct comparisons of pairs of ranks. While six pairwise comparisons are possible, only four are of interest. (We are not interested in comparing correct lumps at time 1 with incorrect lumps at time 2 or vice versa) The Wilcoxon matched-pairs is used for the four comparisons, and the Bonferroni correction is .05/4 or .0125.

In the first comparison, the numbers of correct and incorrect lumps detected at time 1 are compared. The subjects found significantly more correct than incorrect lumps at time 1 ($p = .000$). They also found more correct than incorrect lumps at time 2 (second comparison, $p = .000$). In the third comparison we see that they found more correct lumps at time 2 versus time 1, which indicates that the training was effective ($p = .000$). They found more incorrect lumps at time 2 than time 1, but this difference was not statistically significant when the Bonferroni correction is used ($p = .023$).

The superscript letters on the printout can be confusing. Look at the first one in Fig. 4-9. This is saying that in 273 of the cases, the subjects rated the number of incorrect lumps lower than the number of correct lumps. Only five subjects found

Wilcoxon Signed Ranks Test

Ranks

		N	Mean rank	Sum of ranks
Lumps Incorrect, time 1; lumps correct, time 1	Negative ranks	273(a)	141.45	38614.50
	Positive ranks	5(b)	33.30	166.50
	Ties	140(c)		
	Total	418		
Lumps incorrect, time 2; lumps correct, time 2	Negative ranks	330(d)	170.09	56130.00
	Positive ranks	5(e)	30.00	150.00
	Ties	85(f)		
	Total	420		
Lumps correct, time 2; lumps correct, time 1	Negative ranks	51(g)	104.18	5313.00
	Positive ranks	226(h)	146.86	33190.00
	Ties	149(i)		
	Total	426		
Lumps incorrect, time 2; lumps incorrect, time 1	Negative ranks	28(j)	39.45	1104.50
	Positive ranks	50(k)	39.53	1976.50
	Ties	330(l)		
	Total	408		

a Lumps incorrect, time 1 < lumps correct, time 1
b Lumps incorrect, time 1 > lumps correct, time 1
c Lumps incorrect, time 1 = lumps correct, time 1
d Lumps incorrect, time 2 < lumps correct, time 2
e Lumps incorrect, time 2 > lumps correct, time 2
f Lumps incorrect, time 2 = lumps correct, time 2
g Lumps correct, time 2 < lumps correct, time 1
h Lumps correct, time 2 > lumps correct, time 1
i Lumps correct, time 2 = lumps correct, time 1
j Lumps incorrect, time 2 < lumps incorrect, time 1
k Lumps incorrect, time 2 > lumps incorrect, time 1
l Lumps incorrect, time 2 = lumps incorrect, time 1

FIGURE 4-9. Computer output, Wilcoxon.

more incorrect lumps than correct lumps. One hundred and forty subjects found an equal number of correct and incorrect lumps. Take a few minutes to look at the remaining superscript letters to be sure you understand their use.

EXAMPLE FROM THE LITERATURE

Tombes and Gallucci (1993) used subjects as their own controls in a study of the effects of hydrogen peroxide rinses on the normal oral mucosa. There were three "rinse" groups: normal saline, quarter-strength hydrogen peroxide, and half-strength hydrogen peroxide. The Friedman test was used to compare the groups. In the hydrogen peroxide groups, significant mucosal abnormalities occurred over time.

Summary of Friedman and Wilcoxon

The Friedman and Wilcoxon techniques are the nonparametric analogs of the repeated measures analysis of variance and the paired *t* test.

SUMMARY

A few of the more commonly reported nonparametric techniques have been presented. It is important for investigators to examine their data before analysis to determine which techniques are appropriate.

Application Exercises and Results

Exercises

Conduct the appropriate nonparametric analyses to answer the research questions. Write a description of your results as it might appear in a manuscript.

1. Do men and women differ in their political affiliation?

2. Does current satisfaction with weight differ significantly from satisfaction with weight at age 18? To answer this question, first use the Recode procedure to create two new variables. Recode both SATCURWT and SATWT18 into new variables where the values of $1 - 5 = 0$, and $6 - 10 = 1$. This will create two dichotomous variables. Conduct your analysis on the dichotomous variables.

3. Does smoking status affect quality of life in the past month?

4. Do the respondents to this survey differ significantly on productivity (IPA9), goals (IPA13), or worry about the future (IPA29)?

Results

1. Exercise Fig. 4-1 contains the results of this analysis. We would report that chi-square was used to answer the research question. Men and women differed significantly in their political affiliation ($p = .025$). More men (24.8%) are Republicans than women (16.9%), and more women (35.1%) than men (28.3%) are Democrats. Men (46.9%) and women (48.0%) are fairly evenly represented in the Independent category.

2. Exercise Fig. 4-2 contains the results. McNemar was used to answer the research question. There is a significant difference between ratings of satisfaction with weight currently and at age 18 ($p = .000$). Zero equals a low level of satisfaction and one a high level. Of the 697 individuals included in the analysis, 168 were dissatisfied at both times (rating = 0), and 324 were satisfied at both times. Of those who changed their ratings over time, 157 who

political affiliation * gender Cross-tabulation

			Gender		Total
			Male	Female	
Political affiliation	Republican	Count	63	73	136
		% within gender	24.8%	16.9%	19.8%
	Democrat	Count	72	152	224
		% within gender	28.3%	35.1%	32.6%
	Independent	Count	119	208	327
		% within gender	46.9%	48.0%	47.6%
Total		Count	254	433	687
		% within gender	100.0%	100.0%	100.0%

Chi-Square Tests

	Value	*df*	Asymp. sig. (2 sided)
Pearson chi-square	7.393(a)	2	.025
Likelihood ratio	7.298	2	.026
Linear-by-linear association	2.234	1	.135
N of valid cases	687		

a 0 cells (.0%) have expected count less than 5. The minimum expected count is 50.28.

EXERCISE FIGURE 4-1. Results for Exercise 1, chi-square.

were satisfied with their weight at age 18 are no longer satisfied, and 48 people who were not satisfied at age 18 are currently satisfied. Therefore, significantly more people reported satisfaction with their weight at age 18 than with their current weight.

3. Exercise Fig. 4-3 contains the results of the analysis. Kruskal-Wallis was used to answer the research question. Smoking status is significantly related to quality of life in the past month ($p = .030$). To test pairwise differences, Mann-Whitney U was used. Because three comparisons were made, the Bonferroni correction was used (0.05/3); thus a p value of .0167 was considered significant. There was no significant difference in quality of life between those who never smoked and those who quit smoking ($p = .971$). Subjects who never smoked rated their quality of life significantly higher than subjects who were still smoking ($p = .010$). Subjects who had quit smoking did not rate their quality of life significantly higher than those who were still smoking ($p = .018$).

McNemar Test

**Satisfaction with current weight recoded &
satisfaction with weight at age 18 recoded**

Satisfaction with current weight recoded	Satisfaction with weight at age 18 recoded	
	0	1
0	168	157
1	48	324

Test Statistics (b)

	Satisfaction with current weight recoded & satisfaction with weight at age 18 recoded
N	697
Chi-Square (a)	56.898
Asymp. Sig.	.000

a Continuity Corrected
b McNemar Test

EXERCISE FIGURE 4-2. Results for Exercise 2, McNemar.

Kruskal-Wallis Test

Ranks

	Smoking history	N	Mean rank
Quality of life in past month	Never Smoked	432	355.00
	Quit smoking	185	354.51
	Still smoking	78	293.81
	Total	695	

EXERCISE FIGURE 4-3. Results for Exercise 3, Kruskal-Wallis and Mann-Whitney U.

Test Statistics (a, b)

	Quality of life in past month
Chi-Square	7.021
df	2
Asymp. Sig.	.030

a Kruskal Wallis Test
b Grouping variable: Smoking history

Mann-Whitney Test

Ranks

	Smoking history	N	Mean rank	Sum of ranks
Quality of life in past month	Never Smoked	432	309.17	133559.50
	Quit smoking	185	308.61	57093.50
	Total	617		

Test Statistics (a)

	Quality of life in past month
Mann-Whitney U	39888.500
Wilcoxon W	57093.500
Z	−.037
Asymp. Sig. (2-tailed)	.971

b Grouping variable: Smoking history

EXERCISE FIGURE 4-3. (*Continued*)

Mann-Whitney Test

Ranks

	Smoking history	N	Mean rank	Sum of ranks
Quality of life in past month	Never Smoked	432	262.33	113326.50
	Still smoking	78	217.67	16978.50
	Total	510		

Test Statistics (a)

	Quality of life in past month
Mann-Whitney U	13897.500
Wilcoxon W	16978.500
Z	−2.576
Asymp. Sig. (2 tailed)	.010

a Grouping variable: Smoking history

Mann-Whitney Test

Ranks

	Smoking history	N	Mean rank	Sum of ranks
Quality of life in past month	Quit smoking	185	138.90	25696.50
	Still smoking	78	115.63	9019.50
	Total	263		

Test Statistics (a)

	Quality of life in past month
Mann-Whitney U	5938.500
Wilcoxon W	9019.500
Z	−2.374
Asymp. Sig. (2-tailed)	.018

a Grouping variable: Smoking history

EXERCISE FIGURE 4-3. (*Continued*)

Friedman Test

Ranks

	Mean rank
Productivity of life	2.50
Defined goals for life	2.04
Worry about future	1.46

Test Statistics (a)

N	698
Chi-Square	472.592
df	2
Asymp. Sig.	.000

a Friedman Test

Wilcoxon Signed Ranks Test

Ranks

		N	Mean rank	Sum of ranks
Defined goals for life— Productivity of life	Negative ranks	341(a)	240.71	82081.00
	Positive ranks	114(b)	189.99	21659.00
	Ties	245(c)		
	Total	700		
Worry about future— Productivity of life	Negative ranks	531(d)	306.75	162882.00
	Positive ranks	61(e)	207.31	12646.00
	Ties	106(f)		
	Total	698		
Worry about future—Definded goals of life	Negative ranks	418(g)	286.91	119928.00
	Positive ranks	131(h)	237.00	31047.00
	Ties	150(i)		
	Total	699		

a defined goals for life < productivity of life
b defined goals for life > productivity of life
c defined goals for life = productivity of life
d worry about future < productivity of life
e worry about future > productivity of life
f worry about future = productivity of life
g worry about future < defined goals for life
h worry about future > defined goals for life
i worry about future = defined goals for life

EXERCISE FIGURE 4-4. Results of Exercise 4, Friedman and Wilcoxon.

Test Statistics (b)

	Defined goals for life—productivity of life	Worry about future—productivity of life	Worry about future—defined goals for of life
Z	−11.070(a)	−18.205(a)	−12.085(a)
Asymp. Sig. (2-tailed)	.000	.000	.000

a Based on positive ranks
b Wilcoxon Signed Ranks Test

EXERCISE FIGURE 4-4. (*Continued*)

4. Exercise Fig. 4-4 contains the results. Friedman was used to answer the main question. There was an overall significant result ($p = .000$) in the comparison of the following ratings: productivity, goals, and worry about the future. Wilcoxon tests with a Bonferroni correction were conducted to test the pairwise comparisons. A p value of 0.0167 was considered significant. All of the pairwise comparisons were significant. Subjects rated their productivity significantly higher than their goals ($p = .000$) and significantly higher than their worry about the future ($p = .000$). They also rated their goals significantly higher than their worry about the future ($p = .000$).

t Tests: Measuring the Differences Between Group Means

Barbara Hazard Munro

Objectives for Chapter 5

After reading this chapter, you should be able to do the following:

1. Determine when the *t* test is appropriate to use.
2. Discuss how mean difference, group variability, and sample size are related to the statistical significance of the *t* statistic.
3. Discuss how the results of the homogeneity of variance test are related to choice of *t* test formula.
4. Select the appropriate *t* test formula (separate, pooled, or correlated) for a given situation.
5. Interpret computer printouts of *t* test analyses.

Many research projects are designed to test the differences between two groups. The *t* test involves an evaluation of means and distributions of each group. The *t* test, or Student's *t* test, is named after its inventor, William Gosset, who published under the pseudonym of Student. Gosset invented the *t* test as a more precise method of comparing groups. He described a set of distributions of means of randomly drawn samples from a normally distributed population. These distributions are the *t* distributions and are detailed in Appendix C.

The shape of the distributions varies depending on the size of the samples drawn from the populations. However, all the *t* distributions have a normal distribution with a mean equal to the mean of the population. Unlike the *z* distributions, which are based on the normal curve and estimate the theoretical population parameters, the *t* distributions are based on sample size and vary according to the degrees of freedom (*df*). Theoretically, when an infinite number of samples of equal size are drawn from a normally distributed population, the mean of the sampling distribution will equal the mean of the population. If the sample sizes were large enough, the shape of the sampling distribution would approximate the normal curve.

RESEARCH QUESTION

When we compare two groups on a particular characteristic, we are asking whether the groups are different. The statistical question asks how different the groups are; that is, is the difference we find greater than that which could occur by chance alone? The null hypothesis for the *t* test states that any difference that occurs between the means of two groups is a difference in the sampling distribution. The means are different not because the groups are drawn from two different theoretical populations, but because of different random distributions of the samples from such a population. The null hypothesis is represented by the *t* distributions constructed by the random sampling of one population. When we use the *t* test to interpret the significance of the difference between groups, we are asking the statistical question, "What is the probability of getting a difference of this magnitude in groups this size if we were comparing random samples drawn from the same population?" In other words, "What is the probability of getting a difference this large by chance alone?"

An example of the *t* test used to compare two groups is the study of Appel, Harrell, and Deng (2002), who compared African American and White southern rural women on physiological variables (Table 5-1). The two groups of women differed significantly on two of the four physiological variables, weight and body mass index (BMI). African American women were significantly heavier and had significantly higher BMIs. The groups of women did not differ on age (*p* = .064) or height (*p* = .0931).

To answer research questions through use of the *t* test, we compare the difference we obtained between our means with the sampling distribution of such differences. In general, the larger the difference between our two means, the more likely it is that the *t* test will be significant. However, two other factors are taken into

TABLE 5-1 *Physiological Variables by Race (n = 1,110)*

| Variables | African American (n = 300) | | | White (n = 810) | | | t | p |
	M	(SD)	Range	M	(SD)	Range		
Age	37.3	(6.9)	24–1	38.2	(6.1)	22–68	−1.85	.64
Weight (kg)	78.5	(17.5)	45.4–158.2	69.0	(15.3)	40.4–168.1	8.05	.001
Height (cm)	163.5	(7.3)	123.1–187.9	164.3	(6.7)	134.6–195.5	−1.6	.0931
BMI (kg/m²)	29.5	(7.0)	15.6–61.7	25.5	(5.6)	14.2–65.6	8.32	<.0001

Note. M = mean; SD = standard deviation; BMI = body mass index.
From Appel, S. J., Harrell, J. S., & Deng, S. (2002). Racial and socioeconomic differences in risk factors for cardiovascular disease among southern rural women. *Nursing Research, 51*(3), 144.

account: the variability and the sample size. An increase in variability leads to an increase in error, and an increase in sample size leads to a decrease in error.

Given the same mean difference, groups with less variability will be more likely to be significantly different than groups with wide variability. This is because in groups with more variability, the error term will be larger. If the groups have scores that vary widely, there is likely to be considerable overlap between the two groups; thus, it will be difficult to ascertain whether a difference exists. Groups with less variability and a real mean difference will have distributions more clearly distinct from each other; that is, there will be less overlap between their respective distributions. With more variability (thus, larger error), we need a larger difference to be reasonably "sure" that a real difference exists.

TYPE OF DATA REQUIRED

For the *t* test, we need one nominal level variable, with two levels as the independent variable. A simpler way to say this is that we must have two groups. The dependent variable should be continuous.

Some people have criticized the use of the term *continuous* rather than specifying the level of measurement of the variable (ordinal, interval, ratio). However, even when data are measured at the ordinal level, they may be appropriate for use in parametric analyses if they approximate the data required to meet the assumptions of a given analysis. Nunnally and Bernstein (1994) consider any measure that can assume 11 or more dichotomous levels as continuous and state that with multi-category items, "somewhat fewer items are needed to qualify" (p. 570). Scales with fewer items are considered discrete. For ease of expression, we use the term continuous to describe scale scores.

The *t* test has been commonly used to compare two groups. The mathematics involved are simpler than those required for analysis of variance, which is discussed in Chapter 6. However, when comparing two groups, it does not matter whether one uses a *t* test or a one-way analysis of variance: The results will be mathematically identical. The *t* statistic (derived from the *t* test formula) is equal to the square root of the *F* statistic (derived from the one-way analysis of variance), or $t^2 = F$.

With the use of the computer, ease of calculation is not an issue, so some people use analysis of variance to compare two groups. Either way is correct. The typical *t* test table has the advantage of clearly presenting the means being compared in the analysis.

ASSUMPTIONS

The three assumptions underlying the *t* test concern the type of data used in the test and the characteristics of the distribution of the variables:

1. The independent variable is categorical and contains two levels; that is, you have two mutually exclusive groups of subjects. Mutually exclusive means that a

subject can contribute just one score to one of the two groups. This is the assumption of independence. When this assumption is violated, as when subjects are measured twice, a correlated or paired *t* test may be appropriate.

2. The distribution of the dependent variable is normal. If the distribution is seriously skewed, the *t* test may be invalid.

3. The variances of the dependent variable for the two groups are similar. This is related to the assumption implied by the null hypothesis that the groups are from a single population. This assumption is called the *requirement of homogeneity of variance*.

Meeting this last assumption protects against type II errors (incorrectly accepting the null hypothesis). When the variances are unequal—that is, when the variation in one sample is significantly greater than the variation in the other—we are less likely to find a significant *t* value. Therefore, we might incorrectly conclude that the groups were drawn from the same population when they were not.

What if the variances are significantly different? Occasionally, groups that we want to compare do not have equal variances. Fortunately, a statistical method approximates the *t* test and can be interpreted in the same way using a different calculation for the standard error.

Actually, three different formulas based on the *t* distribution can be used to compare two groups:

1. The *basic formula*, sometimes called the *pooled formula*, is used to compare two groups when the three assumptions for the *t* test are met.

2. When the variances are unequal, the *separate formula* is used. This takes into account the fact that the variances are not alike and is a more conservative measure.

3. When the two sets of scores are not independent (assumption 1)—that is, there is correlation between the data taken from the two groups—adjustment must be made for that relationship. That formula often is called the *correlated t test* or the *paired t test*. Comparing a group of subjects on their pretest and posttest scores is an example of when this technique would be used. Because these are not two independent groups, but rather one group measured twice, the scores will most likely be correlated. Another example is when the two groups consist of matched pairs. If the pairs are carefully matched, their scores will correlate, and the standard *t* test would not be appropriate.

When checking the assumptions, the first step is to be sure that each subject contributes only one score to one of the groups. In a randomized clinical trial with angioplasty patients (Sulzbach, Munro, & Hirshfeld, 1995), some patients who had been enrolled in the study in one of the two groups returned to the hospital for a second angioplasty. They could not be reentered into the study without violating the principles underlying the notion of mutual exclusivity.

Next, examine the frequency distribution of the dependent variable. Is it normally distributed? Remember that you divide the skewness by the standard error of the skewness to make this determination. Values that are greater than ±1.96 are considered skewed. Alternatives for dealing with skewed data include data transformations, categorizing the variable, or using a nonparametric (distribution free) test. If data transformation is selected and successful, then the *t* test can still be used. If the variable is categorized, then a chi-square would be appropriate. The Mann-Whitney U is an appropriate nonparametric test.

For the test of homogeneity of variance, the analysis is run and the results are examined. The computer produces a test of the assumption, the results of two *t* tests, the pooled or equal variance formula, and the separate or unequal variance formula. An example is given after the discussion of sample size considerations.

SAMPLE SIZE CONSIDERATIONS AND POWER

How many subjects do you need for a *t* test? Cohen (1987) provides tables for determining sample size based on power and effect size determinations, or a computerized program can be used. To enter the tables, we must first decide whether we will be conducting a one- or two-tailed test and what our alpha or probability level will be. If there is sufficient theoretical rationale and we can hypothesize that one group will score significantly higher than the other, we will be using a one-tailed test. If we simply want to answer a question such as, "Is there a difference between the experimental and control groups on the outcome measure?" then we will use a two-tailed test. When planning a study, the sample size is set based on the planned analysis that will require the highest number of subjects. If you were going to run three *t* tests and one would be two tailed, you would base your sample on that, because it requires more subjects than the one-tailed tests.

The power of the test of the null hypothesis is "the probability that it will lead to the rejection of the null hypothesis" (Cohen, 1987, p. 4). A power of 0.80 means, therefore, that there is an 80% chance of rejecting the null hypothesis. The higher the desired power, the more subjects required. Cohen (1987) suggests that for the behavioral scientist, a power of 0.80 is reasonable, given no other basis for selecting the desired level.

The effect size should be based on previous work, if it exists, rather than simply picking a "moderate" effect from the Cohen (1987) tables. The effect size for the *t* test is simply the difference between the means of the two groups divided by the standard deviation for the measure. Cohen's moderate effect size is set at 0.5, which means half of a standard deviation unit. As an example, the graduate record examinations (GRE) have a mean of 500 and a standard deviation of 100. Half of a standard deviation unit on that measure would be 50 (100/2). Thus, a moderate effect would be a difference of 50 points on the GRE between two groups.

In a test of the model of transitional nursing care (Brooten et al., 1995), the LaMonica-Oberst Patient Satisfaction Scale was used. A 17-point difference was found between the experimental and control groups. The standard deviation on the scale was 24. If we were going to use that scale again in a similar experiment, what

TABLE 5-2   n *to Detect d by* t *Test*

| Power | \multicolumn{11}{c}{$a_2 = .05 \; (a_1 = .025)$} |
	.10	.20	.30	.40	.50	.60	.70	.80	1.00	1.20	1.40
.25	332	84	38	22	14	10	8	6	5	4	3
.50	769	193	86	49	32	22	17	13	9	7	5
.60	981	246	110	62	40	28	21	16	11	8	6
2/3	1144	287	128	73	47	33	24	19	12	9	7
.70	1235	310	138	78	50	35	26	20	13	10	7
.75	1389	348	155	88	57	40	29	23	15	11	8
.80	1571	393	175	99	64	45	33	26	17	12	9
.85	1797	450	201	113	73	51	38	29	19	14	10
.90	2102	526	234	132	85	59	44	34	22	16	12
.95	2600	651	290	163	105	73	54	42	27	19	14
.99	3675	920	409	231	148	103	76	58	38	27	20

| Power | \multicolumn{11}{c}{$a_1 = .05 \; (a_2 = .10)$ — d} |
	.10	.20	.30	.40	.50	.60	.70	.80	1.00	1.20	1.40
.25	189	48	21	12	8	6	5	4	3	2	2
.50	542	136	61	35	22	16	12	9	6	5	4
.60	721	181	81	46	30	21	15	12	8	6	5
2/3	862	216	96	55	35	25	18	14	9	7	5
.70	942	236	105	60	38	27	20	15	10	7	6
.75	1076	270	120	68	44	31	23	18	11	8	6
.80	1237	310	138	78	50	35	26	20	13	9	7
.85	1438	360	160	91	58	41	30	23	15	11	8
.90	1713	429	191	108	69	48	36	27	18	13	10
.95	2165	542	241	136	87	61	45	35	22	16	12
.99	3155	789	351	198	127	88	65	50	32	23	17

From Cohen, J. (1987). *Statistical power analysis for the behavior sciences* (Rev. ed.). Hillsdale, NJ: Lawrence Erlbaum Assoc. pp. 54–55.

would our expected effect size be? Divide the difference between the means of 17 by the standard deviation of 24 (17/24), which gives an effect size of .71.

    Table 5-2 gives a section of Cohen's tables. The top section has the table for a two-tailed test (a_2) at the .05 level (or a one-tailed test at the .025 level). Given an effect size of .70 (numbers across top of table) and a power of .80 (numbers down the left side of the table), we would need 33 subjects in each of our groups. If we had used the moderate effect (defined by Cohen as .50), we would need 64 subjects in each of our groups at the same power level. The larger effect size indicates a larger difference between the mean scores and can be detected by fewer subjects.

Now look at the lower section, which includes a one-tailed test at the 0.05 level ($a_1 = .05$). Given an effect size of .70 and a power of .80, we would need 26 subjects per group. Thus, we can see that a one-tailed test is more powerful; that is, we need fewer subjects to detect a significant difference.

To summarize, for sample size with the *t* test, you must determine:

- One tailed versus two tailed
- Alpha level
- Effect size
- Power

You must also estimate how many subjects will be "lost" during data collection and oversample to be sure of having the appropriate numbers for analysis.

COMPUTER ANALYSIS

Dr. Robin Wood (1997) collected data from women in Massachusetts and Georgia. To compare these two groups of women on their years of education, a *t* test was used. Figure 5-1, produced by SPSS for Windows, contains the results. Author comments have been added and appear in a shaded box. The first table contains the group statistics. We see that 99 women were from Massachusetts and 333 from Georgia. The Massachusetts group on average completed 12.6 years of school, whereas the Georgia group averaged 10 years.

The second table, titled Independent Samples Test, contains Levene's test for equality of variances. This is a test of the equality of variance assumption. The test is not significant ($p = .787$), indicating that the variances are equal. We can see in the table of Group Statistics that the standard deviations for the two groups were 4.19946 and 4.19624. The Levene's test tells us that these numbers are equivalent, and that the equal variance or pooled formula *t* test is appropriate.

The computer produces the equal (pooled) variance formula and the unequal (equal variances not assumed or separate) variance formula. Always look first at Levene's test. If the significance level exceeds .05, report the equal variance (pooled) results; if the significance level is less than .05, report the unequal (separate) variance results. In this example, we report the equal variance formula.

The Independent Samples Test table contains both results. Since the variances were equal, we would report a *t* of 5.435, *df* = 430, and *p* = .000. Our analysis indicates that the women from Massachusetts had significantly more years of education (mean = 12.6) than did the women from Georgia (mean = 10.0). The computer printed out the two-tailed significance. For a one-tailed significance, simply divide the *p* value by 2.

T-Test

Group Statistics

What is the highest grade or year of school that you completed?	State	N	Mean	Std. deviation	Std. error mean
	MA	99	12.6111	4.19946	.42206
	GA	333	10.0000	4.19624	.22995

Independent Samples Test

		Levene's test for equality of variances		t test for equality of means					95% confidence interval of the difference	
		F	Sig.	t	df	Sig. (2 tailed)	Mean difference	Std. error difference	Lower	Upper
What is the highest grade or year of school that you completed?	Equal variances assumed	.073	.787	5.435	430	.000	2.6111	.48044	1.66681	3.55541
	Equal variances not assumed			5.433	160.638	.000	2.6111	.48064	1.66192	3.56030

AUTHOR COMMENTS

If Levene's test for equality of variances is not significant (p > .05) report the equal variance results. If Levene's test is significant (p < .05) report the separate ("equal variances not assumed") results.
For a one-tailed t test, divide the two-tailed significance by 2.

FIGURE 5-1. Computer output, independent *t* tests.

TABLE 5-3 *Racial Differences in Sample Characteristics by Chi-Square and* t *Test*

Variable (Categorical)	Whites (n = 598) N (%)	Blacks (n = 44) N (%)	p	Odds Ratio (95% CI)
Insured by Medicare, Medicaid, city welfare, or none	76 (12.8)	11 (25.0)	.041	2.27 (1.10, 4.68)
Diabetes	174 (29.1)	23 (52.3)	.001	2.67 (1.44, 4.95)
Chronic renal failure	64 (10.7)	12 (27.3)	.002	3.13 (1.54, 6.38)
Current smoking	180 (31.0)	21 (48.8)	.016	2.12 (1.14, 3.96)
Pulmonary edema	100 (16.7)	17 (38.6)	.001	3.14 (1.65, 5.97)
Nonwhite physician	25 (4.2)	12 (27.3)	.000	8.58 (3.95, 18.62)
Noncardiac physician	192 (32.1)	26 (59.1)	.001	3.05 (1.64, 5.71)
Variable (Continuous)	**Whites (n − 598) Mean (SD)**	**Blacks (n − 44) Mean (SD)**	**p**	
Age	66.99 (12.65)	61.39 (13.40)	.005	

Note. CI = confidence interval.
From Funk, M., Ostfeld, A. M., Chang, V. M. & Lee, F. A. (2002). Racial differences in the use of cardiac procedures in patients with acute myocardial infarction. *Nursing Research, 51*(3), p. 149.

EXAMPLE FROM A PUBLISHED STUDY

Funk and colleagues (2002) studied the racial differences in the use of cardiac procedures in patients with acute myocardial infarctions. First, they compared the two racial groups on various demographic characteristics. They used chi-square for the categorical variables and *t* test for the continuous variable. Table 5-3 contains the results of their comparison of the ages of the two groups. There was a significant difference in age between the Black and Whites in their study (p = .005). Whites were significantly older (mean age = 67) than Blacks (mean age = 61).

CORRELATED OR PAIRED *t* TEST

If the two groups being compared are matched or paired on some basis, the scores are likely to be similar. The chance differences between the two groups will not be as large as when they are drawn independently. In the correlated *t* test, a correction is made that has the effect of increasing *t*, thus making it more likely to find a significant difference if one exists.

Figure 5-2 contains a computer printout produced by SPSS for Windows, using data collected by Wood (1997). Subjects were tested on their knowledge of breast self-examination at two points in time. There was a significant change over time with

T-Test

Paired Samples Statistics

		Mean	N	Std. deviation	Std. error mean
Pair 1	Knowledge score time 1	50.0683	439	20.53497	.98008
	Knowledge score time 2	71.0706	439	22.83537	1.08987

Paired Samples Correlations

		N	Correlation	Sig.
Pair 1	Knowledge score time 1 & % of total Knowledge score, time 2	439	.441	.000

Paired Samples Test

		Paired differences					t	df	Sig. (2 tailed)
					95% confidence interval of the difference				
		Mean	Std. deviation	Std. error mean	Lower	Upper			
Pair 1	Knowledge score time 1 & % of total Knowledge score, time 2	−21.0023	23.01275	1.09834	−23.1609	−18.8436	−19.122	438	.000

FIGURE 5-2. Computer output, paired *t* test.

subjects scoring significantly higher ($p = .000$) at the second testing (mean $= 71$) than at the first testing (mean $= 50$). The correlation between the two scores, presented in the second table, was .441, significant at the .000 level. The Paired Samples Test table shows that the means differed by 21.0023. The *t* value of -19.122, with $df = 438$, has a two-tailed significance of .000 (at least less than .001).

SUMMARY

The *t* test is a statistical method for comparing differences between two groups. The test requires a continuous dependent variable on which the groups are being compared. The test assumes that the variable is normally distributed in the populations from which the samples are drawn and that the samples have equivalent variances. The *t* test is particularly useful in experimental and quasi-experimental designs in which an experimental and a control group are compared.

Application Exercises and Results

Exercises

Answer the following research questions by running the appropriate *t* tests and writing up the results.

1. Do people who have never smoked differ significantly from those who are still smoking on positive psychological attitudes (total IPPA score)?

2. Do current ratings of quality of life differ significantly from ratings of quality of life at age 18?

Results

1. An independent *t* test should be used to answer this question. On the SMOKE variable, only two groups are selected, those who never smoked (0) and those who are still smoking (2). Exercise Fig. 5-1 contains the results.

   Which *t* test should be reported? Because Levene's test for equality of variances is significant ($p = .000$), the equal variances not assumed (separate) formula should be reported. We would report that people who never smoked scored significantly higher ($p = .004$) on the total IPPA score (mean $= 154.67$) than did those who are still smoking (mean $= 141.35$). It should be noted that there was a large difference in the size of the two groups.

2. There was no significant difference ($p = .251$) between the ratings of quality of life in the past month (mean $= 4.27$) and at age 18 (mean $= 4.22$). The correlation between the two measures was .331 ($p = .000$). Exercise Fig. 5-2 contains the printout.

T-Test

Group Statistics

	Smoking history	N	Mean	Std. deviation	Std. error mean
TOTAL	Never smoked	410	154.6683	26.41131	1.30436
	Still smoking	71	141.3521	36.57013	4.34008

Independent Samples Test

		Levene's test for equality of variances		t test for equality of means					95% confidence interval of the difference	
		F	Sig.	t	df	Sig. (2 tailed)	Mean difference	Std. error difference	Lower	Upper
TOTAL	Equal variances assumed	14.086	.000	3.683	479	.000	13.3162	3.61540	6.21219	20.42017
	Equal variances not assumed			2.938	83.100	.004	13.3162	4.53184	4.30268	22.32968

EXERCISE FIGURE 5-1. Results of Exercise 1, independent samples *t* test.

T-Test

Paired Samples Statistics

		Mean	N	Std. deviation	Std. error mean
Pair 1	Quality of life in past month	4.27	697	1.043	.039
	Quality of life at age 18	4.22	697	1.123	.043

Paired Samples Correlations

		N	Correlation	Sig.
Pair 1	Quality of life in past month & quality of life at age 18	697	.331	.000

Paired Samples Test

		Paired differences							
					95% confidence interval of the difference				
		Mean	Std. deviation	Std. error mean	Lower	Upper	t	df	Sig. (2-tailed)
Pair 1	Quality of life in past month—quality of life at age 18	0.5	1.254	0.47	−.04	.15	1.148	696	.251

EXERCISE FIGURE 5-2. Results of Exercise 2, paired samples t test.

Differences Among Group Means: One-Way Analysis of Variance

Barbara Hazard Munro

Objectives for Chapter 6

After reading this chapter, you should be able to do the following:

1. Determine when analysis of variance is appropriate to use.
2. Interpret a computer printout of a one-way analysis of variance.
3. Describe between-group, within-group, and total variance.
4. Explain the use of posthoc tests and a priori comparisons.
5. Report the results of one-way analysis of variance in a summary table.

Many times, a clinical research question involves a comparison of several groups on a particular measure. In Chapter 5, we discussed the *t* test as a method for examining the difference between two groups. The basic *t* test compares two means in relation to the distribution of the differences between pairs of means drawn from a random sample. When we have more than two groups and are interested in the differences among the set of groups, we are dealing with different combinations of pairs of means. If we choose to analyze the differences by *t* test analysis, we would need to do a number of *t* tests. Suppose that we had four different groups—A, B, C, and D—that we wanted to compare on a particular variable. If we were interested in the differences among the four groups, we would need to do a *t* test for each of the possible pairs that exist in the four groups. We would have A versus B, A versus C, A versus D, B versus C, B versus D, and C versus D. In all, we would have six separate comparisons, each requiring a separate analysis.

The problem with conducting such multiple-group comparisons relates to the underlying concept of statistical analysis. Each test is based on the probability that the null hypothesis is true. Therefore, each time we conduct a test, we are running the risk of a type I error. The probability level we set as the point at which we reject the null hypothesis also is the level of risk with which we are comfortable. If that level is 0.05, we are accepting the risk that 5 of 100 times, our rejection of the null hypothesis will be in error. However, when we calculate multiple *t* tests on independent samples that are being measured on the same variable, the rate of error increases exponentially by the number of tests conducted. For example, with our four-group problem, the error rate increases to 18 of 100 times, a substantial increase. The calculation of the rate of type I errors is determined by the following formula:

$$1 - (1 - a)^t$$

where a = the level of significance for the tests and *t* = the number of test comparisons used. In our example, the calculation would give us:

$$1 - (1 - 0.05)^4 = 0.18.$$

Instead of using a series of individual comparisons, we examine the differences among the groups through an analysis that considers the variation across all groups at once. This test is the *analysis of variance* (ANOVA).

STATISTICAL QUESTION IN ANALYSIS OF VARIANCE

The statistical question using ANOVA is based on the null hypothesis: the assumption that all groups are equal and drawn from the same population. Any difference comes from a random sampling difference. The question answered by the ANOVA test is whether group means differ from each other.

TYPE OF DATA REQUIRED

With ANOVA, the independent variable(s) are at the nominal level. A one-way ANOVA means that there is only one independent variable (often called *factor*). That independent variable has two or more levels. Gender would be a variable with two levels, whereas race, religion, and so forth may have varying numbers of levels depending on how the variable is defined. Two-way ANOVA indicates two independent variables, and *n*-way ANOVA indicates that the number of independent variables is defined by *n*. The dependent variable must be continuous and meet the assumptions described in the next section.

For example, Anderson and Helms (1998) used analysis of variance to compare hospitals grouped by size (small, medium, large, and very large) on their scores on the Referral Data Inventory (RDI), which "measures the amount and type of information an ECF (extended care facility) receives upon referral of an elderly patient from a hospital, as well as the organizational and medical factors associated with interorganizational communication" (p. 388). Table 6-1 contains an edited version of the results from the study. The RDI scores can range between 0 and 40, with higher scores indicating more data sent from hospital to extended care facility. Looking at the mean scores, we can see that large hospitals sent the least data (mean = 30.02), and very large hospitals sent the most (36.06). The *F* ratio is significant at p < .0001. The Scheffe posthoc test was

TABLE 6-1 *Summary of ANOVA for Size of Referring Hospital (N = 455)*

	Total Score
Hospital Size	(0–40) M (SD)
Small (Sm) (n = 50)	32.66 (2.37)
Medium (Med) (n = 126)	32.41 (2.46)
Large (Lg) (n = 257)	30.02 (3.06)
Very Large (Vlg) (n = 22)	36.06 (3.22)
SS (Between Grp.)	1171.85
SS (Within Grp.)	3661.43
df (Between [Within])	3 [451]
MS (Between Grp.)	390.61
MS (Within Grp.)	8.11
F ratio	48.11**
Scheffe	Lg < others
	Vlg > others

$**p < .0001$.
Adapted from Anderson, M. A., & Helms, L. B. (1998). Extended care referral after hospital discharge. *Research in Nursing & Health, 21*(5), 385–394.

used to determine which pairs of scores were significantly different. There are six pairwise comparisons that can be made, small with medium, small with large, small with very large, medium with large, medium with very large, and large with very large. You wouldn't expect the small- and medium-sized hospitals to be significantly different, given the closeness of their mean scores. The authors have reported the significant results at the bottom of the column. Large (with the lowest mean score) is reported as significantly less than the other three groups, and Very Large (with the highest mean score) is reported as significantly higher than the other three groups.

ASSUMPTIONS

ANOVA has been shown to be fairly *robust*. This means that even if the researchers do not rigidly adhere to the assumptions, the results may still be close to the truth. The assumptions for ANOVA are the same as those for the *t* test; that is, the dependent variable should be a continuous variable that is normally distributed, the groups should be mutually exclusive (independent of each other), and the groups should have equal variances (homogeneity of variance requirement).

TABLE 6-2 *Sample Size Determination*											

	$\dfrac{u = 4}{f}$										
Power	.05	.10	.15	.20	.25	.30	.35	.40	.50	.60	.70	.80
.10	74	19	9	6	4	3	2	2	—	—	—	—
.50	514	129	58	33	21	15	11	9	6	5	4	3
.70	776	195	87	49	32	22	17	13	9	6	5	4
.80	956	240	107	61	39	27	20	16	10	8	6	5
.90	1231	309	138	78	50	35	26	20	13	10	7	6
.95	1486	372	166	94	60	42	31	24	16	11	9	7
.99	2021	506	225	127	82	57	42	33	21	15	11	9

Adapted from Cohen, J. (1987). *Statistical power analysis for the behavioral sciences* (Rev. ed.). Hillsdale, NJ: Lawrence Erlbaum Assoc.

SAMPLE SIZE CONSIDERATIONS AND POWER

The principles relating to considerations of sample size and power are based on those outlined in Chapter 5, where two means were compared through use of the *t* test. Using means and standard deviations from previous work, we can calculate expected effect sizes, either by using the formulas provided in Cohen (1987) or by one of the software programs available. Given an expected effect size, desired power, and alpha level, we can determine sample size. For example, Table 6-2 contains an excerpt from Cohen's Table 8.44 (p. 384). It is used to determine appropriate sample size when alpha is .05 and the degrees of freedom (*df*, u) equal 4. Because the *df* is one less than the number of groups, this table is used when there are five groups. The effect sizes are indicated by *f* across the top of the table, and the power values are listed down the left side. Suppose we calculated an effect size of .30. (Cohen defines a moderate effect size as .25, which with two groups is still half of a standard deviation unit.) If we desired a power of .80, how many subjects would we need in each group, and how many would we need overall? We would need 27 subjects in each group, and because there are 5 groups, we would need a total of 135 subjects.

SOURCE OF VARIANCE

According to the null hypothesis, all groups are from the same population, and each of their scores comes from the same population of measures. Any variability of scores can be seen in two ways: First, the scores vary from each other in their own group; and second, the groups vary from each other. The first variation is called *within-group variation*; the second variation is called *between-group variation*. Together, the two types of variation add up to the total variation.

Students often are confused when we say that ANOVA tells us whether the means of groups differ significantly and then proceed to talk about analyzing variance. The *t* test was clearly a test of mean difference, because the difference between the two means was contained in the numerator of the *t* test formula. It is important to understand how analyzing the variability of groups on some measure can tell us whether their measures of central tendency (means) differ.

With ANOVA, the variance of each group is measured separately; all the subjects are then lumped together, and the variance of the total group is computed. If the variance of the total group (total variation) is about the same as the average of the variances of the separate groups (within-group variation), the means of the separate groups are not different. This is because if total variation is the sum of within-group variation and between-group variation, and if within-group variation and total variation are equal, there is no between-group variation. This should become more clear in the diagrams that follow. However, if the variance of the total group is much larger than the average variation within the separate groups, a significant mean difference exists between at least two of the subgroups. In that case, the within-group variation does not equal the total variation. The difference between them must equal the between-group variation.

To visualize the difference in the types of variation, consider three groups exposed to three different experimental conditions. Suppose that the three conditions yielded such widely different scores that there was no overlap among the three groups in terms of the outcome measure (Fig. 6-1). We could then represent our three

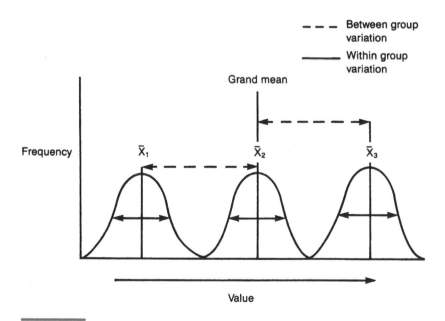

FIGURE 6-1. Between-group and within-group variation: The case of no overlap.

groups in terms of their relationship to each other and in terms of a total group. Each group would then have its own mean and its own distribution around its mean. At the same time, there would be a *grand mean*, which is a mean for all the groups combined. As shown in Figure 6-1, we can look at the variation within the groups and between the groups. The combination of the within-group and between-group variation equals the total variation.

The ANOVA test examines the variation and tests whether the between-group variation exceeds the within-group variation. When the between-group variance is greater (statistically greater) than the within-group variance, the means of the groups must be different. However, when the within-group variance is approximately the same as the between-group variance, the group's means are not importantly different. This relationship between the difference among groups and the different types of variance is shown in Figure 6-2.

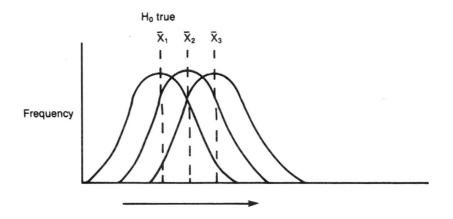

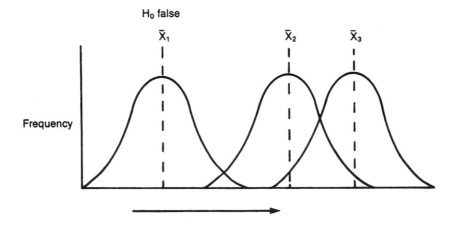

FIGURE 6-2. Relationship of variation to null hypothesis.

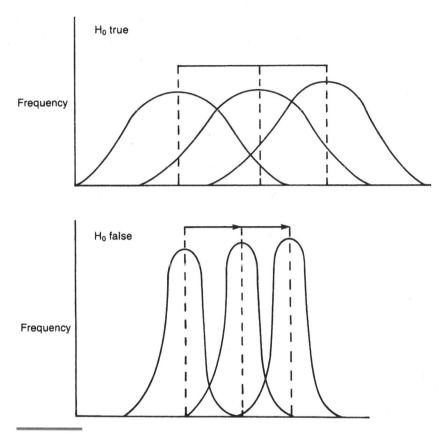

FIGURE 6-3. Effect of within-group variation on null hypothesis.

When the null hypothesis (H_o) is true, the groups overlap to a large extent, and the within-group variation exceeds the between-group variation. When the null hypothesis is false, the groups show little overlapping, and the distance between group is greater. In the lower portion of Fig. 6-2, we see that group 1 overlaps very little with group 2 and not at all with group 3. Groups 2 and 3 do overlap. In that case, it may be that group 1 scored significantly lower than groups 2 and 3, and that groups 2 and 3 do not differ significantly from each other. Thus, the group variation and the deviation between group means determine the likelihood that the null hypothesis is true.

Figure 6-3 illustrates the fact that when the variation within a group or groups is great, the difference between the groups must be greater than when the distribution within groups is narrow to reject the null hypothesis. In the same way, when the group distributions are narrow (low within-group variance), relatively small between-group differences will be significant.

MEASURE OF VARIANCE: SUMS OF SQUARES

The kinds of variation of scores within groups has an intuitive and a statistical meaning. We have discussed the intuitive meaning as the extent to which the scores

TABLE 6-3 *Calculation of Sum of Squares*		
	Group 1	*Group 2*	*Group 3*
	1	4	6
	2	5	8
	3	3	5
	2	4	5
	—	—	—
$\bar{X}_s$	2	4	6

Total Sum of Squares

	Raw Scores	Deviations from Grand Mean	Squared Deviation
	1	$1 - 4 = -3$	9
	2	$2 - 4 = -2$	4
	3	$3 - 4 = -1$	1
	2	$2 - 4 = -2$	4
	4	$4 - 4 = 0$	0
	5	$5 - 4 = 1$	1
	3	$3 - 4 = -1$	1
	4	$4 - 4 = 0$	0
	6	$6 - 4 = 2$	4
	8	$8 - 4 = 4$	16
	5	$5 - 4 = 1$	1
	5	$5 - 4 = 1$	1
	Grand Mean = 4	Sum = 0	42

Total sum of squares = 42

Within Sum of Squares

	Group 1		
	Raw Scores	Deviations from Group Mean	Squared Deviations
	1	$1 - 2 = -1$	1
	2	$2 - 2 - 0$	0
	3	$3 - 2 = 1$	1
	2	$2 - 2 = 0$	0
	$\bar{X} = 2$	Sum = 0	Sum = 2

(continued)

TABLE 6-3 *(Continued)*

Group 2

	Raw Scores	Deviations from Group Mean	Squared Deviations
	4	$4 - 4 = \ \ 0$	0
	5	$5 - 4 = \ \ 1$	1
	3	$3 - 4 = -1$	1
	4	$4 - 4 = \ \ 0$	0
	$\overline{X} = 4$	Sum = 0	Sum = 2

Group 3

	6	$6 - 6 = \ \ 0$	0
	8	$8 - 6 = \ \ 2$	4
	5	$5 - 6 = -1$	1
	5	$5 - 6 = -1$	1
	$\overline{X} = 6$	Sum = 0	Sum = 6

Within sum of squares = 2 + 2 + 6 = 10

Between Sum of Squares

Deviations of Group Means from Grand Mean	Squared Deviations	Number in Group
Group 1 $2 - 4 = -2$	4	4
Group 2 $4 - 4 = \ \ \ 0$	0	4
Group 3 $6 - 4 = \ \ \ 2$	4	4

Between Sum of Squares = (4)(4) + (4)(0) + (4)(4) = 32

Summary Table

Source of Variance	SS	df	MS	F	p
Between group	32	2	16	14.41	<.01
Within group	10	9	1.11		
Total	42	11			

within a group vary from each other and the extent to which the groups vary from each other. The statistical concept of this variation involves a quantification of the amount of variation of scores around the mean. We have already defined and used this concept with the term *sum of squares.*

The sum of squares is the sum of the squared deviations of each of the scores around a respective mean. In ANOVA, the sum of squares is used to measure the total variation, between-group variation, and within-group variation. Table 6-3 contains an example of the calculation of the sums of squares using the formulas based on the deviations of the scores from their respective means. The data consist of four scores in each of three groups. The means for the three groups are 2, 4, and 6, respectively.

Sum of Squares for Total Variation

The total sum of squares is equal to the sum of the squared deviations of each score in all groups from the grand mean. In our example, the grand mean (mean of the nine scores) is 4. The sum of the deviations around the mean equals zero, and the sum of the squared deviations equals 42. This total sum of squares represents the basis of the null hypothesis that all the subjects belong to one population, which is described by the grand mean.

Sum of Squares for within-Group Variation

The within-group variation is the total of the variation that occurs in each subgroup. It is calculated by finding the sum of squares for each group separately and then summing the results. The sums of the squared deviations for the three groups are 2, 2, and 6, and the sum across the three groups is 10.

Sum of Squares for between-Group Variation

The between-group variation examines how each of the groups varies from the grand mean. For this calculation, we use group means as representative of the individual groups. The between-group variation examines the variation of the group means from the grand mean. In Table 6-3, the mean for group 1 is two less than the grand mean. The sum of the deviations around the grand mean is (as always) zero, and the squared deviations are 4, 0, and 4, respectively. Because the weight of the difference of any mean from the grand mean is influenced by the number of the scores in the group, we weight the squared deviations by the number in the group. The weighted squared deviations are then summed to provide the between sum of squares (32).

In summary, these three sums of squares define the three different kinds of variation that exist when subjects are members of different groups and are measured on a single variable. They include the total variation of each of the scores around the grand mean, the variation of scores within their respective groups, and the deviation between groups measured by the deviation of group means from the grand mean.

DISPLAYING THE RESULTS: SUMMARY OF ANALYSIS OF VARIANCE

The results of the calculations leading to the *F* ratio are summarized in a table form that is standard for presenting ANOVA results. This presentation of the results is called the *summary of ANOVA table*. In Table 6-3, *SS* stands for sum of squares, *df* for degrees of freedom, *MS* for mean square, *F* for the statistic generated, and *p* for the probability level.

Degrees of Freedom

The *df* for the between-group variance is equal to the number of groups minus one. In our example, this is $3 - 1 = 2$. The *df* for the within-group variance is equal to the total number of subjects minus the number of groups, or $12 - 3 = 9$. The *df* for the total variance is equal to the number of subjects minus one ($12 - 1 = 11$). The mean square is the sum of squares divided by its *df*. Thus, the between-group sum of squares, 32, divided by 2 results in a mean square of 16.

Testing the Difference among Groups: The *F* Ratio

To determine whether the between-group difference is great enough to reject the null hypothesis, we compare it statistically to the within-group variance. The *F* represents the ratio of between to within variance and is calculated as the between mean square divided by the within mean square, or $16/1.11 = 14.41$. The *F* value is compared to the values obtained when the null hypothesis is true, and the scores are randomly selected from one population. To make the interpretation, we use the table that presents the *F* distributions (Appendix D). We locate the critical values for comparison by using the *df* for the between and within mean squares.

In the example, the between *df* was 2 and the within df was 9. We locate the between *df* on the row across the top of the table, and we locate the within *df* on the column on the left side of the table. With these points as coordinates, we locate two critical values for *F*. The top value (in light print) is 4.26. This is the value required to reject the null hypothesis at a probability level of 0.05 (given a one-tailed test). The value below (in bold print) is 8.02, the value required to reject the null hypothesis at the 0.01 level. The value of 14.41 is greater than the value required to reach an alpha of 0.01. Therefore, we can reject the null hypothesis at the 0.01 level. We say we have reached a probability level of "less than 0.01." In summary, we obtained an *F* value of 14.41. We therefore rejected the null hypothesis that there were no differences between the groups, and we concluded that the groups were different.

In other standard presentations of ANOVA summary tables, the within variance is sometimes called the *error variance* or *error term*. This terminology reflects the assumption of the ANOVA that the within difference is sampling error or random difference.

In addition to the summary table, often it is helpful to include a table in your results section that shows the means and standard deviations for the scores of each group. One can then see which group scored higher and by how much. Without further analysis, however, we do not know which pairs of means differ significantly. A posthoc analysis would allow us to compare group 1 with group 2, group 1 with group 3, and group 2 with group 3. Before discussing such contrasts in detail, however, we first present another example with a computer analysis of the data.

ONE-WAY ANALYSIS OF VARIANCE

We have one independent categorical variable with *n* levels and one continuous dependent variable that meets the assumptions, that is that it is normally distributed and that the variance is equal across the groups. To demonstrate, we used data from

One way

Descriptives

CONCERTS

	N	Mean	Std. deviation	Std. error	95% confidence interval for mean		Minimum	Maximum
					Lower bound	Upper bound		
Private home	195	5.4103	4.26879	.30569	4.8073	6.0132	.00	10.00
Apartment	86	5.6047	4.37447	.47171	4.6668	6.5425	.00	10.00
Elder housing	139	4.1079	4.56466	.38717	3.3424	4.8735	.00	10.00
Total	420	5.0190	4.42704	.21602	4.5944	5.4437	.00	10.00

Test of Homogeneity of Variances

CONCERTS

Levene statistic	df1	df2	Sig.
2.218	2	417	.110

AUTHOR COMMENTS
The assumption of homogeneity of variance has been met.

ANOVA

CONCERTS

	Sum of squares	*df*	Mean square	*F*	Sig.
Between groups	174.729	2	87.364	4.533	.011
Within groups	8037.119	417	19.274		
Total	8211.848	419			

AUTHOR COMMENTS
The overall analysis is significant (p = .011).

FIGURE 6-4. Computer output of one-way analysis of variance with posthoc comparisons.

Posthoc Tests

Multiple Comparisons

Dependent Variable: CONCERTS

Scheffé

(I) Living recoded	(J) Living recoded	Mean difference (I-J)	Std. error	Sig.	95% confidence interval	
					Lower bound	Upper bound
Private home	Apartment	−.1944	.56829	.943	−1.5904	1.2016
	Elder housing	1.3023(*)	.48734	.029	.1052	2.4995
Apartment	Private home	.1944	.56829	.943	−1.2016	1.5904
	Elder housing	1.4967(*)	.60231	.047	.0171	2.9763
Elder housing	Private home	−1.3023(*)	.48734	.029	−2.4995	−.1052
	Apartment	−1.4967(*)	.60231	.047	−2.9763	−.0171

* The mean difference is significant at the .05 level.

AUTHOR COMMENTS
The elder housing group scored significantly lower than the other two groups.
There was no significant difference between the private home and apartment groups.

FIGURE 6-4. (*Continued*)

Dr. Wood's study on promoting breast self-examination (1997). The housing of her subjects can be described by three categories: private home, apartment, and elder housing. Subjects were asked to rate the desirability of certain things that could be offered to them for participation in the study. One choice was concert tickets. Participants rated this choice from 0 = undesirable to 10 = very attractive. The research question is whether the three housing groups differ significantly in their rating of the desirability of receiving concert tickets.

COMPUTER ANALYSIS

To answer the research question, the data were submitted to analysis by the one-way program in SPSS for Windows. This program handles one-way ANOVA (one independent variable) and posthoc tests necessary to compare pairs of means. Figure 6-4 contains the computer output. Author comments have been added to ease interpretation and appear in a shaded box.

The dependent variable is the rating of the desirability of concert tickets, and the independent variable is housing group with three levels: private home, apartment, and elder housing. The descriptive statistics are given first. The groups are somewhat unequal with the smallest number living in apartments (86) and the largest number living in private homes (195). Looking at the mean scores, we see that on a scale of 0 to 10, the groups are about in the middle. The elder housing group has the lowest mean rating (4.11), and the apartment group gave it the highest rating (5.60). The standard deviations and standard errors are listed. Based on the standard errors, 95% confidence intervals (CI) also are listed. For the private home group, the 95% CI is 4.8073 to 6.0132. This means that if 100 similar samples were drawn, in 95 out of 100 tests, the mean would fall between 4.8 and 6.0. The minimum and maximum scores for each group also are listed. For each group, the entire potential range of scores was covered, that is, all three groups had low scores of zero and high scores of 10.

The assumption of homogeneity of variance is met ($p = .110$). The ANOVA summary table is typical of what is reported in the literature. The variance is reported as between groups, within groups, and total. "Between groups" indicates the differences among the three groups, "within groups" is the error term, and "total" is the total variance in the dependent variable.

Sums of squares are reported first. Because there are three groups, $df = 2$ (number of groups minus one). Dividing the sum of squares by its associated df gives the mean square value. For example, for between groups, $174.729/2 = 87.364$. The F is the ratio of between to within variance, or $87.364/19.274 = 4.533$. This number is significant at the .011 level.

Because the overall F is significant, we want to know which pairs of means are significantly different. The Scheffé posthoc procedure, which will be described in the next section, was requested. All possible pairwise comparisons are tested. We see that there is a significant difference between the elder housing group and both of the other two groups. For the comparison with the private home group $p = .029$ and for the apartment group $p = .047$. The private home and apartment groups did not differ from each other ($p = .943$). Looking at the means to describe the results, we would say that the group that lived in elder housing rated the desirability of concert tickets (mean = 4.11) significantly lower than the private home group (mean = 5.41) and the apartment group (mean = 5.60).

MULTIPLE GROUP COMPARISONS

Two types of comparisons can be made among group means. The most commonly reported are posthoc (after the fact) comparisons and a priori (planned) comparisons, based on hypotheses stated before the analysis.

Posthoc Tests

When a significant F test is obtained, the null hypothesis that all the groups are from the same population or that all the populations are equal is rejected; that is, we can state that there is a difference among the groups. However, when more than two groups are being compared, we cannot determine from the F test alone which groups differ from each other. In other words, a significant F test does not mean that every group in the analysis is different from every other group. Many patterns of difference are possible. Some of the groups may be similar, forming a cluster that is different from another select group; depending on the number of groups being compared, there may be wide deviation between each pair of the groups.

To determine where the significant differences lie, further analysis is required. Therefore, we must compare group means. However, if we decide to use the standard *t* test, we are confronted with the possibility of an increased rate of type I errors. To prevent this, secondary analyses following the computation of the *F* ratio are available to pinpoint the source of the difference.

Many techniques exist. A complete discussion of each is beyond the scope of this book, but the aim of all is to decrease the likelihood of making a type I error when making multiple comparisons. For more details on posthoc tests following ANOVA, we suggest Klockars and Sax (1991), and Toothaker (1993).

The *Scheffé test* is reported frequently. The formula is based on the usual formula for the calculation of a *t* test or *F* ratio. The critical value used for determining whether the resulting *F* statistic is significant is different. In other words, the *F* associated with comparing the two means is the same as if they had been compared in the usual ANOVA, but the critical value is changed based on the number of comparisons. The new critical value is simply the usual value multiplied by the number of groups being compared minus one. In our example in Fig. 6-4, the critical value at the 0.05 level with 2 and 417 *df* is 3.02 (see Appendix D). Multiplying that by 2 (the number of groups minus one) results in a critical value of 6.04. Thus, the critical value is twice as stringent when making all possible comparisons among three groups than it was for the overall analysis. The Scheffé test is stringent, but it can be used with groups of equal and unequal size.

The *Bonferroni correction* has been explained previously. The desired alpha is divided by the number of comparisons. For example, with an alpha of 0.05 and four comparisons, the significance level would have to be equal to or less than 0.0125 for the paired comparison to be significant.

The *Duncan test* is computed in the same way as the student Newman-Keuls, but the critical value is less stringent.

The *Least Significant Difference test* is equivalent to multiple *t* tests. The modification is that a pooled estimate of variance is used rather than variance common to groups being compared.

Student Newman-Keuls is similar to Tukey's honestly significant difference (HSD) but the critical values do not stay the same. They reflect the variables being compared.

Tukey's honestly significant difference (HSD) is the most conservative comparison test and as such is the least powerful. The critical values for Tukey remain the same for each comparison, regardless of the total number of means to be compared.

Tukey's wholly significant difference uses critical values that are the average of those used in Tukey's HSD and Student Newman-Keuls. It is therefore intermediate in conservatism between those two measures.

EXAMPLE FROM THE LITERATURE

Look again at Table 6-1 that contains the table from Anderson and Helms (1998). They used the Scheffe test for pairwise comparisons. Their *F* ratio (48.11) was significant at

$p < .0001$. It was, therefore, appropriate to use a posthoc test. It should be noted that even when the overall F is significant, it is possible that none of the pairwise comparisons will be significant. This is because the posthoc tests protect against a type I error by being more stringent. Given the four groups of hospitals, six posthoc comparisons could be made. The authors tell us that large hospitals differed significantly from the other three, as did the very large hospitals. That means that the only comparison that was not significant was between small and medium hospitals. Here is the breakdown of possible comparisons. An asterisk indicates significant differences. Take a moment to look at Table 6-1 and this outline to be sure you understand it.

Comparisons by hospital size:

Small with Medium
Small with Large*
Small with Very Large*
Medium with Large*
Medium with Very Large*
Large with Very Large*

Basically, since Large and Very Large are reported as significantly different from all other groups, any comparison that they are in is significant.

Planned Comparisons

Planned comparisons, or a priori contrasts, are based on hypotheses stated before data are collected. When you hypothesize ahead of time, you can use more powerful statistical tests. One way to do this is through the development of prespecified contrasts that are *orthogonal* to each other. Orthogonal means that the hypothesis tests are unrelated to each other; that is, knowing one result tells you nothing about the other. For an overview of planned comparisons versus omnibus tests, refer to Wu and Slakter (1990). Here we demonstrate how orthogonal contrasts can be developed and analyzed in SPSS for Windows. To have comparisons that are independent, only $n - 1$ comparisons can be made. In our three-group living arrangements example (Fig. 6-4), therefore, there could be only two orthogonal contrasts. In our example, we might want to test the hypothesis that the two independent living (private home and apartment) groups will score significantly higher on desire for concert tickets than the elder housing group and that there will be no difference between the apartment and private home groups. Table 6-4 contains the vectors necessary to code such a contrast. On vector 1 (V1), subjects in both independent living groups receive a -1, and the elder housing subjects receive a 2. This contrast tests the difference between the desirability of a concert ticket mean score for all the independent living subjects and the mean for the elder housing subjects. The second contrast is given in vector 2 (V2). The two independent living groups are compared. The elder housing group is not considered in the second contrast. (Note, in building the contrasts, you must list the groups in the order in which they are in the dataset. In our dataset, the values are 1 = Private home, 2 = Apartment, and 3 = Elder housing.)

TABLE 6-4 *Orthogonal Coding*		
	Vectors	
Groups	V1	V2
Private home	−1	1
Apartment	−1	−1
Elder housing	+2	0

To ensure that hypothesized contrasts are orthogonal, three tests must be applied:

1. There must be only $n - 1$ contrasts.
2. The sum of each vector must equal zero. In the example, the sum of V1 is $(-1) + (-1) + 2 = 0$, and the sum of V2 is $1 + (-1) + 0 = 0$.
3. The sum of the cross-products must equal zero. In the example, $(-1 \times 1) + (-1 \times -1) + (2 \times 0) + = 0$.

Table 6-5 provides other examples of possible contrasts, given three groups. Are they all orthogonal? The vectors X1 and X2 reflect an orthogonal contrast, as do the vectors Y1 and Y2. Vectors Z1 and Z2 do not reflect an orthogonal contrast; group 1 is compared to group 2 and to group 3. The sum of the cross-products does not equal zero $(-1 \times 1) - (0 \times -1) + (1 \times 0) = -1$.

We now demonstrate the use of the contrasts specified in Table 6-4 in a computer analysis of these data. See Fig. 6-5 for the computer output of the a priori contrasts. In the first analysis (see Fig. 6-4), we requested a posthoc test and determined that the elder housing group scored significantly lower than the other two groups.

In the analysis in Fig. 6-5, we are testing a priori orthogonal contrasts. Since the Descriptives, Test of Homogeneity of Variance, and ANOVA table are the same as those in Fig. 6-4, they are not repeated here. Author's comments have been added

TABLE 6-5 *Contrasts*						
	Pairs of Vectors					
Groups	X1	X2	Y1	Y2	Z1	Z2
1	2	0	−1	1	−1	1
2	−1	1	2	0	0	−1
3	−1	−1	−1	−1	1	0

Contrast Coefficients

Contrast	Type of living quarters		
	Private home	Apartment	Elder housing
1	−1	−1	2
2	1	−1	0

AUTHOR COMMENTS
The first contrast tests the difference between the two independent living groups (each given a coefficient of −1) and the elder housing group (coefficient = 2).
The second contrast tests the difference between the two independent living groups.

Contrast Tests

		Contrast	Value of Contrast	Std. Error	t	df	Sig. (2-tailed)
Coupon for concerts	Assume equal variances	1	−2.7991	.93680	−2.988	417	.003
		2	−.1944	.56829	−.342	417	.732
	Does not assume equal variances	1	−2.7991	.95685	−2.925	259.302	.004
		2	−.1944	.56210	−.346	159.093	.730

AUTHOR COMMENTS
Because the homogeneity of variance assumption was met, the equal variance contrasts are appropriate. Only the first contrast is significant.

———
FIGURE 6-5. Computer output containing a priori contrasts.

to increase clarity and appear in a shaded box. This is a more powerful analysis; that is, it is more likely to find a significant difference among groups. This is because the contrasts are stated a priori and are restricted to orthogonal contrasts. In the case of posthoc tests, the overall F value must be significant before we can test pairwise comparisons. When using orthogonal contrasts, these contrasts can be examined even when the overall F is not significant. The first contrast (read across the row) compares the means of the two independent living groups with the elder housing group. The second contrast compares the two independent living groups.

The equal variance estimate is appropriate because the assumption of homogeneity of variance has been met (see Fig. 6-4, Levene test, $p = .110$). We hypothesized that the first contrast would be significant, but that the second would not. Our hypotheses have been supported. The first contrast is significant ($p = .003$), thus the independent living groups did differ significantly from the elder housing group.

Looking at the means, we see that as hypothesized the independent living groups rated the desirability of concert tickets significantly higher than did the elder housing group. The private home and apartment groups did not differ significantly ($p = .732$). In this example, the a priori and posthoc tests resulted in the same findings. This is not always the case.

A priori contrasts must be based on firm theoretical grounds.

EXAMPLE FROM THE LITERATURE

In a study of Australian nurses' experiences and attitudes in the "do not resuscitate" decision, Manias (1998) used a priori planned contrasts, although not orthogonal contrasts, to test specific contrasts. Nurses from four practice areas (intensive care, coronary care, acute medical, acute surgical) were compared on their experiences in decision making. The a priori contrasts showed that intensive care nurses considered themselves to be less effective in influencing a "do not resuscitate" order compared to the other three groups.

SUMMARY

One-way ANOVA is used to compare the means of two or more groups. When the overall F is significant and more than two groups are being compared, posthoc tests are necessary to determine which pairs of means differ from each other. Also, when directional hypotheses are appropriate, a priori contrasts may be specified and tested.

Application Exercises and Results

Exercises

Run the appropriate analyses to answer the question and test the hypotheses. Write a description of the results.

1. Do the three smoking groups differ significantly in their quality of life during the past month?

2. Test the following hypotheses:

   a. The smoking group will score significantly lower on quality of life during the past month than the other two groups.

   b. There will be no significant difference in quality of life between the group that quit smoking and the group that never smoked.

Results

1. To answer this question, a one-way ANOVA was run and the Scheffé posthoc test was requested. Exercise Fig. 6-1 contains the output.

   Looking at the descriptives, we see that the group that is still smoking had the lowest mean score (4.01) on the 6-point scale that ranged from a low of 1 (very dissatisfied, unhappy most of the time) to a high of 6 (extremely happy, could not be more pleased). The other two groups' scores were almost identical (4.31 and 4.30). The assumption of homogeneity of variance has been met ($p = .300$). The overall F is not significant ($p = .067$). Since the overall F is not significant, it is not appropriate to report the Scheffé test results.

2. One-way ANOVA with a priori contrasts was used to test the two hypotheses. Since the overall analysis is the same as the one in Exercise 1, Exercise Fig. 6-2 contains only the a priori contrasts. From Exercise 1, we know that the assumption of equality of variance has

One Way

Descriptives

Quality of life in past month

	N	Mean	Std. deviation	Std. error	95% confidence interval for mean		Minimum	Maximum
					Lower bound	Upper bound		
Never smoked	432	4.31	1.046	.050	4.21	4.40	1	6
Quit smoking	185	4.30	1.018	.075	4.15	4.44	1	6
Still smoking	78	4.01	1.026	.116	3.78	4.24	1	6
Total	695	4.27	1.039	.039	4.19	4.35	1	6

Test of Homogeneity of Variances

Quality of life in past month

Levene statistic	$df1$	$df2$	Sig.
1.205	2	692	.300

ANOVA

Quality of life in past month

	Sum of squares	df	Mean square	F	Sig.
Between groups	5.843	2	2.921	2.720	.067
Within groups	743.302	692	1.074		
Total	749.145	694			

EXERCISE FIGURE 6-1. One-way analysis of variance with posthoc test, Exercise 1.

been met (Levene's $p = .300$), and the overall F is not significant ($p = .067$). The first contrast tests whether the still-smoking group differs significantly from the other two groups. The second contrast tests whether the two nonsmoking groups differ from each other.

Because the homogeneity of variance assumption has been met, we use the equal variance contrasts. We would report that the first hypothesis was supported ($p = .000$). The group that is still smoking scored significantly lower on their quality of life score (mean 5 =.01) than the other two groups combined. The second hypothesis was also supported ($p = .928$). There was no significant difference between the two nonsmoking groups on their reported quality of life. Thus, the a priori results indicate significant differences, whereas the posthoc did not.

Contrast Coefficients

Contrast	Smoking history		
	Never smoked	Quit smoking	Still smoking
1	1	−1	2
2	1	−1	0

Contrast Tests

		Contrast	Value of Contrast	Std. error	t	df	Sig. (2 tailed)
Quality of life in past month	Assume equal variances	1	8.03(a)	.252	31.913	692	.000
		2	.01	.091	.091	692	.928
	Does not assume equal variances	1	8.03(a)	.249	32.246	101.477	.000
		2	.01	.090	.092	356.918	.927

a The sum of the contrast coefficients is not zero.

EXERCISE FIGURE 6-2. One-way analysis of variance with a priori contrasts, Exercise 2.

Differences Among Group Means: Multifactorial Analysis of Variance

Barbara Hazard Munro

Objectives for Chapter 7

After reading this chapter, you should be able to do the following:

1. Discuss the advantages of testing for interactions.
2. Interpret computer output from a two-way analysis of variance.
3. Determine when it is appropriate to use a multivariate analysis of variance.

TWO-WAY ANALYSIS OF VARIANCE

Research Question

We have discussed the use of analysis of variance (ANOVA) with one categorical independent variable (with two or more levels) and one continuous dependent variable. This chapter discusses the use of ANOVA with more than one independent variable. We then extend the discussion to an analysis that includes more than one dependent variable. Such an analysis, usually called multivariate analysis of variance (MANOVA), allows the researcher to look for relationships among dependent and independent variables.

There are great advantages in having more than one independent variable in an ANOVA. One advantage is economy: Many hypotheses can be tested for almost the same cost. The other is the ability to test for interactions. Although it is interesting and valuable to learn whether one approach works better than another, it may be even more important to find out whether the effect of an approach varies depending on the group of subjects. Testing for an interaction allows us to determine whether the results of a treatment vary depending on the groups or conditions in which it is applied.

Table 7-1 illustrates a fictitious example of a test of two methods for teaching statistics. This is an example of a 2×2 design, often called a 2×2 factorial design.

TABLE 7-1 *Example of an Interaction (Numbers Represent Group Means)*

	Type of Instruction		
	Computer Tutorial	Classroom Instruction	Row Means
Computer Ability			
Computer whiz	90	82	86
Computer novice	80	88	84
Column means	85	85	

Diagonals: Computer whiz taught by computer and computer novice taught in classroom, mean = 89. Computer whiz taught in classroom and computer novice taught by computer, mean = 81.

Each of the two independent variables (or factors) has two levels. The first between-subject factor is type of instruction, with two groups: one that used a computer tutorial program, and one that received usual classroom instruction. The second factor (independent variable) is computer ability, with two groups (computer whizzes and computer novices). The outcome measure is the grade on the final examination.

If we analyzed each independent variable separately, we would not derive the information that is provided by studying the interaction effect in the two-way ANOVA. If we compared those taught by computer versus those taught in the classroom, we would find no difference, because the means for both groups are the same (85). If we compared computer whizzes with computer novices, we would find no statistically significant difference (means = 86 and 84). Looking at the cells in the table, however, we can see that the computer whizzes did better when taught by computer (mean = 90), and the computer novices did better when taught in the classroom (mean = 88). The test of the interaction is the statistical comparison of the diagonal means, 89 versus 81.

In the example provided, three research questions (or hypotheses) can be addressed:

1. Is there a significant difference between those taught by computer and those taught in the classroom?
2. Is there a significant difference between computer whizzes and computer novices?
3. Is there a significant interaction between type of instruction and computer ability of the subject?

Testing of the interaction provides information about whether effects are altered by other factors. This allows us to investigate differences among groups of subjects in relation to an outcome measure.

TABLE 7-2 *Summary Results of Three-Way Analysis of Variance*	
Source of Variation	$F_{(1,631)}$
Main Effects	
Country (US vs. Mexico)	63.7*
Profession (physicians vs. nurses)	79.1*
Gender (men vs. women)	0.45
Two-Way Interactions	
Country–profession	5.4[†]
Country–gender	0.81
Profession–gender	0.09
Three-Way Interaction	
Country–Gender–Profession	0.04

*$p < .01$; [†]$p < .05$.
Source: From Hojat et al. (2001). Attitudes toward physician-nurse collaboration: A cross-cultural study of male and female physicians and nurses in the United States and Mexico. *Nursing Research, 50*(2), p. 127.

Type of Data Required

This is simply an extension of the one-way ANOVA. The independent variables are nominal (categorical), and the dependent variable is continuous. For example, Hojat and colleagues (2001) used a three-way analysis of variance to study attitudes toward physician-nurse collaboration. They had three independent variables (factors): country, with two levels, U.S. and Mexico; profession, with two levels, physicians and nurses; and gender, with two levels. Because there were three main effects (independent variables) they tested three 2-way interactions (country × profession, country × gender, and profession × gender). They also tested one 3-way interaction (country × gender × profession). The results are shown in Table 7-2. There was a main effect for country with U.S. professionals reporting more positive attitudes toward physician-nurse collaboration than Mexican professionals. There was also a significant main effect for profession, with nurses reporting more positive attitudes toward collaboration than physicians. Men did not differ from women in their attitudes. There was one significant interaction between country and profession. Posthoc comparisons showed that U.S. nurses had significantly more positive attitudes than any of the other groups. Their mean score was 55.2, whereas Mexican nurses was 48.3, U.S. physicians 48.2, and Mexican physicians 44.8.

Assumptions

The assumptions are the same as those for the one-way ANOVA. The independent variables must be made up of mutually exclusive groups. The dependent variable must be normally distributed and must demonstrate homogeneity of variance across groups.

Power

We have described the relationships among alpha level, effect size, power, and sample size for the *t* test and the one-way ANOVA. To test for an interaction, you must calculate the expected effect size for the interaction and for the independent variables to determine the appropriate sample size. You can request effect and power calculations as part of the output in ANOVA programs.

Example of a Computer Printout of a Two-Way Analysis of Variance

Figure 7-1, produced by SPSS for Windows, was derived from Dr. Robin Wood's data collected in a study of the effectiveness of models for demonstrating breast self-examination (Wood, 1997). Author comments have been added for clarity.

In this analysis there are two independent variables (main effects or factors). One is what the subjects like to read. There are four levels: books, magazines, newspapers, and the Bible. The second independent variable is whether or not they like gospel music, scored as yes or no. The outcome variable is their ability to count backward from 100 by 7s (a measure frequently used to test mental ability). That variable is normally distributed, thus meeting the assumption for the analysis. The questions to be addressed are:

1. Do the four reading groups differ significantly in their ability to count backward?
2. Do subjects who like gospel music differ significantly from those who do not in their ability to count backward?
3. Is there an interaction between reading preference and music preference in relation to counting backward?

We can see in the table of between-subjects factors that more of our subjects like to read books (n = 101) than any of the other alternatives. More people like to listen to gospel music (n = 167) than do not (n = 118). The assumption of homogeneity of variance has been met ($p = .240$).

In the ANOVA table labeled "Tests of Between-Subjects Effects," READMOST indicates the reading preferences (four groups) and is significant at the .000 (<.001) level. MUSIC2 indicates the whether or not they like gospel music and is not significant ($p = .059$). The interaction is indicated by READMOST * MUSIC2 and is significant ($p = .021$). Because there is a significant difference for the reading groups, we look at the post-hoc tests (Scheffé), which are labeled "Multiple Comparisons." We see that the group that likes to read the Bible the most is significantly different from the other three groups. None of the other pairwise comparisons are significant. Looking at the means for these four groups in the table titled "2. What do you like to read most?", we see that the group that preferred to read the Bible scored significantly lower (mean = 1.580) on their ability to count backward by 7s from 100 than did the other three groups (means of 3.020 to 3.268). The interaction was also significant, so we examine the means in the table titled, "4. What do you like to read the most? * my favorite music is gospel." We also examine the plot of the means, titled "Estimated

(text continues on page 180)

Univariate Analysis of Variance

Between-Subjects Factors

		Value Label	N
What do you	1.00	Books	101
like to read	2.00	Magazines	47
the most?	3.00	Newspapers	47
	4.00	Bible	90
my favorite			
music is	.00	No	118
gospel	1.00	Yes	167

Levene's Test of Equality of Error Variances (a)

Dependent Variable: Count backward from 100 by subtracting 7, Interviewer stops at 5 answers. Score # correct answers before 1st mistake.

F	df1	df2	Sig.
1.321	7	277	.240

Tests the null hypothesis that the error variance of the dependent variable is equal across groups.
a Design: Intercept+READMOST+MUSIC2+READMOST * MUSIC2

AUTHOR COMMENTS
The assumption of homogeneity of variance has been met, since Levene's Test has a significance level greater than .05.

Tests of Between-Subjects Effects

Dependent Variable: Count backward from 100 by subtracting 7. Interviewer stops at 5 answers. Score # correct answers before 1st mistake.

Source	Type III Sum of Squares	df	Mean Square	F	Sig.	Partial Eta Squared	Noncent. Parameter	Observed Power(a)
Corrected Model	242.224(b)	7	34.603	9.130	.000	.187	63.912	1.000
Intercept	1690.714	1	1690.714	446.101	.000	.617	446.101	1.000
READMOST	105.946	3	35.315	9.318	.000	.092	27.954	.997
MUSIC2	13.638	1	13.638	3.598	.059	.013	3.598	.472
READMOST * MUSIC2	37.344	3	12.448	3.284	.021	.034	9.853	.748
Error	1049.825	277	3.790					
Total	3271.000	285						
Corrected Total	1292.049	284						

a Computed using alpha = .05
b R Squared = .187 (Adjusted R Squared = .167)

FIGURE 7-1. Computer printout of a two-way ANOVA.

Estimated Marginal Means

1. Grand Means

Dependent Variable: Count backward from 100 by subtracting 7. Interviewer stops at 5 answers. Score # correct answers before 1st mistake.

Mean	Std. Error	95% Confidence Interval	
		Lower Bound	Upper Bound
2.773	.131	2.514	3.031

2. What do you like to read the most?

Dependent Variable: Count backward from 100 by subtracting 7. Interviewer stops at 5 answers. Score # correct answers before 1st mistake.

What do you like to read the most?	Mean	Std. Error	95% Confidence Interval	
			Lower Bound	Upper Bound
Books	3.268	.194	2.885	3.650
Magazines	3.223	.286	2.661	3.786
Newspapers	3.020	.284	2.461	3.579
Bible	1.580	.275	1.038	2.122

3. my favorite music is gospel

Dependent Variable: Count backward from 100 by subtracting 7. Interviewer stops at 5 answers. Score # correct answers before 1st mistake.

my favorite music is gospel	Mean	Std. Error	95% Confidence Interval	
			Lower Bound	Upper Bound
No	3.022	.199	2.630	3.413
Yes	2.524	.171	2.186	2.861

4. What do you like to read the most? * my favorite music is gospel

Dependent Variable: Count backward from 100 by subtracting 7. Interviewer stops at 5 answers. Score # correct answers before 1st mistake.

What do you like to read the most?	my favorite music is gospel	Mean	Std. Error	95% Confidence Interval	
				Lower Bound	Upper Bound
Books	No	3.407	.265	2.886	3.929
	Yes	3.128	.284	2.569	3.687
Magazines	No	2.923	.382	2.171	3.675
	Yes	3.524	.425	2.688	4.360
Newspapers	No	3.957	.406	3.157	4.756
	Yes	2.083	.397	1.301	2.866
Bible	No	1.800	.503	.810	2.790
	Yes	1.360	.225	.917	1.803

FIGURE 7-1. (*Continued*)

Posthoc Tests

What do you like to read the most?

Multiple Comparisons

Dependent Variable: Count backward from 100 by subtracting 7. Interviewer stops at 5 answers. Score # correct answers before 1st mistake.

Scheffe

(I) What do you like to read the most?	(J) What do you like to read the most?	Mean Difference (I-J)	Std. Error	Sig.	95% Confidence Interval	
					Lower Bound	Upper Bound
Books	Magazines	.09	.344	.996	−.88	1.05
	Newspapers	.28	.344	.885	−.69	1.24
	Bible	1.84(*)	.282	.000	1.05	2.64
Magazines	Books	−.09	.344	.996	−1.05	.88
	Newspapers	.19.	402	.973	−.94	1.32
	Bible	1.76(*)	.350	.000	.77	2.74
Newspapers	Books	−.28	.344	.885	−1.24	.69
	Magazines	−.19	.402	.973	−1.32	.94
	Bible	1.57(*)	.350	.000	.58	2.55
Bible	Books	−1.84(*)	.282	.000	−2.64	−1.05
	Magazines	−1.76(*)	.350	.000	−2.74	−.77
	Newspapers	−-1.57(*)	.350	.000	−2.55	−.58

Based on observed means
* The mean difference is significant at the .05 level.

FIGURE 7-1. (*Continued*)

Profile Plots

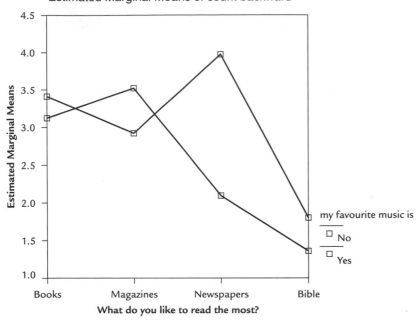

Estimated Marginal Means of count backward

AUTHOR COMMENTS
The largest discrepancy was in the newspaper group.

FIGURE 7-1. (*Continued*)

Marginal Means of count backward." Those who like to read the Bible the most and who like gospel music have the lowest mean score (1.360) on counting backward, and those who like to read newspaper the most and don't like gospel music have the highest (3.957). We can also see that for three of the reading groups (all but magazines), those who do not like gospel music scored higher on the outcome measure than those who did like gospel music. Looking at the graph, we see that the largest discrepancy is for those who like to read newspapers. If they like gospel music, their mean score is 2.083, whereas if they do not like gospel music, their mean is 3.957 (the highest mean score). It is important to point out here that when you "play around" with data in order to have some examples (ie, have no theory driving the question), there is no real relevance to these results. Now, look back at the ANOVA table at the measures of effect size and power. SPSS for Windows provides a partial eta-squared statistic as a measure of effect size. Eta-squared is used to describe the proportion of variance explained by the differences among groups. It is the ratio of the between-groups sum of squares and the total sum of squares (SPSS, 1999b). Generally, power of about 0.80 is considered acceptable. We see that for the two main effects, the power is .997 and .472, and for the interaction, it is .748.

Interactions

With two or more variables in an ANOVA, we can test for interactions. To understand the meaning of an interaction, one generally plots the means of the groups. As Hinkle, Wiersma, and Jurs (1998) summarized, "A nonsignificant interaction is illustrated by nearly parallel lines that connect the cell means. A significant interaction is ordinal when the lines do not intersect within the plot; an interaction is disordinal when they do intersect" (p. 437).

Figure 7-2 contains examples of plots of means. Part (a) plots the means contained in Table 7-1, when we compared methods for teaching statistics, factoring in the computer capabilities of the subjects. In that case there were no significant main effects, but there was a significant disordinal interaction; that is, computer novices did better when taught in the classroom, and computer whizzes did better with computer instruction. In part (b), we see an ordinal interaction. Here the computer whiz group's means are consistent across the two types of instruction, but the computer novice group does much better with classroom instruction and much worse with the computer training. Part (c) contains an example of a significant main effect. There the computer whizzes do better regardless of type of instruction, and the computer novices do worse. In part (d) there is also a significant main effect. There, students score significantly higher in the computer group than in the classroom group.

MULTIVARIATE ANALYSIS OF VARIANCE

Type of Data Required

Often we are interested in more than one outcome. For example, Anderson, Hsieh, and Su (1998) compared two groups of nursing homes (those with the best and worst resident outcomes) on structure and allocation of human and financial resources. Given the number of outcomes measured, they chose to use MANOVA. The two groups of nursing homes did not differ significantly on any of the outcome measures.

Although MANOVA techniques were developed in the 1930s and 1940s, it was only when computer software that could handle the technique became readily available that they began to be reported in the social science literature. Today, MANOVA can be performed on a personal computer. Because in the health professions we are usually interested in more than one outcome, MANOVA is being reported with increasing frequency in research publications.

Advantages of Multivariate Analysis of Variance

Health care outcomes measures, including physiologic, psychological, and sociologic ones, often are correlated. MANOVA includes the interrelation among the outcome measures, whereas separate ANOVAs (one for each dependent variable) do not. Conducting one overall analysis protects against type I errors. An alternative would be to use a Bonferroni correction, but that would ignore any relationships among the dependent variables. MANOVA is more powerful than separate ANOVAs, and the interpretation of the results may be improved by considering the outcome

Final Exam Scores

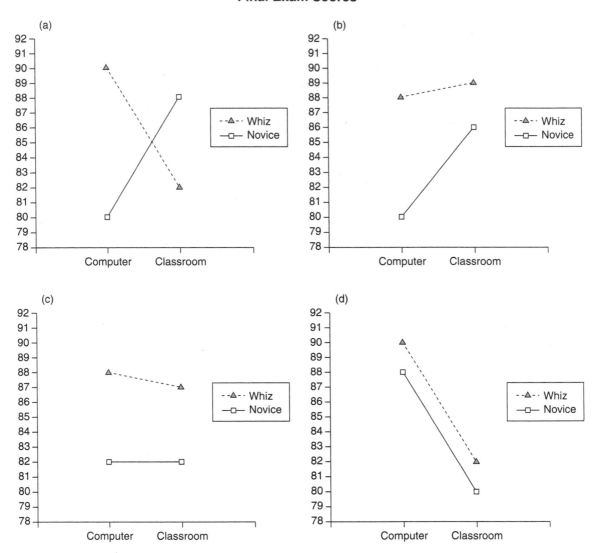

FIGURE 7-2. Plots of mean scores.

measures simultaneously. If the outcome measures are not correlated, however, there is no advantage to conducting a MANOVA.

Assumptions

For ANOVA, the assumptions include random sample, normal distribution, and equal variances across the groups on the dependent variable. When this is extended to MANOVA, not only should the univariate assumptions hold, but the dependent variable should also have a multivariate normal distribution with the same variance covariance matrix in each group (SPSS, 1999a). To meet the assumption of multivariate normal distribution, each dependent variable must have a normal distribution, but this does not ensure that the overall measure of the dependent variables taken together will be normally distributed. Thus, the multivariate assumption needs to be tested. Box's M is a measure of the multivariate test for homogeneity of variance and can be requested as part of the MANOVA program in SPSS for Windows. Although widely used, Box's M is sensitive to departures from normality, and data must be submitted to preliminary checks for meeting the underlying assumptions of normal distribution and the like before the analysis is conducted.

Statistical Power

It is difficult to ascertain the power when planning a MANOVA study because of the number of parameters to be estimated. Increasing the number of dependent variables requires an increase in sample size to maintain a given level of power. Because it is now possible to request power and effect measurements as part of the output from statistical analyses, prior work should be used for estimates on which to base sample size determinations.

Results of Multivariate Analysis of Variance

The first step in assessing the results is to look at the overall MANOVA. This is similar to looking at the F in the ANOVA. It tells whether there is an overall significant result. If there is, it indicates that there is a difference in at least one of the dependent variables. There is only one outcome measure for ANOVA, F, but there are four outcome measures for MANOVA:

1. Wilks' lambda
2. Pillai-Bartlett trace
3. Roy's greatest characteristic root
4. Hotelling-Lawley trace.

Wilks' lambda is also explained in the sections on canonical correlation and discriminant analysis. It represents the product of the unexplained variances—that is, the error variance. Thus, a small value indicates significance.

Pillai-Bartlett trace is the sum of the explained variances; therefore, a large value indicates significance.

Roy's greatest characteristic root is based on the first discriminant variate (see the section on discriminant function analysis for further detail).

Hotelling-Lawley trace is the sum of the ratio of the between- and within-sums of squares for each of the discriminant variates.

Any of these statistics might be used to test the overall multivariate hypothesis. Wilks' lambda is historically the most widely used, and Pillai-Bartlett trace has been found to be the most robust. If the overall MANOVA is significant, you want to determine where the differences lie: Do the groups differ on all the dependent variables or only one? Generally, investigators have conducted univariate analyses after a multivariate significant result; that is, they conduct an ANOVA for each dependent variable. The danger of type I error is "protected" by the overall significant MANOVA. Although some statisticians criticize this approach, it is commonly used and reported.

Computer Output of a Multivariate Analysis of Variance

To demonstrate a MANOVA analysis, we once again use data provided by Wood (1997) from her study of techniques for promoting breast self-examination. There are subjects from two states, Massachusetts and Georgia, and three living conditions (private home, apartment, elder housing). Thus, we have two independent variables (factors, main effects), one is state of residence with two levels and the other is living arrangement with three levels. There are two dependent (outcome) variables, the ability to count backward from 100 by 7s and a knowledge score on breast self-examination (BSE) taken before the subjects were exposed to any treatment. The knowledge scores range from 0 to 100. Both of these outcome measures are normally distributed. The research questions are:

1. Do residents of Massachusetts and Georgia differ significantly from each other in their ability to count backward and their knowledge of BSE?
2. Do the three living groups differ significantly from each other in their ability to count backward and their knowledge of BSE?
3. Is there an interaction between state of residence and living arrangement in relation to counting backward and knowledge of BSE?

Figure 7-3 contains the output (we have eliminated some tables to save space). Author Comments have been added to increase clarity.

Note that the groups are unequal in size. More of the subjects (326) come from Georgia than from Massachusetts (99), and apartment dwellers (87) are the smallest of the three living groups. The assumption of multivariate equality of covariance matrices has been met (p value for Box's M = .363). The multivariate tests are presented first. Remember that rather than one statistic (F in ANOVA), we get four multivariate tests. The multivariate tests of the main effect "state" are all significant (p = .000). The multivariate tests of the main effect, "living," are given next. They are also all significant (p values of .004 to .019). The multivariate tests of the interaction are not significant (p = .253 to .521). If the multivariate results are significant, we can then examine the relevant univariate results. In this case, we would examine the univariate results for the two factors, state and living. We would not examine the univariate effects for the interaction, because the multivariate results were not significant.

The test of homogeneity of variance for the outcome variable "count" was not met (Levene's p = .000). Therefore, those results should be interpreted with caution. Because ANOVA is fairly robust, we will continue to examine the results for "count." The homogeneity of variance test for "knowledge score" was met (p = .135).

The univariate results are labeled "Between-Subjects Effects." There are two dependent variables: count and knowledge. The univariate results tell us whether the significant multivariate results apply to one or both dependent variables.

(text continues on page 189)

General Linear Model

Between-Subjects Factors

		Value Label	N
State	1.00	MA	99
	2.00	GA	326
Type of living	1.00	Private home	197
quarters	2.00	Apartment	87
	3.00	Elder housing	141

Box's Test of Equality of Covariance Matrices(a)

Box's M	16.631
F	1.086
df1	15
df2	66814.139
Sig.	.363

Tests the null hypothesis that the observed covariance matrices of the dependent variables are equal across groups.
a Design: Intercept+STATE+LIVING+STATE * LIVING

AUTHOR COMMENTS
The assumption of multivariate equality of covariance matrices has been met (p = .363).

Multivariate Tests(d)

Effect		Value	F	Hypothesis df	Error df	Sig.	Partial Eta Squared	Noncent. Parameter	Observed Power(a)
Intercept	Pillai's Trace	.832	1035.538(b)	2.000	418.000	.000	.832	2071.076	1.000
	Wilks' Lambda	.168	1035.538(b)	2.000	418.000	.000	.832	2071.076	1.000
	Hotelling's Trace	4.955	1035.538(b)	2.000	418.000	.000	.832	2071.076	1.000
	Roy's Largest Root	4.955	1035.538(b)	2.000	418.000	.000	.832	2071.076	1.000
STATE	Pillai's Trace	.098	22.692(b)	2.000	418.000	.000	.098	45.384	1.000
	Wilks' Lambda	.902	22.692(b)	2.000	418.000	.000	.098	45.384	1.000
	Hotelling's Trace	.109	22.692(b)	2.000	418.000	.000	.098	45.384	1.000
	Roy's Largest Root	.109	22.692(b)	2.000	418.000	.000	.098	45.384	1.000
LIVING	Pillai's Trace	.028	2.949	4.000	838.000	.019	.014	11.798	.792
	Wilks' Lambda	.972	2.957(b)	4.000	836.000	.019	.014	11.830	.793
	Hotelling's Trace	.028	2.965	4.000	834.000	.019	.014	11.862	.795
	Roy's Largest Root	.026	5.519(c)	2.000	419.000	.004	.026	11.038	.851
STATE * LIVING	Pillai's Trace	.008	.808	4.000	838.000	.520	.004	3.233	.260
	Wilks' Lambda	.992	.807(b)	4.000	836.000	.521	.004	3.228	.260
	Hotelling's Trace	.008	.806	4.000	834.000	521	.004	3.224	.260
	Roy's Largest Root	.007	1.378(c)	2.000	419.000	.253	.007	2.756	.296

a Computed using alpha = .05
b Exact statistic
c The statistic is an upper bound on F that yields a lower bound on the significance level.
d Design: Intercept+STATE+LIVING+STATE * LIVING

FIGURE 7-3. Computer output, MANOVA.

AUTHOR COMMENTS

Multivariate results are examined first. Here we see that both main effects, state and living, are significant. The interaction between the two independent variables is not significant.

Levene's Test of Equality of Error Variances (a)

	F	df1	df2	Sig.
Count backward from 100 by subtracting 7. Interviewer stops at 5 answers. Score # correct answers before 1st mistake.	5.269	5	419	.000
Knowledge score, time 1	1.691	5	419	.135

Tests the null hypothesis that the error variance of the dependent variable is equal across groups.
a Design: Intercept+STATE+LIVING+STATE * LIVING

AUTHOR COMMENTS

The assumption of homogeneity of variance has not been met for the count variable (p = .000), but has been met for the knowledge score (p = .135).

Tests of Between-Subjects Effects

Source	Dependent Variable	Type III Sum of Squares	df	Mean Square	F	Sig.	Partial Eta Squared	Noncent. Parameter	Observed Power(a)
Corrected Model	Count backward from 100 by subtracting 7. Interviewer stops at 5 answers. Score # correct answers before 1st mistake.	332.302(b)	5	66.460	17.451	.000	.172	87.254	1.000
	knowledge score, time 1	2665.249(c)	5	533.050	1.270	.276	.015	6.352	.451
Intercept	Count backward from 100 by subtracting 7. Interviewer stops at 5 answers. Score # correct answers before 1st mistake.	2211.645	1	2211.645	580.722	.000	.581	580.722	1.000
	knowledge score, time 1	689410.341	1	689410.341	1643.075	.000	.797	1643.075	1.000
STATE	Count backward from 100 by subtracting 7. Interviewer stops at 5 answers. Score # correct answers before 1st mistake.	171.582	1	171.582	45.053	.000	.097	45.053	1.000
	knowledge score, time 1	621.780	1	621.780	1.482	.224	.004	1.482	.229

FIGURE 7-3. (*Continued*)

Source	Dependent Variable	Type III Sum of Squares	df	Mean Square	F	Sig.	Partial Eta Square	Noncent Parameter	Observed Power(a)
LIVING	Count backward from 100 by subtracting 7. Interviewer stops at 5 answers. Score # correct answers before 1st mistake.	41.096	2	20.548	5.395	.005	.025	10.791	.843
	knowledge score, time 1	609.802	2	304.901	.727	.484	.003	1.453	.173
STATE * LIVING	Count backward from 100 by subtracting 7. Interviewer stops at 5 answers. Score # correct answers before 1st mistake.	8.846	2	4.423	1.161	.314	.006	2.323	.255
	knowledge score, time 1	326.647	2	163.324	.389	.678	.002	.778	.113
Error	Count backward from 100 by subtracting 7. Interviewer stops at 5 answers. Score # correct answers before 1st mistake.	1595.735	419	3.808					
	knowledge score, time 1	175806.280	419	419.585					
Total	Count backward from 100 by subtracting 7. Interviewer stops at 5 answers. Score # correct answers	4632.000	425						
	knowledge score, time 1	1252000.000	425						
Corrected Total	Count backward from 100 by subtracting 7. Interviewer stops at 5 answers. Score # correct answers before 1st mistake.	1928.038	424						
	knowledge score time 1	178471.529	424						

a Computed using alpha = .05
b R Squared = .172 (Adjusted R Squared = .162)
c R Squared = .015 (Adjusted R Squared = .003)

AUTHOR COMMENTS

Since the two main effects were significant at the multivariate level, we examine the univariate results for those two factors. For both main effects, the groups differed significantly on counting backward, but not on their knowledge score.

FIGURE 7-3. (*Continued*)

Estimated Marginal Means

1. Grand Mean

Dependent Variable	Mean	Std. Error	95% Confidence Interval	
			Lower Bound	Upper Bound
Count backward from 100 by subtracting 7. Interviewer stops at 5 answers. Score # correct answers before 1st mistake.	2.911	.121	2.673	3.148
knowledge score, time 1	51.388	1.268	48.896	53.880

2. State

Dependent Variable	State	Mean	Std. Error	95% Confidence Interval	
				Lower Bound	Upper Bound
Count backward from 100 by subtracting 7. Interviewer stops at 5 answers. Score # correct answers before 1st mistake.	MA	3.721	.212	3.304	4.139
	GA	2.100	.115	1.873	2.326
knowledge score, time 1	MA	52.931	2.228	48.551	57.311
	GA	49.845	1.210	47.466	52.223

3. Type of living quarters

Dependent Variable	Type of living quarters	Mean	Std. Error	95% Confidence Interval	
				Lower Bound	Upper Bound
Count backward from 100 by subtracting 7. Interviewer stops at 5 answers. Score # correct answers before 1st mistake.	Private home	3.361	.157	3.053	3.669
	Apartment	2.909	.231	2.454	3.363
	Elder housing	2.462	.231	2.008	2.916
knowledge score, time 1	Private home	51.838	1.645	48.603	55.072
	Apartment	53.171	2.426	48.401	57.941
	Elder housing	49.155	2.423	44.393	53.917

FIGURE 7-3. (*Continued*)

4. State * Type of living quarters

Dependent Variable	State	Type of living quarters	Mean	Std. Error	95% Confidence Interval Lower Bound	Upper Bound
Count backward from 100 by subtracting 7. Interviewer stops at 5 answers. Score # correct answers before 1st mistake.	MA	Private home	4.000	.268	3.473	4.527
		Apartment	3.640	.390	2.873	4.407
		Elder housing	3.524	.426	2.687	4.361
	GA	Private home	2.722	.163	2.403	3.042
		Apartment	2.177	.248	1.690	2.665
		Elder housing	1.400	.178	1.050	1.750
Knowledge score, time 1	MA	Private home	54.717	2.814	49.186	60.248
		Apartment	53.600	4.097	45.547	61.653
		Elder housing	50.476	4.470	41.690	59.262
	GA	Private home	48.958	1.707	45.603	52.314
		Apartment	52.742	2.601	47.628	57.855
		Elder housing	47.833	1.870	44.158	51.509

AUTHOR COMMENTS
These are cell means and would be examined if an interaction had been significant.

FIGURE 7-3. (*Continued*)

For the state groups, the univariate results indicate that residents of the two states differed significantly on count ($p = .000$) but not on knowledge ($p = .224$). The three living groups differed significantly on count ($p = .005$), but not on knowledge ($p = .484$). Because the multivariate results were not significant for the interaction, we do not examine those univariate results.

For the state measure, we did not request posthoc tests, as there are only two groups. We simply need to look at the means in the table titled, "2. State." Because the only significant result was for count, we look at those means. We see that subjects from Massachusetts scored significantly higher in their ability to count backward (mean = 3.721) than did subjects from Georgia (mean = 2.100). The three living groups also differed significantly on count, but not on knowledge, life purpose, and satisfaction. Because there are three groups, we had requested Scheffé posthoc tests. Looking at the table of "Multiple Comparisons," we see that those in elder housing differed significantly from the other two groups ($p = .000$ and .004). There was no difference between home and apartment dwellers. Looking at the table of means titled "3. Type of living quarters," we see that those who lived in elder housing scored significantly lower (mean = 2.462) than those in the other two groups.

Posthoc Tests
Type of living quarters

Multiple Comparisons

Scheffe

Dependent Variable	(I) Type of living quarters	(J) Type of living quarters	Mean Difference (I-J)	Std. Error	Sig.	95% Confidence Interval	
						Lower Bound	Upper Bound
Count backward from 100 by subtracting 7. Interviewer stops at 5 answers. Score # correct answers before 1st mistake.	Private home	Apartment	.47	.251	.177	−.15	1.09
		Elder housing	1.35(*)	.215	.000	.82	1.88
	Apartment	Private home	−.47	.251	.177	−1.09	.15
		Elder housing	.88(*)	.266	.004	.23	1.53
	Elder housing	Private home	−1.35(*)	.215	.000	−1.88	−.82
		Apartment	−.88(*)	.266	.004	−1.53	−.23
Knowledge score, time 1	Private home	Apartment	−2.4809	2.63680	.643	−8.9582	3.9965
		Elder housing	2.2807	2.25957	.601	−3.2700	7.8314
	Apartment	Private home	2.4809	2.63680	.643	−3.9965	8.9582
		Elder housing	4.7616	2.79260	.235	−2.0985	11.6216
	Elder housing	Private home	−2.2807	2.25957	.601	−7.8314	3.2700
		Apartment	-4.7616	2.79260	.235	−11.6216	2.0985

Based on observed means.
* The mean difference is significant at the .05 level.

> **AUTHOR COMMENTS**
> *Each group is compared with every other group. We only examine the comparisons for counting backward, as the groups didn't differ significantly on knowledge score. We can see that the elder housing group differed significantly from the private home group (p = .000) and from the apartment group (p = .004). The private home and apartment groups did not differ (p = .177).*

FIGURE 7-3. (*Continued*)

Example from the Published Literature

Table 7-3 is an edited version of the results of the study by Anderson and colleagues (1998). They created two groups of nursing homes, those with the best resident outcomes and those with the worst. Then they compared the two groups on structure, human resource allocation, and financial resource allocation variables. They ran three MANOVAs, none of which was significant, indicating that resident outcomes were not related to structure or allocation of resources.

SUMMARY

ANOVA is a powerful, robust test that allows us to test for relationships between categorical independent variables and a continuous (measured at the interval or ratio

TABLE 7-3 *Multivariate Analysis of Variance for Comparison Groups: Best and Worst Average Resident Outcomes and Most and Least Improvement in Resident Outcomes*

Development Variables	df	Grouped by Average Resident Outcomes		
		Λ	F	η^2
Structure				
Full model	3	.97	0.16	.025
Owner status	1		0.36	.002
No. of licensed beds	1		2.41	.012
% private pay	1		2.51	.013
Human Resource Allocation				
Full model	2	.99	0.74	.008
RN pattern score	1		0.08	.000
LVN pattern score	1		1.45	.007
Financial Resource Allocation				
Full model	3	.98	0.72	.011
Admin/care costs	1		1.35	.007
Expense/day	1		0.12	.001
Salary pattern score	1		0.24	.001

*$p < .05$.
From Anderson, R. A., Hsieh, P.-C., & Su, H. F. (1998). Resource allocation and resident outcomes in nursing homes: Comparison between the best and the worst. *Research in Nursing & Health, 21*(4), 307.

level) dependent variable. Testing for interactions between the independent variables is particularly useful when we want to determine whether the effects of some intervention will be the same for all types of people or conditions. ANOVA may be extended to the use of more than one dependent variable in a given analysis. This analysis, usually called MANOVA, allows the researcher to look for relationships among dependent and many independent variables.

Application Exercises and Results

Exercises

1. Recode the depression variable into a new variable where 0 = rarely depressed and 1 = sometimes, often, or routinely depressed.

   Run the appropriate analysis to answer the following questions, and write up the results:

a. Do the three smoking groups differ significantly in worrying about the future (IPA29)?

b. Do people who are rarely depressed differ from those who are sometimes to routinely depressed in worrying about the future?

c. Is there an interaction between smoking status and level of depression in relation to worrying about the future?

2. Add a second dependent variable, reaction to pressure (IPA2), to the analysis in Exercise 1. Run the analysis, and write up the results.

Results

1. A two-way ANOVA was used to answer the questions. Exercise Figure 7-1 contains the output. The two independent variables were smoking history, with three levels, never smoked, quit smoking, and still smoking; and depression, with two levels, rarely and sometimes to routinely. The smoking groups are unequal in size. The dependent variable was worry about the future, which was measured on a 7-point scale and recoded so that 1 = all the time, and 7 = never. (The IPPA scale measures positive psychological attitudes, so after recoding items that are negatively weighted, a high score on all items indicates positive psychological attitudes.) This variable is normally distributed. The assumption of homogeneity of variance was met ($p = .062$). The three smoking groups do not differ significantly in reported quality of life ($p = .102$). Looking at the means, we see that the mean scores for the three groups varied from 3.9 to 4.2. The two depressed groups did differ significantly on worry about the future ($p = .000$). There was no interaction between smoking status and level of depression in relation to worry about the future ($p = .626$).

Univariate Analysis of Variance

Between-Subjects Factors

		Value Label	N
Smoking History	0	Never Smoked	431
	1	Quit Smoking	184
	2	Still Smoking	79
Depression recoded	.00	Rarely	358
	1.00	Sometimes to Routinely	336

Levene's Test of Equality of Error Variances (a)

Dependent Variable: Worry about future

F	df1	df2	Sig.
2.117	5	688	.062

Tests the null hypothesis that the error variance of the dependent variable is equal across groups.
a Design: Intercept+SMOKE+DEPREC+SMOKE * DEPREC

EXERCISE FIGURE 7-1. Results of Exercise 1, two-way ANOVA.

Tests of Between-Subjects Effects

Dependent Variable: Worry about future

Source	Type III Sum of Squares	df	Mean Square	F	Sig.
Corrected Model	202.593(a)	5	40.519	15.965	.000
Intercept	6717.973	1	6717.973	2647.048	.000
SMOKE	11.649	2	5.825	2.295	.102
DEPREC	98.918	1	98.918	38.976	.000
SMOKE * DEPREC	2.381	2	1.190	.469	.626
Error	1746.083	688	2.538		
Total	13173.000	694			
Corrected Total	1948.676	693			

a R Squared = .104 (Adjusted R Squared = .097)

Estimated Marginal Means

1. Grand Mean

Dependent Variable: Worry about future

Mean	Std. Error	95% Confidence Interval	
		Lower Bound	Upper Bound
4.069	.079	3.914	4.224

2. Smoking History

Dependent Variable: Worry about future

Smoking History	Mean	Std. Error	95% Confidence Interval	
			Lower Bound	Upper Bound
Never Smoked	3.892	.078	3.739	4.044
Quit Smoking	4.169	.118	3.938	4.401
Still Smoking	4.147	.191	3.772	4.521

3. Depression Recoded

Dependent Variable: Worry about future

Depression Recorded	Mean	Std. Error	95% Confidence Interval	
			Lower Bound	Upper Bound
Rarely	4.563	.124	4.320	4.806
Sometimes to Routinely	3.575	.098	3.382	3.769

EXERCISE FIGURE 7-1. (*Continued*)

4. Smoking History * depression recoded

Dependent Variable: Worry about future

Smoking History	Depression Recoded	Mean	Std. Error	95% Confidence Interval	
				Lower Bound	Upper Bound
Never Smoked	Rarely	4.472	.101	4.273	4.670
	Sometimes to Routinely	3.311	.118	3.080	3.543
Quit Smoking	Rarely	4.679	.174	4.337	5.020
	Sometimes to Routinely	3.660	.159	3.347	3.973
Still Smoking	Rarely	4.538	.312	3.925	5.152
	Sometimes to Routinely	3.755	.219	3.325	4.184

EXERCISE FIGURE 7-1. (*Continued*)

2. A MANOVA was used for this analysis. Exercise Figure 7-2 contains the output. There were two independent variables, smoking status and level of depression, and two dependent variables, worry about the future and reaction to pressure. Both of these variables are measured on a 7-point scale where a high score indicates a positive psychological attitude. Both variables are normally distributed. The assumption of equality of covariance matrices has been met (Box's M, $p = .229$).

At the multivariate level, the first main effect, smoke, is not significant. The second main effect, depression, is significant ($p = .000$). The interaction is not significant. The assumption of homogeneity of variance has also been met for both dependent variables. For reaction to pressure, Levene's $p = .575$, and for worry about the future, Levene's $p = .053$.

Because depression was significant at the multivariate level, we examine the univariate results. The depression groups differed significantly on both of the outcome measures. Because this is a dichotomous (2-group) variable, we only need to examine the means to interpret the results. We see that on both outcome variables, the group that reports being sometimes to routinely depressed scored significantly lower than the group that reported being rarely depresssed.

General Linear Model

Between-Subject Factors

		Value Label	N
Smoking History	0	Never Smoked	428
	1	Quit Smoking	183
	2	Still Smoking	78
Depression recoded	.00	Rarely	357
	1.00	Sometimes to Routinely	332

Box's Test of Equality of Covariance Matrices (a)

Box's M	18.920
F	1.245
df1	15
df2	126109.31
	2
Sig.	.229

Tests the null hypothesis that the observed covariance matrices of the dependent variables are equal across groups.
a Design: Intercept+SMOKE+DEPREC+SMOKE * DEPREC

Multivariate Tests (c)

Effect		Value	F	Hypothesis df	Error df	Sig.
Intercept	Pillai's Trace	.858	2053.477(a)	2.000	682.000	.000
	Wilks' Lambda	.142	2053.477(a)	2.000	682.000	.000
	Hotelling's Trace	6.022	2053.477(a)	2.000	682.000	.000
	Roy's Largest Root	6.022	2053.477(a)	2.000	682.000	.000
SMOKE	Pillai's Trace	.008	1.405	4.000	1366.000	.230
	Wilks' Lambda	.992	1.405(a)	4.000	1364.000	.230
	Hotelling's Trace	.008	1.405	4.000	1362.000	.230
	Roy's Largest Root	.008	2.595(b)	2.000	683.000	.075
DEPREC	Pillai's Trace	.068	25.050(a)	2.000	682.000	.000
	Wilks' Lambda	.932	25.050(a)	2.000	682.000	.000
	Hotelling's Trace	.073	25.050(a)	2.000	682.000	.000
	Roy's Largest Root	.073	25.050(a)	2.000	682.000	.000
SMOKE * DEPREC	Pillai's Trace	.001	.228	4.000	1366.000	.923
	Wilks' Lambda	.999	.228(a)	4.000	1364.000	.923
	Hotelling's Trace	.001	.228	4.000	1362.000	.923
	Roy's Largest Root	.001	.457(b)	2.000	683.000	.633

a Exact statistic
b The statistic is an upper bound on F that yields a lower bound on the significance level.
c Design: Intercept+SMOKE+DEPREC+SMOKE * DEPREC

EXERCISE FIGURE 7-2. Results of Exercise 2, MANOVA.

Levene's Test of Equality of Error Variances (a)

	F	df1	df2	Sig.
Reaction to Pressure	.765	5	683	.575
Worry about Future	2.201	5	683	.053

Tests the null hypothesis that the error variance of the dependent variable is equal across groups.
a Design: Intercept+SMOKE+DEPREC+SMOKE * DEPREC

Tests of Between-Subjects Effects

Source	Dependent Variable	Type III Sum of Squares	df	Mean Square	F	Sig.
Corrected Model	Reaction to Pressure	106.661(a)	5	21.332	7.679	.000
	Worry about Future	203.786(b)	5	40.757	15.989	.000
Intercept	Reaction to Pressure	6798.294	1	6798.294	2447.082	.000
	Worry about Future	6661.988	1	6661.988	2613.566	.000
SMOKE	Reaction to Pressure	5.680	2	2.840	1.022	.360
	Worry about Future	11.512	2	5.756	2.258	.105
DEPREC	Reaction to Pressure	60.541	1	60.541	21.792	.000
	Worry about Future	99.900	1	99.900	39.192	.000
SMOKE * DEPREC	Reaction to Pressure	.114	2	5.703E-02	.021	.980
	Worry about Future	2.328	2	1.164	.457	.634
Error	Reaction to Pressure	1897.458	683	2.778		
	Worry about Future	1740.969	683	2.549		
Total	Reaction to Pressure	13318.000	689			
	Worry about Future	13073.000	689			
Corrected Total	Reaction to Pressure	2004.119	688			
	Worry about Future	1944.755	688			

a R Squared = .053 (Adjusted R Squared = .046)
b R Squared = .105 (Adjusted R Squared = .098)

Estimated Marginal Means

1. Grand Mean

Dependent Variable	Mean	Std. Error	95% Confidence Interval	
			Lower Bound	Upper Bound
reaction to pressure	4.106	.083	3.943	4.269
worry about future	4.065	.080	3.908	4.221

EXERCISE FIGURE 7-2. (*Continued*)

2. Smoking History

Dependent Variable	Smoking History	Mean	Std. Error	95% Confidence Interval	
				Lower Bound	Upper Bound
Reaction to Pressure	Never Smoked	3.970	.082	3.810	4.130
	Quit Smoking	4.098	.124	3.855	4.340
	Still Smoking	4.250	.200	3.857	4.643
Worry about Future	Never Smoked	3.887	.078	3.733	4.040
	Quit Smoking	4.163	.118	3.930	4.395
	Still Smoking	4.144	.192	3.768	4.521

3. Depression Recoded

Dependent Variable	Depression Recoded	Mean	Std. Error	95% Confidence Interval	
				Lower Bound	Upper Bound
Reaction to Pressure	Rarely	4.493	.130	4.239	4.748
	Sometimes to Routinely	3.718	.104	3.515	3.922
Worry about Future	Rarely	4.562	.124	4.318	4.806
	Sometimes to Routinely	3.567	.099	3.372	3.762

4. Smoking History * depression recoded

Dependent Variable	Smoking History	Depression recoded	Mean	Std. Error	95% Confidence Interval	
					Lower Bound	Upper Bound
Reaction to Pressure	Never Smoked	Rarely	4.377	.106	4.168	4.585
		Sometimes to Routinely	3.564	.124	3.320	3.807
	Quit Smoking	Rarely	4.488	.182	4.131	4.845
		Sometimes to Routinely	3.707	.168	3.378	4.036
	Still Smoking	Rarely	4.615	.327	3.974	5.257
		Sometimes to Routinely	3.885	.231	3.431	4.338
Worry about Future	Never Smoked	Rarely	4.470	.102	4.270	4.669
		Sometimes to Routinely	3.304	.119	3.071	3.537
	Quit Smoking	Rarely	4.679	.174	4.337	5.021
		Sometimes to Routinely	3.646	.160	3.331	3.962
	Still Smoking	Rarely	4.538	.313	3.924	5.153
		Sometimes to Routinely	3.750	.221	3.315	4.185

EXERCISE FIGURE 7-2. (*Continued*)

Analysis of Covariance

Barbara Hazard Munro

In the preceding chapters, the statistical methods of analysis of variance (ANOVA)—one way and complex—were described as techniques used to investigate differences among group means. Those tests are used when we are interested in the effects of categorical (independent) variables on "continuous" (dependent) measures.

This chapter presents another ANOVA technique: the analysis of covariance (ANCOVA). This technique combines the ANOVA with regression to measure the differences among group means. The advantages that ANCOVA has over other techniques are the ability to reduce the error variance in the outcome measure and the ability to measure group differences after allowing for other differences between subjects. The error variance is reduced by controlling for variation in the dependent measure that comes from separate measurable variables that influence all the groups being compared. Such a separate variable is considered to be neither independent nor dependent in the ANOVA. However, it contributes to the variation and reduces the magnitude of the differences among groups. In ANCOVA, the variation from this variable is measured and extracted from the within (or error) variation. The effect is the reduction of error variance and therefore an increase in the power of the analysis. Power is the likelihood of correctly rejecting the null hypothesis. With ANCOVA, the control of the extraneous variation provides a more accurate estimate of the real difference among groups. For example, if one knows that length of time since diagnosis has an effect on adherence to treatment regimen, the effect of time on adherence could be measured and accounted for before intervention groups were compared.

RESEARCH QUESTION

In general, ANCOVA answers the same research question as ANOVA: Do the experimental groups differ to a greater degree than we would expect by chance alone? However, with ANOVA, two sets of variables are involved in the analysis: the independent variables and the dependent variable. With ANCOVA, a third type of variable is included: the covariate. The covariate may be entered because it is known to have an effect on the dependent variable and removal of its effect decreases the error term. It also may be entered to "equate" the groups. For example, Wood and colleagues (2002) tested an educational intervention to promote breast self-examination (BSE) in older women. In their quasi-experimental design, subjects were not randomly assigned to groups and it was found that, prior to the intervention, the control group differed significantly from the experimental group in knowledge and skill related to BSE. Therefore, those variables were entered into the analyses as covariates. If the investigators had not done that, they could not have determined whether significant differences between the two groups after the intervention were due to the intervention or to the initial differences between the groups.

When subjects are not randomly assigned to groups, it is very important to compare the groups on important variables before the analyses are conducted. Even with random assignment, one cannot assume group equality, especially when the groups are small. ANCOVA has been used when random assignment has not "worked" to measure and control for initial differences.

Although ANCOVA has been widely used for such statistical equalization of groups, it is not a cure-all and should be used with caution. Some authors condemn its use for anything but the intent to remove another source of variation from the dependent variable; they do not believe that it should be used to equate groups. To use ANCOVA with dissimilar groups, one would have to be able to assert that the groups were essentially equivalent except for the variable(s) being used as covariate(s). This is virtually impossible to know for certain. For more information, see the article by Owens and Froman (1998).

TYPE OF DATA REQUIRED

As with ANOVA, one or more categorical variables are independent variables, and the dependent variable is continuous and meets the requirements of normal distribution and equality of variance across groups. In addition, the covariate should be a continuous variable. This is discussed in further detail in the following section.

ASSUMPTIONS

To ensure a valid interpretation of ANCOVA results, several assumptions should be met. These assumptions are based on requirements necessary for the validity of the regression and the ANOVA components of the test. The first three assumptions are those associated with ANOVA:

1. The groups should be mutually exclusive.
2. The variances of the groups should be equivalent (homogeneity of variance).
3. The dependent variable should be normally distributed.

There are three additional assumptions for ANCOVA.

4. The covariate should be a continuous variable. If a variable is at the nominal level, it cannot be used as a covariate. (However, a nominal variable may be included as an additional independent variable in ANOVA, rather than as a covariate.)
5. The covariate and the dependent variable must show a linear relationship. When this assumption is violated, the analysis will have little benefit, because there will be little reduction in error variance. The test is most effective when that relationship lies above $r = 0.30$. The stronger the relationship, the more effective the ANCOVA analysis will be; that is, the more the two variables are related, the greater is the reduction in error variance by controlling for the covariate. If the relationship between the covariate and the dependent variable is not linear, one appropriate test would be the complex ANOVA, with the levels of the covariate as another independent variable. Another possibility would be mathematical transformation of the variables to achieve a linear relationship. The transformed variables could then be used in ANCOVA.

   Consider an example that demonstrates a violation of this assumption. Suppose we wished to study the effects of two different teaching methods on student performance. Suppose also the investigator wanted to control for the effects of anxiety. Previous research implies there is a U-shaped relationship between anxiety and performance; that is, performance seems to be enhanced by moderate levels of anxiety, but at high and low levels, performance is hampered. This is depicted in Figure 8-1. Therefore, ANCOVA analysis with level of anxiety as a covariate would violate the assumption of a linear relationship between the covariate and the outcome variable.

   One appropriate analysis in this case would be a complex ANOVA with three levels of anxiety as one main effect variable and types of teaching as a second main effect. Another approach would be to use curvilinear regression analysis, in which the anxiety scores could be treated as continuous rather than categorical data. For further information on curvilinear regression, see Pedhazur and Schmelkin (1991, Chapter 18).
6. The direction and strength of the relationship between the covariate and the dependent variable must be similar in each group. We call this requirement

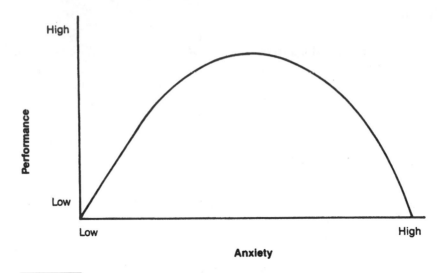

FIGURE 8-1. Possible relationship between performance and anxiety.

homogeneity of regression across groups. When there is homogeneity of regression, the regression lines will be parallel. When this assumption is violated, the chance of a type I error is increased. This assumption can be expressed in another way: The independent variable should not have an effect on the relationship between the covariate and the dependent variable. Another way to say this is that the covariate has the same effect on the dependent variable in all the groups.

Figure 8-2 demonstrates a violation of the assumption of homogeneity of regression. The lines are not parallel, indicating that the interventions affected the covariate-dependent relationship differentially. Quantitative ability is the covariate (varying from low to high), and the score on the statistics final examination is the outcome measure. There are two groups: one taught by the lecture method and one by programmed instruction. The covariate, quantitative ability, does not have the same relationship with the dependent variable in these two groups. In the programmed instruction group, students with higher quantitative ability scored lower on the statistics examination (a negative correlation). In the lecture group, the opposite was true: students with higher quantitative ability scored higher on the examination.

RELATION OF ANOVA AND REGRESSION TO ANCOVA

To understand the rationale behind the mathematical operations involved in ANCOVA, it is necessary to understand the concept of the residual. In the chapter on correlation (Chapter 10, this volume), we explain that squaring the correlation coefficient results in a quantity, r^2, known as a *coefficient of determination*. This coefficient is often used as a measure of the meaningfulness of r because it is a measure

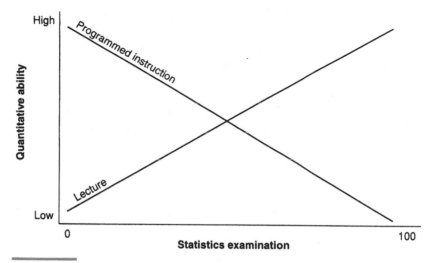

FIGURE 8-2. Lack of homogeneity of regression across two groups.

of the variance shared by the two variables. To calculate the proportion of variance that is not shared by the two variables, we would subtract r^2 from 1. For example, if the correlation between two variables is 0.50, then r^2 is 0.25, and 1 minus r^2 is 0.75. We could then state that 25% of the variance was shared by the two variables and 75% was not shared. This 75% is called the *variance of the residual*. Regression analysis is concerned with the regression sum of squares and the residual sum of squares. With ANOVA, the within sum of squares, or the error term, is analogous to the residual sum of squares in regression. Thus, the residual variance is the variation not explained by the variables in the study. With ANCOVA, we use the residuals to determine whether groups differ *after* the effect of some other variable has been removed.

POWER OF THE ANALYSIS

With ANCOVA, one must determine power based on the number of cells in the analysis and on the covariate. Because the covariate reduces the error term, it increases the power of the test. When determining sample size, the investigator must include the expected impact of the covariate on the effect size. Effect and power calculations can be requested with ANCOVA procedures.

EXAMPLE OF A COMPUTER PRINTOUT

The data for this example came from Wood's (1997) study of the efficacy of an intervention to teach BSE. The question to be addressed is: After controlling for years of education, do the four groups defined by location and treatment differ significantly in their knowledge of BSE? Because one would expect that years of education

(HIGHED) would be related to scores on a knowledge examination, it makes sense to control for that variable, thus reducing the error term. Years of education is normally distributed and ranges from no education to 20 years. The four groups are included in the variable labeled NEWSITE and include the experimental group in Massachusetts, the experimental group in Georgia, the control group in Massachusetts, and the control group in Georgia. The outcome measure is knowledge of BSE. It is normally distributed and ranges from a low of 0 to a high of 100.

Before running the analysis, the assumption of homogeneity of regression must be checked. To adjust for a covariate, the difference between the score of an individual on the covariate and the grand mean of the covariate is weighted by a common regression coefficient (b). Use of such a common regression coefficient is based on the assumption that there is no interaction between the covariate and the independent variable. If such an interaction exists, ANCOVA should not be used.

The question is whether there is an interaction between the independent variable (NEWSITE) and the covariate (HIGHED). We need to build a model that will test this interaction before carrying out the ANCOVA. In SPSS for Windows, descriptions of how to conduct the test of the assumption are included in a chapter on the univariate analysis of variance (SPSS, 1999b).

Because it is important that this assumption be checked, we will walk you through the steps in the process. In this example, in SPSS for Windows, we first selected the Analyze menu, then General Linear Model, and then Univariate. After identifying The % correct of knowledge score as the dependent variable, NEWSITE as the factor (independent variable), and HIGHED as the covariate, we selected Model and within this menu selected Custom. Under Build Terms, we highlighted Main Effects. We then clicked on HIGHED and NEWSITE and moved them to the space for the model on the right side. Next, we changed the Build Terms to Interaction, again highlighted HIGHED and NEWSITE, and moved them over together as an interaction term. The resulting model looked like this:

HIGHED
NEWSITE
NEWSITE * HIGHED

Figure 8-3 contains the results of this analysis. Of interest is the interaction between the main effect, NEWSITE, and the covariate, HIGHED. The F associated with the interaction is 2.606 ($p = .051$). Because the p value is greater than .05 (although close), there is no significant interaction between the independent variable and the covariate. Thus, the assumption is met, and it is appropriate to conduct the ANCOVA. If the interaction had been significant, one could study the effect of education on knowledge of BSE in each of the four groups.

With the assumptions met, we go back to the Model menu and select Full Factorial. We can then run the ANCOVA. The output is shown in Figure 8-4. Look at the means for the four groups in the Descriptive Statistics table. These are the original group means. They have not been adjusted for the covariate. Note that the control groups have the lower scores (45.3571 and 46.3121), and the experimental groups have the higher scores (56.7606 and 51.1979). The assumption of homogeneity of variance for the outcome measure has been met (Levene's test, $p = .645$).

Between-Subjects Factors

		Value Label	N
Group by Site	1.00	Experimental group in MA	71
	2.00	Experimental group in Georgia	192
	3.00	Control group in MA	28
	4.00	Control group in Georgia	141

Tests of Between-Subjects Effects

Dependent Variable: % correct of knowledge score

Source	Type III Sum of Squares	df	Mean Square	F	Sig.
Corrected Model	17987.318(a)	7	2569.617	6.635	.000
Intercept	37304.623	1	37304.623	96.326	.000
HIGHED	6078.758	1	6078.758	15.696	.000
NEWSITE	3618.765	3	1206.255	3.115	.026
NEWSITE * HIGHED	3027.420	3	1009.140	2.606	.051
Error	164204.349	424	387.274		
Total	1268200.000	432			
Corrected Total	182191.667	431			

a R Squared = .099 (Adjusted R Squared = .084)

AUTHOR COMMENTS
The interaction between the independent variable (main effect), NEWSITE, and the covariate, HIGHED, is not significant (p = .051). Thus, the assumption of homogeneity of regression is met.

FIGURE 8-3. Computer output test of assumption of homogeneity of regression.

HIGHED, the covariate, is significant ($F = 22.792$ $p = .000$). After controlling for the covariate, the main effect, NEWSITE, is significant ($F = 2.902$, $p = .035$).

With ANCOVA, the effect of the covariate is removed before the means are compared. Look at the means contained in the Estimates table. The means listed there are the *adjusted* means (ie, means adjusted for the covariate). Compare the adjusted means with the unadjusted means (Descriptive Statistics table). For three of the groups, the adjusted means are lower than the original means. The control group in Georgia is the only group in which the adjusted mean is higher than the original mean. These adjusted means do differ significantly from each other; therefore, we would state that after controlling for years of education, the four groups differed significantly in their knowledge of BSE. Because there are four groups, pairwise comparisons are necessary to determine where the differences lie. Look at the Pairwise Comparisons table. All the comparisons are listed. The experimental

Descriptive Statistics

Dependent Variable: % correct of knowledge score

Group by Site	Mean	Std. Deviation	N
Experimental group in MA	56.7606	19.84041	71
Experimental group in Georgia	51.1979	19.97701	192
Control group in MA	45.3571	21.85510	28
Control group in Georgia	46.3121	20.61246	141
Total	50.1389	20.56012	432

Levene's Test of Equality of Error Variances (a)

Dependent Variable: % correct of knowledge score

F	df1	df2	Sig.
.554	3	428	.645

Tests the null hypothesis that the error variance of the dependent variable is equal across groups.
a Design: Intercept+HIGHED+NEWSITE

Tests of Between-Subjects Effects

Dependent Variable: % correct of knowledge score

Source	Type III Sum of Squares	df	Mean Square	F	Sig.
Corrected Model	14959.898(a)	4	3739.975	9.549	.000
Intercept	64366.754	1	64366.754	164.350	.000
HIGHED	8926.338	1	8926.338	22.792	.000
NEWSITE	3410.001	3	1136.667	2.902	.035
Error	167231.769	427	391.643		
Total	1268200.000	432			
Corrected Total	182191.667	431			

a R Squared = .082 (Adjusted R Squared = .074)

AUTHOR COMMENTS
After controlling for the covariate HIGHED, the four groups (NEWSITE) differ significantly on knowledge of BSE.

Estimated Marginal Means

1. Grand Mean

Dependent Variable: % correct of knowledge score

Mean	Std. Error	95% Confidence Interval	
		Lower Bound	Upper Bound
49.160(a)	1.243	46.718	51.603

a Covariates appearing in the model are evaluated at the following values: What is the highest grade or year of school that you completed? = 10.5984.

FIGURE 8-4. Computer output of analysis of covariance.

Estimates

Dependent Variable: % correct of knowledge score

Group by Site	Mean	Std. Error	95% Confidence Interval	
			Lower Bound	Upper Bound
Experimental group in MA	54.651(a)	2.390	49.954	59.349
Experimental group in Georgia	50.790(a)	1.431	47.978	53.602
Control group in MA	42.753(a)	3.780	35.325	50.182
Control group in Georgia	48.447(a)	1.726	45.055	51.838

a Covariates appearing in the model are evaluated at the following values: What is the highest grade or year of school that you completed? = 10.5984.

Pairwise Comparisons

Dependent Variable: % correct of knowledge score

(I) Group by Site	(J) Group by Site	Mean Difference (I-J)	Std. Error	Sig.(a)	95% Confidence Interval for Difference(a)	
					Lower Bound	Upper Bound
Experimental group in MA	Experimental group in Georgia	3.862	2.772	.164	−1.587	9.310
	Control group in MA	11.898(*)	4.417	.007	3.215	20.581
	Control group in Georgia	6.205(*)	3.014	.040	.281	12.129
Experimental group in Georgia	Experimental group in MA	−3.862	2.772	.164	−9.310	1.587
	Control group in MA	8.036(*)	4.030	.047	.116	15.957
	Control group in Georgia	2.343	2.259	.300	−2.096	6.782
Control group in MA	Experimental group in MA	−11.898(*)	4.417	.007	−20.581	−3.215
	Experimental group in Georgia	−8.036(*)	4.030	.047	−15.957	−.116
	Control group in Georgia	−5.693	4.213	.177	−13.974	2.588
Control group in Georgia	Experimental group in MA	−6.205(*)	3.014	.040	−12.129	−.281
	Experimental group in Georgia	−2.343	2.259	.300	−6.782	2.096
	Control group in MA	5.693	4.213	.177	−2.588	13.974

Based on estimated marginal means
* The mean difference is significant at the .05 level.
a Adjustment for multiple comparisons: Least Significant Difference (equivalent to no adjustments).

FIGURE 8-4. (*Continued*)

TABLE 8-1 *Analyses of Covariance Summary Table for the Corrected Model after Removal of Covariate Influence*

Scale	F	p
Post-test		
Knowledge	19.1	0.000
Breast self-examination skill	27.2	0.000
Lump detection	12.8	0.000

From Wood, R. Y., Duffy, M. E., Morris, S. J., & Carnes. J. E. (2002). The effect of an educational intervention on promoting breast self-examination in older African American and Caucasian women. *Oncology Nursing Forum, 29*(7), p. 1087.

group in Massachusetts scored significantly higher on the knowledge score than the two control groups ($p = .007$ and $.040$). The experimental group in Georgia scored significantly higher than the control group in Massachusetts ($.047$), but not higher than the control group in Georgia ($p = .300$).

EXAMPLE FROM THE LITERATURE

In the study described earlier in this chapter and the one from whom we borrowed the data used in the previous example, Wood and colleagues (2002) used ANCOVA to control for variables on which the experimental and control groups differed. They found that the control and experimental groups differed significantly on pretest scores for "knowledge, BSE skill, and lump detection. Therefore, these variables became covariates in subsequent analyses" (p. 1086). In Table 8-1, we see the comparisons on the posttests with the effect of the pretest scores removed. Even with the initial differences, the groups still differed significantly on the outcome measures with the experimental group showing significantly more knowledge and skill in BSE.

SUMMARY

ANCOVA is an extension of ANOVA that allows us to remove additional sources of variation from the error term, thus enhancing the power of our analysis. This technique is not a cure-all for difficulties with unequal groups and should be used only after careful consideration has been given to meeting the underlying assumptions. It is especially important to check for homogeneity of regression, because if that assumption is violated, ANCOVA can lead to improper interpretation of results.

Application Exercises and Results

Exercises

Run the analysis, and describe the results for the following research question: After controlling for years of education, does one's choice about how to spend a $500,000 gift relate to positive psychological attitudes? Hints: Only three groups have adequate numbers of subjects in the "gift" variable. Check the assumption of homogeneity of regression.

Results

To answer the research question, we ran an ANCOVA. The covariate was years of education. The independent variable was how one would spend a $500,000 gift with three levels: invest with a broker, buy a vacation home, and pay off mortgage. The dependent variable was the total score on the IPPA, in which the potential range of scores is 30 to 210.

First, we checked the assumption of homogeneity of regression. The output is contained in Exercise Figure 8-1. We tested to see whether there was an interaction between the covariate (EDUC) and the independent variable (USEGIFT). Because the interaction was not significant ($p = .316$), the assumption was met.

Next, we ran the ANCOVA. The output is contained in Exercise Figure 8-2. In the table of descriptive statistics, we see that the group who would invest the money with a broker had the highest mean score on positive psychological attitudes, and those who would pay off the mortgage had the lowest. The assumption of homogeneity of variance was met ($p = .166$).

In the analysis, we see that the covariate education was significantly related to positive psychological attitudes ($p = .001$) and there was a significant main effect (ie, the three groups did differ on their positive psychological attitude scores after controlling for their level of education, $p = .004$). The table of means entitled "Estimates" lists the adjusted means. The pairwise comparisons indicate that after controlling for years of education, the group who would invest the money (mean = 157.097) scored significantly higher on the IPPA than did the group who would pay off the mortgage (mean = 148.710).

Univariate Analysis of Variance

Between-Subjects Factors

		Value Label	N
How use gift?	1.00	invest	246
	2.00	vacation home	130
	3.00	mortgage	221

Tests of Between-Subjects Effects

Dependent Variable: TOTAL

Source	Type III Sum of Squares	df	Mean Square	F	Sig.
Corrected Model	19885.356(a)	5	3977.071	5.385	.000
Intercept	411271.596	1	411271.596	556.827	.000
EDUC	6151.284	1	6151.284	8.328	.004
USEGIFT	1739.655	2	869.827	1.178	.309
USEGIFT * EDUC	1705.817	2	852.908	1.155	.316
Error	436511.874	591	738.599		
Total	14400070.000	597			
Corrected Total	456397.229	596			

a R Squared = .044 (Adjusted R Squared = .035)

EXERCISE FIGURE 8-1. Test of the assumption of homogeneity of regression.

Univariate Analysis of Variance

Between-Subjects Factors

		Value Label	N
How use gift?	1.00	invest	246
	2.00	vacation home	130
	3.00	mortgage	221

Descriptive Statistics

Dependent Variable: TOTAL

How use gift?	Mean	Std. Deviation	N
invest	157.6138	26.79478	246
vacation home	150.6231	26.89436	130
mortgage	148.7964	28.39109	221
Total	152.8275	27.67250	597

EXERCISE FIGURE 8-2. Analysis of covariance.

Levene's Test of Equality of Error Variances (a)

Dependent Variable: TOTAL

F	df1	df2	Sig.
1.799	2	594	.166

Tests the null hypothesis that the error variance of the dependent variable is equal across groups.
a Design: Intercept+EDUC+USEGIFT

Tests of Between-Subjects Effects

Dependent Variable: TOTAL

Source	Type III Sum of Squares	df	Mean Square	F	Sig.
Corrected Model	18179.539(a)	3	6059.846	8.200	.000
Intercept	417976.090	1	417976.090	565.609	.000
EDUC	8320.990	1	8320.990	11.260	.001
USEGIFT	8336.148	2	4168.074	5.640	.004
Error	438217.691	593	738.984		
Total	14400070.000	597			
Corrected Total	456397.229	596			

a R Squared = .040 (Adjusted R Squared = .035)

Estimated Marginal Means

1. Grand Mean

Dependent Variable: TOTAL

Mean	Std. Error	95% Confidence Interval	
		Lower Bound	Upper Bound
152.518(a)	1.157	150.245	154.792

a Covariates appearing in the model are evaluated at the following values: education in years = 16.53.

EXERCISE FIGURE 8-2. (*Continued*)

2. How use gift?

Estimates

Dependent Variable: TOTAL

How use gift?	Mean	Std. Error	95% Confidence Interval	
			Lower Bound	Upper Bound
invest	157.097(a)	1.740	153.679	160.514
vacation home	151.748(a)	2.408	147.020	156.477
mortgage	148.710(a)	1.829	145.118	152.302

a Covariates appearing in the model are evaluated at the following values: education in year = 16.53.

Pairwise Comparisons

Dependent Variable: TOTAL

(I) How use gift?	(J) How use gift?	Mean Difference (I-J)	Std. Error	Sig.(a)	95% Confidence Interval Difference(a)	
					Lower Bound	Upper Bound
invest	vacation home	5.348	2.988	.074	−.520	11.217
	mortgage	8.387(*)	2.523	.001	3.432	13.341
vacation home	invest	−5.348	2.988	.074	−11.217	.520
	mortgage	3.038	3.026	.316	−2.905	8.982
mortgage	invest	−8.387(*)	2.523	.001	−13.341	−3.432
	vacation home	−3.038	3.026	.316	−8.982	2.905

Based on estimated marginal means
* The mean difference is significant at the .05 level.
a Adjustment for multiple comparisons: Least Significant Difference (equivalent to no adjustments).

EXERCISE FIGURE 8-2. (*Continued*)

Repeated Measures Analysis of Variance

Barbara Hazard Munro

Objectives for Chapter 9

After reading this chapter, you should be able to do the following:

1. Describe the two major ways in which repeated measures analysis of variance (ANOVA) is used.
2. Explain the assumption of compound symmetry.
3. Interpret a repeated measures ANOVA computer printout.
4. Discuss difficulties that may arise with the use of this technique.

Repeated measures ANOVA is an approach that helps us deal with individual differences. These differences usually are part of the error term. Because they increase the error term, they decrease the likelihood of finding a significant result. Although individual differences reflect actual differences among subjects, they also reflect the person's state when the instrument was administered (eg, tired, bored, angry), environmental factors (eg, noise, heat, cold), and response styles (eg, unwillingness to check extreme value). With repeated measures ANOVA, we may be able to measure, and thus control, some of this variation.

RESEARCH QUESTION

There are two main types of repeated measures designs (also called within-subjects designs). One type involves taking repeated measures of the same variable(s) over time on a group or groups of subjects. For example, if we were studying hypertension, we would probably want more than one blood pressure reading on our subjects.

The other main type of repeated measures design involves exposing the same subjects to all levels of the treatment. This is often called using subjects as their own controls. Suppose we wanted to test medications to reduce nausea during chemotherapy. We could randomly assign patients to one of the following three conditions: medication 1, medication 2, or control.

However, if our subjects varied widely in the amount of nausea they experienced, the within-subject variability would be large. Because the F statistic is based on the ratio of between-group variance to within-group variance, there would have to be a very large between-group difference to attain a significant result; that is, the large variability among the subjects could obscure any real differences between the groups. This would be especially true if the groups were small. One way to remove these individual differences would be to assign each subject to all treatments. Each subject would be exposed to medication 1, medication 2, and the control condition in random order. Each subject would serve as his or her own control, and the within or error variance would be decreased. This would result in a more powerful test and would decrease the number of subjects needed for the study.

TYPE OF DATA REQUIRED

The between-subjects factors meet the same requirements as other ANOVA models; that is, the categories of each independent variable are mutually exclusive. The within-subjects factors contain repeated measures and are often presented as time 1, time 2, and so forth. This means that we have more than one measure on each subject. The dependent variable must be continuous and must meet the assumptions described in the next section.

In a study of the effects of cognitive-behavioral interventions on adolescents' pain following spinal fusion surgery, LaMontagne and colleagues (2003) used repeated measures ANOVA. They randomly assigned subjects to one of four groups. The groups were: information only, coping only, information plus coping, and control. The repeated measures were measures of postoperative pain taken at days two and four. At day four, the control group reported the highest levels of pain.

An example of a within-subjects design in which subjects are used as their own control is a study of the measurement of specific gravity in infants' urine by Lybrand, Medoff-Cooper, and Munro (1990). The urine was collected by two different methods (a collecting bag and aspiration from the diaper) from each baby and measured at three different times. The specific gravity was measured after the infant voided, one hour after voiding, and two hours after voiding. Thus, we have a design with two within-subjects measures. One is the method of collection, with two levels, bag and diaper, and the other is time, with three measurements. There were no significant differences for either of the two effects, and there was no interaction between method and time. Thus, whether the urine is measured from the collecting bag or from the diaper, the resulting specific gravity measure is the same, and the measure does not change if it is measured one or two hours after the infant has voided, and the method of collection has no effect on measures over time.

ASSUMPTIONS

The basic assumptions for the *t* test and ANOVA also are necessary here. The dependent variable should be normally distributed, and the homogeneity of variance requirement should be met.

There is one major difference, however. With ANOVA, the observations are independent of each other. This is achieved by randomly assigning subjects to mutually exclusive groups. With repeated measures, however, there is correlation between the measures because they are from the same people. Therefore, the assumption of compound symmetry must be met.

There are two parts to this assumption. The first part is the assumption that the correlations across the measurements are the same. Suppose you measured a variable three times. You could then calculate the correlation between the first measure and the second, between the first and the third, and between the second and the third. All three of these correlations should be about the same, or $r_{12} = r_{13} = r_{23}$.

The second part of the assumption is that the variances should be equal across measurements. With three measurements, the variance of 1 = variance of 2 = variance of 3. The assumption of compound symmetry is critical. The general robustness of the ANOVA model does not withstand much violation of this assumption.

If, however, the compound symmetry requirement is not met, there are alternative approaches. One is to report the multivariate results rather than the univariate results. Although less restrictive, the multivariate approach is not as powerful as the univariate approach. In the multivariate approach, the within-subjects factor is treated as multiple dependent variables rather than as an independent variable. Another approach is to adjust the degrees of freedom in the univariate approach to decrease the likelihood of type I error. This is done through the use of an epsilon correction for the within-subjects factor(s). Epsilon is multiplied by the degrees of freedom in the numerator and denominator of the within-subjects factor(s), and the new degrees of freedom are used to test the *F* value for significance. These approaches are demonstrated in the computer printouts.

POWER AND SAMPLE SIZE CONSIDERATION

Because repeated measures generally reduce the error term, they enhance the power of the analysis, resulting in the need for fewer subjects.

REPEATED MEASURES OVER TIME

The simplest example of such an analysis was presented in Chapter 5, in which we discussed the use of the correlated *t* test to compare knowledge about breast self-examination as two points in time, before and after an intervention was instituted. Because the two measures of knowledge were taken from the same subjects, the two scores were correlated. The correlated *t* test was appropriate because it removes

		Treatment group			
		Drug therapy	Relaxation therapy	Control	Row means
Time	1 week	A			
	1 month				
	3 months				
	6 months				
	Column means				

FIGURE 9-1. A mixed design.

from the comparison of the two group means the correlation between the two measures. This increases the power of the comparison of the two means. We can extend this concept to situations with more than one group and to situations in which subjects are measured several times on the same variable.

Suppose that instead of one group measured twice, we had a true experimental design with subjects assigned randomly to an experimental group and to a control group. If we measured these subjects two or more times on the same variable, we could no longer use the correlated *t* test. We would now have two groups that were measured repeatedly. This is called a *mixed design* because we have between- and within-subjects measures. First, we have two different groups: the experimental and the control group. These two groups constitute the between-group measure. Comparing these groups answers the question of whether the experimental condition had an effect on the outcome. The second part of the design, the within-group component, concerns the fact that each group is measured two or more times on the same variable. The question answered here is whether there is a difference across the different measures and, specifically, whether there are pairwise differences between these measures. Because there are two independent variables, we also would have an interaction effect (ie, is there an interaction between study group and time?).

Another example of a mixed design is presented in Figure 9-1. We want to study the effectiveness of various treatment modalities on hypertension, and we want to examine the effects over time. We randomly assign patients with hypertension to one of three groups: drug therapy, relaxation therapy, or control. Each subject is in only one group. Blood pressure is measured in all subjects at 1 week, 1 month, 3 months, and 6 months.

If we were to use regular one-way ANOVA to analyze these data, we would have to calculate four ANOVAs, one for each time the blood pressure was measured. With four analyses we would increase the likelihood of a type I error, and we would not be able to determine whether there was an interaction effect, such as one group doing better over time and another doing worse.

If we use repeated measures ANOVA, we have two independent variables. One independent variable is a between-subjects factor, treatment group, with three levels. The other independent variable is a within-subjects factor, time, with four levels. With the repeated measures approach, we can answer three main questions:

1. Do the three groups have significantly different blood pressures after treatment? All blood pressure recordings would be included here; that is, the time component is ignored, and the question is answered by comparing the three column means (ie, the means for drug therapy, relaxation therapy, and control). If the overall *F* is significant, posthoc tests would be used to find differences between pairs of scores.
2. Are there significant differences in blood pressure across the four time periods? Treatment group is ignored here, and the mean blood pressure is calculated for each of the time periods. In our example, the row means would be compared.
3. Is there an interaction between treatment type and time? Twelve cell means would be compared to answer this question (three levels of first independent variable times and four levels of second). In Figure 9-1, those means are shown in the cells. For example, A is the mean for the drug therapy group at week one. This would tell us whether different approaches worked better at one point than another.

EXAMPLE OF COMPUTER ANALYSIS

Figure 9-2 contains the output produced by SPSS for Windows. The data were collected by Capasso (2000) in her study of wound healing. There are two groups, one had their ulcers treated with normal saline (wet-to-dry), and the other had their ulcers treated with hydrogel dressings. The wounds were measured four times in squared centimeters (BWDAREA, WDAREA2, WDAREA3, WDAREA4). The questions to be addressed are:

1. Do the two treatment groups differ significantly in wound size over time?
2. Does wound size differ significantly across the four time periods?
3. Is there an interaction between treatment and time in relation to wound size?

In the table of descriptive statistics, comparing the totals for the four measures, we see that overall, the size of the ulcers decreased over time (from 6.5714 to 1.5850).

Box's test of equality of covariance matrices is given as the test to determine whether the variance–covariance matrices are equal across all levels of the between-subjects factor. It is the assumption underlying the multivariate approach. The *p* value of .551 indicates that the assumption has been met.

At first glance, the output from a repeated measures ANOVA can be confusing. For the within-subjects effects, first multivariate results are presented, then a test of sphericity, then within-subjects effects. Before deciding which results to report for the within-subjects effects, we need to determine whether the assumption of compound symmetry has been met. Look at Mauchly's test of sphericity. The significance level in this example is given as .000; that is, the test is significant, indicating that the assumption of compound symmetry has not been met. When the assumption is met, the univariate results are reported, not the multivariate results, which are less powerful.

(text continues on page 223)

General Linear Model

Within-Subjects Factors

Measure: MEASURE_1

TIME	Dependent Variable
1	BWDAREA
2	WDAREA2
3	WDAREA3
4	WDAREA4

Between-Subjects Factors

		Value Label	N
Dressing	1	normal saline wet-to-dry	25
	2	hydrogel dressing	25

Descriptive Statistics

	Dressing	Mean	Std. Deviation	N
Baseline Wound Area (cm2)	normal saline wet-to-dry	6.9576	6.04477	25
	hydrogel dressing	6.1852	4.60874	25
	Total	6.5714	5.33409	50
Time 2: Wound Area (cm2)	normal saline wet-to-dry	3.8305	3.25539	25
	hydrogel dressing	3.8152	3.89244	25
	Total	3.8229	3.55129	50
Time 3: Wound Area (cm2)	normal saline wet-to-dry	2.7197	2.98085	25
	hydrogel dressing	2.4398	3.01098	25
	Total	2.5798	2.96859	50
Time 4: Wound Area (cm2)	normal saline wet-to-dry	1.8123	2.50870	25
	hydrogel dressing	1.3578	2.19000	25
	Total	1.5850	2.34187	50

FIGURE 9-2. Computer output, repeated measures ANOVA, mixed design.

Box's Test of Equality of Covariance Matrices (a)

Box's M	9.675
F	.880
df1	10
df2	11015.139
Sig.	.551

Tests the null hypothesis that the observed covariance matrices of the dependent variables are equal across groups.
a Design: Intercept+DRESSING Within-Subjects Design: TIME

Multivariate Tests (b)

Effect		Value	F	Hypothesis df	Error df	Sig.
TIME	Pillai's Trace	.535	17.646(a)	3.000	46.000	.000
	Wilks' Lambda	.465	17.646(a)	3.000	46.000	.000
	Hotelling's Trace	1.151	17.646(a)	3.000	46.000	.000
	Roy's Largest Root	1.151	17.646(a)	3.000	46.000	.000
TIME * DRESSING	Pillai's Trace	.020	.308(a)	3.000	46.000	.820
	Wilks' Lambda	.980	.308(a)	3.000	46.000	.820
	Hotelling's Trace	.020	.308(a)	3.000	46.000	.820
	Roy's Largest Root	.020	.308(a)	3.000	46.000	.820

a Exact statistic
b Design: Intercept+DRESSING Within-Subjects Design: TIME

Mauchly's Test of Sphericity (b)

Measure: MEASURE_1

Within-Subjects Effect	Mauchly's W	Approx. Chi-Square	df	Sig.	Epsilon(a)		
					Greenhouse-Geisser	Huynh-Feldt	Lower Bound
TIME	.199	75.463	5	.000	.530	.557	.333

Tests the null hypothesis that the error covariance matrix of the orthonormalized transformed dependent variables is proportional to an identity matrix.
a May be used to adjust the degrees of freedom for the averaged tests of significance. Corrected tests are displayed in the Tests of Within-Subjects Effects table.
b Design: Intercept+DRESSING Within-Subjects Design: TIME

AUTHOR COMMENTS
Because Mauchly's test is significant (ie, assumption of compound symmetry has not been met), either the multivariate results or the univariate results with an epsilon correction is reported.

FIGURE 9-2. (*Continued*)

Tests of Within-Subjects Effects

Measure: MEASURE_1

Source		Type III Sum of Squares	df	Mean Square	F	Sig.
TIME	Sphericity Assumed	698.674	3	232.891	38.108	.000
	Greenhouse-Geisser	698.674	1.591	439.193	38.108	.000
	Huynh-Feldt	698.674	1.671	418.167	38.108	.000
	Lower-bound	698.674	1.000	698.674	38.108	.000
TIME * DRESSING	Sphericity Assumed	3.782	3	1.261	.206	.892
	Greenhouse-Geisser	3.782	1.591	2.377	.206	.763
	Huynh-Feldt	3.782	1.671	2.264	.206	.774
	Lower-bound	3.782	1.000	3.782	.206	.652
Error(TIME)	Sphericity Assumed	880.042	144	6.111		
	Greenhouse-Geisser	880.042	76.359	11.525		
	Huynh-Feldt	880.042	80.199	10.973		
	Lower-bound	880.042	48.000	18.334		

Levene's Test of Equality of Error Variances (a)

	F	df1	df2	Sig.
Baseline Wound Area (cm2)	2.455	1	48	.124
Time 2: Wound Area (cm2)	.148	1	48	.702
Time 3: Wound Area (cm2)	.008	1	48	.929
Time 4: Wound Area (cm2)	.415	1	48	.522

Tests the null hypothesis that the error variance of the dependent variable is equal across groups.
a Design: Intercept+DRESSING Within-Subjects Design: TIME

AUTHOR COMMENTS
Levene's Test indicates that variances for are equivalent for the four measures.

Tests of Between-Subjects Effects

Measure: MEASURE_1

Transformed Variable: Average

Source	Type III Sum of Squares	df	Mean Square	F	Sig.
Intercept	2649.574	1	2649.574	69.816	.000
DRESSING	7.240	1	7.240	.191	.664
Error	1821.626	48	37.951		

FIGURE 9-2. (*Continued*)

Estimated Marginal Means

1. Grand Mean

Measure: MEASURE_1

Mean	Std. Error	95% Confidence Interval	
		Lower Bound	Upper Bound
3.640	.436	2.764	4.516

2. Dressing

Estimates

Measure: MEASURE_1

Dressing	Mean	95% Confidence Interval		
		Std. Error	Lower Bound	Upper Bound
normal saline wet-to-dry	3.830	.616	2.591	5.069
hydrogel dressing	3.450	.616	2.211	4.688

Univariate Tests

Measure: MEASURE_1

	Sum of Squares	df	Mean Square	F	Sig.
Contrast	1.810	1	1.810	.191	.664
Error	455.407	48	9.488		

The F tests the effect of Dressing. This test is based on the linearly independent pairwise comparisons among the estimated marginal means.

3. TIME

Estimates

Measure: MEASURE_1

TIME	Mean	Std. Error	95% Confidence Interval	
			Lower Bound	Upper Bound
1	6.571	.760	5.043	8.100
2	3.823	.507	2.803	4.843
3	2.580	.424	1.728	3.432
4	1.585	.333	.915	2.255

FIGURE 9-2. (*Continued*)

Pairwise Comparisons

Measure: MEASURE_1

(I) TIME	(J) TIME	Mean Difference (I-J)	Std. Error	Sig.(a)	95% Confidence Interval for Difference (a)	
					Lower Bound	Upper Bound
1	2	2.749(*)	.550	.000	1.642	3.855
	3	3.992(*)	.615	.000	2.755	5.228
	4	4.986(*)	.694	.000	3.592	6.381
2	1	−2.749(*)	.550	.000	−3.855	−1.642
	3	1.243(*)	.330	.000	.580	1.906
	4	2.238(*)	.385	.000	1.463	3.012
3	1	−3.992(*)	.615	.000	−5.228	−2.755
	2	−1.243(*)	.330	.000	−1.906	−.580
	4	.995(*)	.219	.000	.555	1.435
4	1	−4.986(*)	.694	.000	−6.381	−3.592
	2	−2.238(*)	.385	.000	−3.012	−1.463
	3	−.995(*)	.219	.000	−1.435	−.555

Based on estimated marginal means
* The mean difference is significant at the .05 level.
a Adjustment for multiple comparisons: Least Significant Difference (equivalent to no adjustments).

4. Dressing * TIME

Measure: MEASURE_1

Dressing	TIME	Mean	Std. Error	95% Confidence Interval	
				Lower Bound	Upper Bound
normal saline	1	6.958	1.075	4.796	9.119
wet-to-dry	2	3.831	.718	2.388	5.273
	3	2.720	.599	1.515	3.924
	4	1.812	.471	.865	2.759
hydrogel	1	6.185	1.075	4.024	8.347
dressing	2	3.815	.718	2.372	5.258
	3	2.440	.599	1.235	3.645
	4	1.358	.471	.411	2.305

FIGURE 9-2. (*Continued*)

Profile Plots

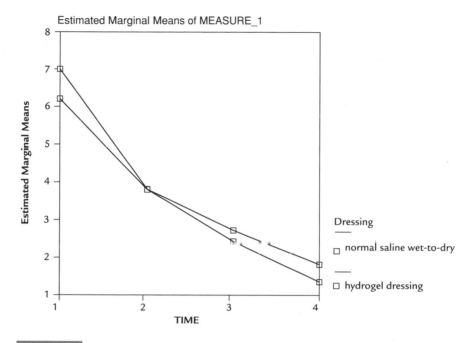

FIGURE 9-2. (*Continued*)

Because the assumption is not met, we should report either the multivariate results, which indicate a significant time effect (*p* = .000) and no significant interaction (*p* = .820); or the univariate results with an epsilon correction. When corrections are made using epsilon, the resulting degrees of freedom are smaller, thus requiring a larger value of *F* for significance. Three epsilon factor corrections are provided by SPSS for Windows: Greenhouse-Geisser, Huynh-Feldt, and lower bound. "The Greenhouse-Geisser epsilon is conservative, especially for a small sample size. The Huynh-Feldt epsilon is an alternative that is not as conservative as the Greenhouse-Geisser epsilon; however, it may be a value greater than 1. . . . The lower-bound epsilon . . . represents the most conservative approach possible, since it indicates the most extreme possible departure from sphericity" (SPSS, 1999a, p. 107).

Look at the Tests of Within-Subjects Effects table. If the assumption of compound symmetry had been met, we would report the Sphericity Assumed results. Because the assumption was not met, we should report one of the corrected results. If you look at the degrees of freedom, you will see that they are smaller for the three epsilon corrections. With smaller degrees of freedom, the value of F must be larger for it to be significant. In this particular case, it really makes no difference, as the results are the same, no matter which correction is used. Generally, one sees Greenhouse-Geisser as the most frequently reported. Using that approach, we would say that there was a significant effect over time (F = 38.108, *df* = 1.591, *p* = .000), and there was no significant interaction effect (F = .206, *df* = 1.591, *p* = .763).

The Levene's Test of Equality of Error Variances table provides the test of the assumption of homogeneity of variance for the between-subjects factor (type of dressing). The two groups have equivalent variance on all four of the measures (ps from .124 to .929). The Tests of Between-Subjects Effects table indicates no significant difference between the two dressing groups ($p = .664$). Looking at the means for the two groups under Dressing in the table labeled Estimates, we see that the means for the two groups were 3.830 and 3.450.

Because there was a significant effect across time, we want to look at the pairwise comparisons. First, look at the means for the four time periods in the table under TIME and labeled Estimates. You can see that the means decreased at each subsequent time. The question is whether or not each of these decreases was significant. The Pairwise Comparisons table indicates that they were all significantly different from each other.

Because the interaction was not significant, we do not need to compare the means over time in the table labeled Dressing * Time. The plot of the means shows that the two treatment groups were quite similar in their response over time.

The questions addressed in this example would be answered as follows:

1. There was no significant difference in healing over time between the two wound treatment groups.
2. The wounds decreased significantly at each of the times.
3. There was no significant interaction between type of dressing and healing over time.

SUBJECTS EXPOSED TO ALL TREATMENT LEVELS

An example is given in Figure 9-3. Ten subjects are exposed to four different methods of pain control. The dependent variable is a rating by the patient of his or her perceived level of pain. This rating is taken four times, once after each treatment. Each cell contains only one score. Subject 1's rating of perceived pain after exposure to drug therapy (6) is the only score in the upper left cell. Because there is only one score in each cell, there is no variability within the cells of this design.

The total variation consists of between-subjects variation and within-subjects variation. Between-subjects variation consists of the differences among the 10 subjects in this design. Testing the significance of that amount of variation would tell us whether the row means differed significantly from each other. We are not interested in this because it tells us only whether the subjects differed from each other; we want to know whether there were differences among the treatments. By calculating the between-people variation, however, we can remove that source of variation from the error term. If the variability among subjects is large, the error term would be substantially reduced.

The second main source of variation is the within-subjects variation. This measures how much each subject's scores varied across the treatment levels. We

Treatments

		Drug therapy	Laughter therapy	Therapeutic touch	Distraction
	1	6	5	8	9
	2	7	8	10	9
	3	4	4	6	7
	4	1	2	4	5
Subjects	5	3	2	3	3
	6	5	6	8	7
	7	2	3	7	6
	8	4	3	8	7
	9	0	1	4	6
	10	5	4	7	5
Col $\bar{X}_s$		3.7	3.8	6.5	6.4

FIGURE 9-3. Within-subjects design.

are interested in this. Do the subjects have lower ratings of pain with some treatments than with others? There are two components to this within-people variation. One is due to the effect of treatment, and the other is due to uncontrolled factors that influence how a subject rates his or her pain at any time.

Example of Computer Analysis of Within-Subjects Design

Figure 9-4 contains the computer output produced by analysis of the data in Figure 9-3. There are four measures, one for each treatment: DRUG, LAUGHTER, TT (therapeutic touch), and DISTRACT (distraction); there is one within-subjects factor with four levels.

Because Mauchly's sphericity test is not significant ($p = .469$), the assumption of compound symmetry has been met, and the univariate test is appropriate (and more powerful).

The univariate tests are contained in the Table titled "Tests of Within-Subjects Effects." Because the assumption of compound symmetry has been met, the Sphericity Assumed results are reported. There is a significant overall difference among the four treatment groups ($p = .000$). Pairwise comparisons were requested. As would be expected from looking at the means, paired comparisons demonstrate that the drug and laughter therapy group means were significantly lower than the means for

General Linear Model

Within-Subjects Factors

Measure: MEASURE_1

RX	Dependent Variable
1	DRUG
2	LAUGHTER
3	TT
4	DISTRACT

Descriptive Statistics

	Mean	Std. Deviation	N
DRUG THERAPY	3.7000	2.21359	10
LAUGHTER THERAPY	3.8000	2.09762	10
THERAPEUTIC TOUCH	6.5000	2.22361	10
DISTRACTION	6.4000	1.83787	10

Multivariate Tests (c)

Effect		Value	F	Hypothesis df	Error df	Sig.	Partial Eta Squared	Noncent. Parameter	Observed Power (a)
RX	Pillai's Trace	.867	15.185(b)	3.000	7.000	.002	.867	45.554	.992
	Wilks' Lambda	.133	15.185(b)	3.000	7.000	.002	.867	45.554	.992
	Hotelling's Trace	6.508	15.185(b)	3.000	7.000	.002	.867	45.554	.992
	Roy's Largest Root	6.508	15.185(b)	3.000	7.000	.002	.867	45.554	.992

a Computed using alpha = .05
b Exact statistic
c Design: Intercept Within-Subjects Design: RX

Mauchly's Test of Sphericity (b)

Measure: MEASURE_1

Within-Subjects Effect	Mauchly's W	Approx. Chi-Square	df	Sig.	Epsilon(a)		
					Greenhouse-Geisser	Huynh-Feldt	Lower bound
RX	.551	4.602	5	.469	.709	.935	.333

Tests the null hypothesis that the error covariance matrix of the orthonormalized transformed dependent variables is proportional to an identity matrix.
a May be used to adjust the degrees of freedom for the averaged tests of significance. Corrected tests are displayed in the Tests of Within-Subjects Effects table.
b Design: Intercept Within-Subjects Design: RX

FIGURE 9-4. Computer output of within-subjects design.

Tests of Within-Subjects Effects

Measure: MEASURE_1

Source		Type III Sum of Squares	df	Mean Square	F	Sig.	Partial Eta Squared	Noncent. Parameter	Observed Power (a)
RX	Sphericity Assumed	73.000	3	24.333	25.269	.000	.737	75.808	1.000
	Greenhouse-Geisser	73.000	2.127	34.319	25.269	.000	.737	53.751	1.000
	Huynh-Feldt	73.000	2.804	26.035	25.269	.000	.737	70.854	1.000
	Lower bound	73.000	1.000	73.000	25.269	.001	.737	25.269	.993
Error (RX)	Sphericity Assumed	26.000	27	.963					
	Greenhouse-Geisser	26.000	19.144	1.358					
	Huynh-Feldt	26.000	25.236	1.030					
	Lower bound	26.000	9.000	2.889					

a Computed using alpha = .05

Estimated Marginal Means

1. Grand Mean

Measure: MEASURE_1

Mean	Std. Error	95% Confidence Interval	
		Lower Bound	Upper Bound
5.100	.607	3.727	6.473

2. RX

Estimates

Measure: MEASURE_1

RX	Mean	Std. Error	95% Confidence Interval	
			Lower Bound	Upper Bound
1	3.700	.700	2.116	5.284
2	3.800	.663	2.299	5.301
3	6.500	.703	4.909	8.091
4	6.400	.581	5.085	7.715

FIGURE 9-4. (*Continued*)

Pairwise Comparisons

Measure: MEASURE_1

(I) RX	(J) RX	Mean Difference (I-J)	Std. Error	Sig.(a)	95% Confidence Interval for Difference(a)	
					Lower Bound	Upper Bound
1	2	−.100	.314	.758	−.811	.611
	3	−2.800(*)	.442	.000	−3.800	−1.800
	4	−2.700(*)	.578	.001	−4.008	−1.392
2	1	.100	.314	.758	−.611	.811
	3	−2.700(*)	.367	.000	−3.529	−1.871
	4	−2.600(*)	.476	.000	−3.677	−1.523
3	1	2.800(*)	.442	.000	1.800	3.800
	2	2.700(*)	.367	.000	1.871	3.529
	4	.100	.407	.811	−.820	1.020
4	1	2.700(*)	.578	.001	1.392	4.008
	2	2.600(*)	.476	.000	1.523	3.677
	3	−.100	.407	.811	−1.020	.820

Based on estimated marginal means
* The mean difference is significant at the .05 level.
a Adjustment for multiple comparisons: Least Significant Difference (equivalent to no adjustments).

AUTHOR COMMENTS
1 = Drug
2 = Laughter
3 = TT
4 = Distract
The first block compares the drug group (1) with the other three groups and shows that the drug group differs significantly from groups 3 and 4, but not from group 2.

FIGURE 9-4. (*Continued*)

therapeutic touch and distraction. Thus, we would report that drug therapy and laughter therapy are related to significantly lower reports of pain than are therapeutic touch and distraction.

PROBLEMS WITH USE OF REPEATED MEASURES

When subjects are exposed to more than one treatment, we need to consider that previous treatments may still be having an effect. In drug trials, for example, time is allowed for one drug to "wash out" before a second drug is tested. Adequate time should be allowed to prevent carryover effects. Pilot testing can be used to determine whether carryover is a problem.

The latency effect is more subtle and involves an interaction with a previous treatment. Would exposure to one treatment have an enhancing or depressing effect on a subsequent treatment?

Repeated exposure to measures may result in an increase in the outcome measure that is related to the subject learning about the measure, rather than a real change. Because subjects are measured repeatedly, such things as sensitization to the instruments may cause difficulties. Scores on an anxiety scale may vary due to repeated exposure to the scale rather than to real changes in anxiety. Even physiologic measures may reflect this. For example, vital signs may increase with a new situation, then decrease with repeated measures. Practice with previous tests may increase scores on later tests. Subjects may be bored by repeated measures and be careless with later tests. Investigators often randomize the order in which the subjects are exposed to the treatments to eliminate effects due to order of treatment.

EXAMPLE FROM THE LITERATURE

Ruth Remington (2002) from Boston College's neighboring school, the University of Massachusetts Lowell, used repeated measures ANOVA in her study of the use of calming music and hand massage with agitated elderly. She used a "four group, repeated measures experimental design to test the effect of a 10-minute exposure to either calming music, hand massage, calming music and hand massage simultaneously, or no intervention (control) on the frequency and type of agitated behaviors in nursing home patients with dementia" (p. 317). Table 9-1 contains the agitation scores by group over time, and Figure 9-5 shows a graph of those means.

TABLE 9-1 *Mean Agitation Scores by Treatment Group over Time*

| Intervention | Mean (SD) | | | | |
	Time 1	Time 2	Time 3	Time 4	n
Calming music	18.41 (11.19)	9.18 (11.11)	7.65 (9.78)	4.65 (7.87)	17
Hand massage	16.47 (9.94)	10.35 (11.20)	7.76 (9.55)	3.06 (5.44)	17
Calming music and hand massage	22.00 (11.94)	8.59 (7.87)	7.06 (7.08)	3.76 (4.40)	17
Control	21.76 (9.09)	21.88 (10.38)	20.88 (8.66)	20.47 (10.90)	17

Note. Results of repeated measures analysis of variance: $F = 6.47$; $df = 3, 9$; $p < .01$.
From Remington, R. (2002). Calming music and hand massage with agitated elderly. *Nurs Res, 51*(5). 317–323.

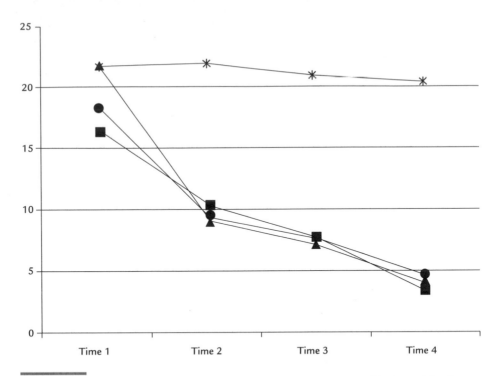

FIGURE 9-5. Mean agitation scores by treatment group over time. [black circle] calming music; [black small square] hand massage; [black up pointing small triangle] calming music and hand massage together; [eight pointed rectilinear black star] control.

From Remington, R. (2002). Calming music and hand massage with agitated elderly. *Nursing Research, 51*(5), p. 321.

Remington reports using the Greenhouse-Geisser epsilon correction because the Mauchley sphericity test was significant. A significant difference in level of agitation over time was found among the four treatment groups. Tukey's HSD procedure was used for pairwise comparisons. The control group was significantly more agitated than the three experimental groups during each treatment period. The three treatment groups did not differ significantly from each other. Thus, both calming music and hand massage worked equally well, and there was no additional effect to providing both of those treatments.

SUMMARY

Repeated measures ANOVA is a particularly interesting technique because health care providers tend to take repeated measures on patients, and it often makes sense to do so with research subjects as well. There are stringent requirements for this analysis, however. If the requirements cannot be met and we have enough subjects, it is possible to use a multivariate approach or the epsilon correction.

Application Exercises and Results

Exercises

1. Run the appropriate analysis to answer the following questions, and write up the results:

    a. Do never-married people rate their quality of life (QOL) differently than married people?

    b. Do people rate their QOL differently now than they did at age 18?

    c. Is there an interaction between marital status and time in relation to QOL rating?

    Hint: Recode MARITAL into a new variable where Never Married = 0, Married = 1, and everyone else is assigned to the missing values category.

2. Are there significant differences in the ratings of the subjects in this study on the following items on the Inventory of Positive Psychological Attitudes scale: reaction to pressure (IPA2), making mistakes (IPA10), defined goals in life (IPA13), and feeling loved (IPA28)?

Results

1. A repeated measures ANOVA was run to answer these questions. The output is contained in Exercise Figure 9-1. There was one between-subjects factor, marital status, with two levels, never married and married, and one within-subjects factor, quality of life, with two levels, QOL18 and QOLCUR.

    Because Mauchly's test of sphericity was not significant, the univariate results are reported. For the within-subjects effects, there was no significant difference between ratings of QOL at the two time points ($p = .173$). Looking at the means, we see that the mean was 4.236 at age 18 and was 4.307 currently. There was no significant interaction between QOL and marital status ($p = .232$).

    The assumption of homogeneity of variance for the between-subjects factors was met for the measure taken in the past month, but not for the measure at age 18. This means that results should be interpreted with caution, and that we might consider other analytic techniques, such as an unequal variance *t* test for making the comparisons at age 18. There is a significant difference between married and never-married people in their reported QOL ($p = .036$). Looking at the means, we see that the never-married group had a significantly lower mean score (4.193) than the married group (4.350), but the difference, although significant, is small, considering that qualify of life was measured on a 6-point scale.

(text continues on page 235)

General Linear Model

Within-Subjects Factors

Measure: MEASURE_1

TIME	Dependent Variable
1	QOL18
2	QOLCUR

Between-Subjects Factors

		Value Label	N
Marital Status	.00	Never married	228
	1.00	Married	346

Box's Test of Equality of Covariance Matrices (a)

Box's M	7.678
F	2.549
df1	3
df2	12435246.149
Sig.	.054

Tests the null hypothesis that the observed covariance matrices of the dependent variables are equal across groups.
a Design: Intercept+MS Within-Subjects Design: TIME

Multivariate Tests (b)

Effect		Value	F	Hypothesis df	Error df	Sig.
TIME	Pillai's Trace	.003	1.862(a)	1.000	572.000	.173
	Wilks' Lambda	.997	1.862(a)	1.000	572.000	.173
	Hotelling's Trace	.003	1.862(a)	1.000	572.000	.173
	Roy's Largest Root	.003	1.862(a)	1.000	572.000	.173
TIME * MS	Pillai's Trace	.002	1.430(a)	1.000	572.000	.232
	Wilks' Lambda	.998	1.430(a)	1.000	572.000	.232
	Hotelling's Trace	.002	1.430(a)	1.000	572.000	.232
	Roy's Largest Root	.002	1.430(a)	1.000	572.000	.232

a Exact statistic
b Design: Intercept+MS Within-Subjects Design: TIME

EXERCISE FIGURE 9-1. Output of a repeated analysis of variance, Exercise 1.

Mauchly's Test of Sphericity (b)

Measure: MEASURE_1

Within-Subjects Effect	Mauchly's W	Approx. Chi-Square	df	Sig	Epsilon(a)		
					Greenhouse-Geisser	Huynh-Feldt	Lower bound
TIME	1.000	.000	0	.	1.000	1.000	1.000

Tests the null hypothesis that the error covariance matrix of the orthonormalized transformed dependent variables is proportional to an identity matrix.

a May be used to adjust the degrees of freedom for the averaged tests of significance. Corrected tests are displayed in the Tests of Within-Subjects Effects table.

b Design: Intercept+MS Within-Subjects Design: TIME

Tests of Within-Subjects Effects

Measure: MEASURE_1

Source		Type III Sum of Squares	df	Mean Square	F	Sig.
TIME	Sphericity Assumed	1.380	1	1.380	1.862	.173
	Greenhouse-Geisser	1.380	1.000	1.380	1.862	.173
	Huynh-Feldt	1.380	1.000	1.380	1.862	.173
	Lower bound	1.380	1.000	1.380	1.862	.173
TIME * MS	Sphericity Assumed	1.060	1	1.060	1.430	.232
	Greenhouse-Geisser	1.060	1.000	1.060	1.430	.232
	Huynh-Feldt	1.060	1.000	1.060	1.430	.232
	Lower bound	1.060	1.000	1.060	1.430	.232
Error(TIME)	Sphericity Assumed	423.933	572	.741		
	Greenhouse-Geisser	423.933	572.000	.741		
	Huynh-Feldt	423.933	572.000	.741		
	Lower bound	423.933	572.000	.741		

Levene's Test of Equality of Error Variances(a)

	F	df1	df2	Sig.
quality of life at age 18	5.327	1	572	.021
quality of life in past month	.724	1	572	.395

Tests the null hypothesis that the error variance of the dependent variable is equal across groups.

a Design: Intercept+MS Within-Subjects Design: TIME

EXERCISE FIGURE 9-1. (*Continued*)

Tests of Between-Subjects Effects

Measure: MEASURE_1

Transformed Variable: Average

Source	Type III Sum of Squares	df	Mean Square	F	Sig.
Intercept	20059.435	1	20059.435	13167.502	.000
MS	6.752	1	6.752	4.432	.036
Error	871.387	572	1.523		

Estimated Marginal Means

1. Grand Mean

Measure: MEASURE_1

Mean	Std. Error	95% Confidence Interval	
		Lower Bound	Upper Bound
4.271	.037	4.198	4.344

2. Marital Status

Measure: MEASURE_1

Marital Status	Mean	Std. Error	95% Confidence Interval	
			Lower Bound	Upper Bound
Never married	4.193	.058	4.079	4.307
Married	4.350	.047	4.258	4.442

3. TIME

Measure: MEASURE_1

TIME	Mean	Std. Error	95% Confidence Interval	
			Lower Bound	Upper Bound
1	4.236	.048	4.142	4.330
2	4.307	.043	4.223	4.391

4. Marital Status * TIME

Measure: MEASURE_1

Marital Status	TIME	Mean	Std. Error	95% Confidence Interval	
				Lower Bound	Upper Bound
Never married	1	4.189	.074	4.043	4.334
	2	4.197	.066	4.067	4.328
Married	1	4.283	.060	4.165	4.402
	2	4.416	.054	4.310	4.522

EXERCISE FIGURE 9-1. (*Continued*)

Profile Plots

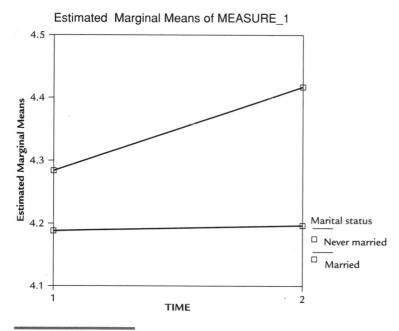

EXERCISE FIGURE 9-1. (*Continued*)

2. A repeated measures ANOVA was run to answer the research question. The outcome is contained in Exercise Figure 9-2. There were no between-subjects factors. There were four within-subjects factors. All items were rated on a 7-point scale.

We see in the table of descriptive statistics that subjects scored themselves lowest on reaction to pressure and highest on feeling loved. Because Mauchly's test of sphericity was significant ($p = .000$), either the multivariate test or the univariate test with an epsilon correction is appropriate. The multivariate tests all result in a p value of .000, indicating that the ratings of the four items differed significantly. The corrected univariate results contained in the Tests of Within-Subjects Effects table give the same result. No matter which epsilon correction is used, the overall F is significant. Looking at the pairwise comparisons, we see that the first item, reaction to pressure, with a mean score of 4.052, was significantly different from the other three measures. The score on item 4, feeling loved, was significantly different from the other three measures. Thus, we would report that our subjects rated themselves significantly lower on their reaction to pressure than in making mistakes, having defined goals for life, and feeling loved. They rated themselves significantly higher on feeling loved than on any of the other three measures.

General Linear Model

Within-Subjects Factors

Measure: MEASURE_1

FACTOR1	Dependent Variable
1	IPA2
2	IPA10
3	IPA13
4	IPA28

Descriptive Statistics

	Mean	Std. Deviation	N
reaction to pressure	4.05	1.704	694
making mistakes	5.04	1.587	694
defined goals for life	5.04	1.650	694
feeling loved	5.85	1.343	694

Multivariate Tests (b)

Effect		Value	F	Hypothesis df	Error df	Sig.
FACTOR1	Pillai's Trace	.480	212.758(a)	3.000	691.000	.000
	Wilks' Lambda	.520	212.758(a)	3.000	691.000	.000
	Hotelling's Trace	.924	212.758(a)	3.000	691.000	.000
	Roy's Largest Root	.924	212.758(a)	3.000	691.000	.000

a Exact statistic
b Design: Intercept Within-Subjects Design: FACTOR1

Mauchly's Test of Sphericity (b)

Measure: MEASURE_1

Within Subjects Effect	Mauchly's W	Approx. Chi-Square	df	Sig.	Greenhouse-Geisser	Huynh-Feldt	Lower bound
					Epsilon(a)		
FACTOR1	.894	77.886	5	.000	.936	.940	.333

Tests the null hypothesis that the error covariance matrix of the orthonormalized transformed dependent variables is proportional to an identity matrix.
a May be used to adjust the degrees of freedom for the averaged tests of significance. Corrected tests are displayed in the Tests of Within-Subjects Effects table.
b Design: Intercept Within-Subjects Design: FACTOR1

EXERCISE FIGURE 9-2. Output of a repeated measures analysis of variance, Exercise 2.

Tests of Within-Subjects Effects

Measure: MEASURE_1

Source		Type III Sum of Squares	df	Mean. Square	F	Sig
FACTOR1	Sphericity Assumed	1127.750	3	375.917	218.916	.000
	Greenhouse-Geisser	1127.750	2.808	401.638	218.916	.000
	Huynh-Feldt	1127.750	2.820	399.845	218.916	.000
	Lower bound	1127.750	1.000	1127.750	218.916	.000
Error(FACTOR1)	Sphericity Assumed	3570.000	2079	1.717		
	Greenhouse-Geisser	3570.000	1945.857	1.835		
	Huynh-Feldt	3570.000	1954.585	1.826		
	Lower bound	3570.000	693.000	5.152		

Estimated Marginal Means

1. Grand Mean

Mesure: MEASURE_1

Mean	Std. Error	95% Confidence Interval	
		Lower Bound	Upper Bound
4.996	.042	4.914	5.078

2. FACTOR1

Estimates

Measure: MEASURE_1

FACTOR1	Mean	Std. Error	95% Confidence Interval	
			Lower Bound	Upper Bound
1	4.052	.065	3.925	4.179
2	5.040	.060	4.922	5.159
3	5.042	.063	4.919	5.165
4	5.850	.051	5.750	5.950

EXERCISE FIGURE 9-2. (*Continued*)

Pairwise Comparisons

Measure: MEASURE_1

(I) FACTOR1	(J) FACTOR1	Mean Difference (I-J)	Std. Error	Sig.(a)	95% Confidence Interval for Difference(a)	
					Lower Bound	Upper Bound
1	2	−.988(*)	.071	.000	−1.129	−.848
	3	−.990(*)	.078	.000	−1.144	−.836
	4	−1.798(*)	.073	.000	−1.941	−1.656
2	1	.988(*)	.071	.000	.848	1.129
	3	−.001	.074	.984	−.147	.144
	4	−.810(*)	.061	.000	−.930	−.690
3	1	.990(*)	.078	.000	.836	1.144
	2	.001	.074	.984	−.144	.147
	4	−.808(*)	.063	.000	−.932	−.685
4	1	1.798(*)	.073	.000	1.656	1.941
	2	.810(*)	.061	.000	.690	.930
	3	.808(*)	.063	.000	.685	.932

Based on estimated marginal means

* The mean difference is significant at the .05 level.

a Adjustment for multiple comparisons: Least Significant Difference (equivalent to no adjustments).

EXERCISE FIGURE 9-2. (*Continued*)

Correlation

Barbara Hazard Munro

RESEARCH QUESTION

Correlational techniques are used to study relationships. They may be used in exploratory studies, in which one intent is to determine whether relationships exist, and in hypothesis-testing studies, in which we test a hypothesis about a particular relationship.

In an examination of the relationships among self-esteem, locus of control, and health perception in African Americans with cancer, Swinney (2002) produced a table of the correlations among these variables. Look at Table 10-1 and try to determine what the correlations indicate. Note that some correlations are positive and some negative.

To interpret correlation coefficients, you must know how the variables are measured. A positive sign indicates that individuals who score high on one of the variables tend to score high on the other and vice versa. For example, in Table 10-1, there is a

TABLE 10-1 *Correlations among the Variables of Self-Esteem, Locus of Control, and Perceived Health Status in African Americans with Cancer ($N = 95$)*

	H Rating	IHLC	CHLC	PHLC	Self-Esteem
H Rating	1.00				
IHLC	.20	1.00			
CHLC	−.19	.10	1.00		
PHLC	.09	.41***	.24*	1.00	
Self-Esteem	.44***	.02	−.26**	.21*	1.00

Note: H Rating, Perceived health status; IHLC, Internal health locus of control; CHLC, External chance health locus of control; PH LC, External Powerful Others health locus of control; Self-Esteem, Total score on the Tennessee Self-Concept Scale.
*$p < 05$, **$p < 01$, ***$p < 001$
From Swinney, J. E. (2002). African Americans with cancer: The relationships among self-esteem, locus of control, and health perception. *Research in Nursing & Health, 25*(5), p. 377.

positive ($r = .44$) correlation between H Rating (perceived health status) and self-esteem. Those with higher self-esteem tend to rate their health status higher, and those with lower self-esteem tend to rate their health status lower. A negative sign indicates that individuals who score high on one of these variables tend to score low on the other. There is a negative correlation ($−.26$) between self-esteem and CHLC (external chance health locus of control), indicating that higher self-esteem is related to a lower score on external chance health locus of control. Those with higher self-esteem are less likely to attribute the cause of their health status to chance.

To judge the strength of the relationship, one must consider the actual value of the correlation coefficient and the associated p value. In Table 10-1 we see that the correlations between H Rating and the locus of control measures (IHLC, CHLC, PHLC) are quite low, from .09 to .20. None of those coefficients was significant. A correlation of .21 (self-esteem and PHLC) was significant at the .05 level, $−.26$ was significant at the .01 level, and .41 was significant at the .001 level. The problem with using only the significance level is that in very large samples, even very small correlation coefficients will be significant. The significance of these coefficients indicates that the value determined in the sample is likely to be the value found in the population, but it does not necessarily mean that the value is of substantive importance. Later in the chapter, we discuss a measure of the meaningfulness of the coefficient and provide more information about the effect of the number of subjects on the p value.

The term *correlation* is used in everyday language. In this chapter, it concerns a relation that can be measured mathematically; we can calculate a number representing the strength of the relationship. However, a correlation that shows that two variables are related does not mean that one variable caused the other. It is a mistake to infer causation from correlation alone. For example, there is a relation between the number of alarms in a fire and the extent of the damage. However, the fire alarms did not cause the damage. Therefore, although a relationship may exist, other factors also may affect the variables under study.

TYPE OF DATA REQUIRED

The Pearson product moment correlation coefficient (r) is the usual method by which the relation between two variables is quantified, and it is the focus of this chapter. A brief description of other formulas, most of which have been derived from the Pearson r, is given. To calculate r, there must be at least two measures on each subject. It is often assumed that both of these measures must be at the interval level. In most cases, however, valid results also may be obtained with ordinal data. Moreover, we can code categorical variables for use with r and with regression equations. Mathematically, it is possible to use any level of data when calculating r, but factors other than the level of the data must be considered when deciding whether a correlation coefficient is appropriate. Sometimes when correlation coefficients are presented, we see the term *zero-order correlation*; this simply means the correlation between two variables. Later we talk about partial and semipartial correlations that are higher-order correlations (ie, more than two variables are involved).

Look again at Table 10-1. Note three additional features of this table:

1. Only the bottom triangle is filled out. If the top portion were filled out, it would duplicate the information contained in the bottom triangle. If you are not familiar with correlation matrices, take a moment to figure out why this is true.
2. There are 1.00s in the diagonal of the table. Sometimes dashes are placed there instead of ones. The indication is that, assuming no measurement error, each variable correlates perfectly with itself. The diagonals become important when we discuss factor analysis and provide information about replacing the diagonals with other numbers.
3. The variable names are repeated across the top of the table. This makes it easier to read the table. Sometimes the variables are numbered and only the number associated with the variable is given across the top. While this simplifies production of the table, it requires checking to see what the numbers represent.

ASSUMPTIONS

Although we can calculate correlations with data at all levels, certain assumptions must be made if we are to generalize beyond the sample statistic; that is, if we are to make inferences about the population itself:

1. The sample must be representative of the population to which the inference will be made.
2. The variables that are being correlated, say X and Y, must each have a normal distribution; that is, the distribution of their scores must approximate the normal curve.
3. For every value of X, the distribution of Y scores must have approximately equal variability. This is called the *assumption of homoscedasticity*. We will demonstrate testing this assumption in Chapter 12.
4. The relationship between X and Y must be linear; that is, when the two scores for each individual are graphed, they should tend to form a straight line. The

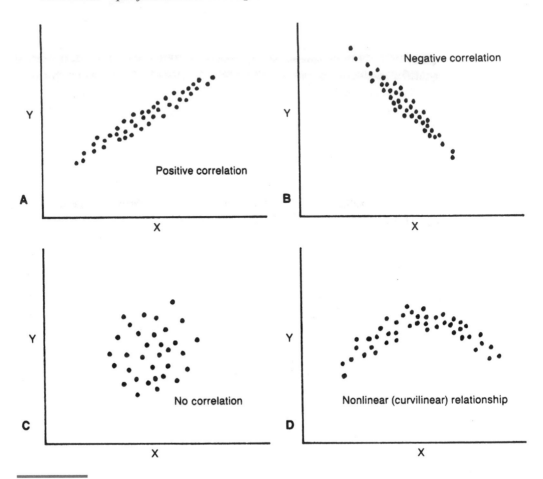

FIGURE 10-1. Linear and nonlinear relationships.

points will not all fall on this line, but they should be scattered closely around it. The technique for graphing the relationship between two variables is demonstrated in the next section of this chapter. In Figure 10-1, *A* and *B* show linear relationships and *D* shows a curvilinear relationship. A technique for measuring curvilinear relationships is presented later in this chapter.

POWER ANALYSIS

Cohen (1987) defines a small effect as a correlation coefficient, *r*, equal to 0.10; a moderate effect as *r* = 0.30; and a large effect as *r* = 0.50. For a two-tailed test with an alpha of 0.05 and a moderate effect size (0.30), we would need 84 subjects for a power of 0.80. A one-tailed test would change the requirement to 68 subjects for the same power.

What happens when we have a small sample (eg, 20 subjects)? For a two-tailed test with an effect size of 0.30 and an alpha of 0.05, our power would only be 0.25. Again, this demonstrates the importance of using adequate numbers of subjects to detect significant results.

CORRELATION COEFFICIENT

The correlation coefficient r allows us to state mathematically the relationship that exists between two variables. The correlation coefficient may range from $+1.00$ through 0.00 to -1.00. A $+1.00$ indicates a perfect positive relationship, 0.00 indicates no relationship, and -1.00 indicates a perfect negative relationship.

The correlation coefficient also tells us the type of relationship that exists, that is, whether the relationship is positive or negative. The relationship between job satisfaction and job turnover has been shown to be negative (we say that an *inverse* relationship exists between them). These terms mean that as one variable increases, the other decreases. People with higher job satisfaction have lower rates of job turnover, and vice versa. Similarly, those with higher grades have lower dropout rates. There is a positive relationship between graduate requirement examination (GRE) scores and graduate grades; that is, those with higher GRE scores usually have higher grades.

If you were to look at scores on two variables, as in Table 10-2, you might observe that those who scored high on one measure tended to score high on the other, and those who did poorly on one measure did poorly on the other. (It is common to use X to designate the independent variable and Y for the dependent variable.)

In addition to "eyeballing" these figures, you might graph the data to see what they look like. Such a graph is called a *scatter diagram* (Fig. 10-2). To draw such a

TABLE 10-2 *Subjects' Scores on Two Measures*

Subjects	X	Y
1	2	1
2	5	6
3	7	9
4	3	2
5	10	8
6	1	3
7	9	10
8	4	3
9	8	9
10	6	7

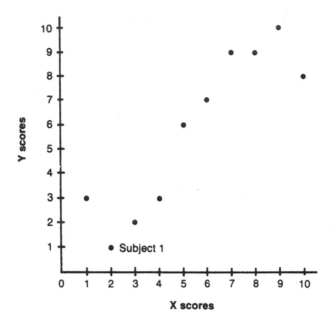

FIGURE 10-2. Graph of scores from Table 10-2.

graph, you plot the pair of scores for each subject. For subject 1, the X score was 2, so you move to 2 on the horizontal scale where the X scores are plotted. The Y score was 1, so you move straight up from the 2 on the horizontal axis to the spot opposite the 1 on the vertical axis where the Y scores are plotted. The dot that represents subject 1's scores is labeled in the graph. All other scores are plotted in the same way. In this example, the scores extend diagonally from the lower-left to the upper-right corner of the graph. Such a configuration indicates a positive relationship between the two scores: Low scores on X tend to go with low scores on Y, and vice versa. If there were a negative relationship—high scores on one variable with low scores on the other—the dots on the graph would go from the upper left to the lower right. When no relationship exists, the dots are scattered in a central cluster like a target (see Fig. 10-1C).

Although the graph indicates a positive relationship between the two variables, it does not tell us how strong the relationship is. To make such a determination, we need to calculate a correlation coefficient, r.

Computer Analysis

Figure 10-3 contains output created by SPSS for Windows through the correlation program. The data were taken from Horowitz (1998). There are four variables: rating of father involvement with mom/baby, family income, parental distress, and the total score on the Beck Depression inventory (bdi total score).

This printout provides three pieces of information: correlation coefficients, levels of significance, and sample size. The table contains redundancy; the correlation

Correlations

Correlations

		How involved is father with mom/baby?	Total income	Psi Parental distress	bdi total score
How involved is father with mom/baby?	Pearson Correlation	1	.233	−.312(*)	−.280(*)
	Sig. (2 tailed)	.	.069	.016	.028
	N		62	59	62
Total income	Pearson Correlation	.233	1	−.325(*)	−.413(**)
	Sig. (2 tailed)	.069	.	.012	.001
	N	62	62	59	62
Psi Parental distress	Pearson Correlation	−.312(*)	−.325(*)	1	.548(**)
	Sig. (2 tailed)	.016	.012	.	.000
	N	59	59	59	59
bdi total score	Pearson Correlation	−.280(*)	−.413(**)	.548(**)	1
	Sig. (2 tailed)	.028	.001	.000	.
	N	62	62	59	62

* Correlation is significant at the 0.05 level (2 tailed).
** Correlation is significant at the 0.01 level (2 tailed).

FIGURE 10-3. Correlation coefficients produced by SPSS for Windows.
Source: Horowitz, J. (1998). *Promoting healthy responsiveness between depressed mothers and their infants.*
Funded by March of Dimes Birth Defects Foundation, 12-FY98-0014.

between each pair of values is given twice. If you were to include this table in a manuscript, you would remove the redundant values (ie, include only the upper or lower triangle). Asterisks are used to indicate values significant at the 0.01 and 0.05 levels, and the actual *p* value is also given right below the correlation coefficient. The *p* values in this table are based on a two-tailed level of significance (you can request one-tailed values). The third number in each box indicates the number of subjects included in each analysis. These numbers are somewhat different because a pairwise deletion was used. That means that subjects were included whenever values were recorded for them on the two variables being correlated. In listwise deletion, subjects would have been excluded if data were missing on any of the four variables in the table.

If our question was which of these variables were significantly related to parental distress, what would the answer be? Take a minute to look at the table. We would say that all of the other three variables were significantly related to parental distress. The father's involvement and total income were both negatively related to parental distress, indicating increased father involvement and increased income are related to lower parental distress. The positive relationship between parental distress and depression (bdi total score) indicates that higher parental distress is related to the

TABLE 10-3 *A Perfect Positive Relationship between Two Variables*					
Subjects	**X**	**Y**	**zX**	**zY**	**zXzY**
1	6	82	−1.42	−1.42	2.0
2	7	86	−0.71	−0.71	0.5
3	8	90	0.00	0.00	0.0
4	9	94	0.71	0.71	0.5
5	10	98	1.42	1.42	2.0

$\bar{X} = 8$, $sd = 1.41$ $\bar{Y} = 90$, $sd = 5.66$ $\Sigma zXzY = 5.00$

$$r = \frac{\Sigma zXzY}{n} = \frac{5.00}{5} = 1$$

mom's higher depression score. The correlation does not indicate whether depression "causes" distress or distress "causes" depression, it just indicates that they are positively related.

Relationships Measured with Correlation Coefficients

When using the formula with z-scores, r is the average of the cross-products of the z-scores. $r = ([\Sigma zXzY]/n)$. (This will be clear when we have taken you through this process.)

A perfect positive relationship, +1.00, is demonstrated in Table 10-3. The five subjects took a quiz, X, on which the scores ranged from 6 to 10 and an examination, Y, on which the scores ranged from 82 to 98. You can see that the subjects have the same rank on both measures. Subject 1 had the lowest score on both tests, subject 2 had the next-lowest scores on both, and so forth.

Because the means and standard deviations (sd) of the two tests are different, we cannot directly compare the scores from the two tests. We can, however, transform the scores to z-scores with a mean of zero and a standard deviation of 1. In Chapter 3, the formula for converting a score to a z-score was given as:

$$z = \frac{X - \bar{X}}{sd}$$

in which X = individual's score
        $\bar{X}$ = mean
        sd = standard deviation.

In Table 10-3, the z-scores for the X variable are listed under zX, and the z-scores for the Y variable are under zY. We can now compare the z-scores for X and Y and see that each subject received matching z-scores for the two tests. This is a perfect positive correlation.

The correlation is the mean of the cross-product of the z-scores for each subject. This is a measure of how much each pair of scores varies together. The

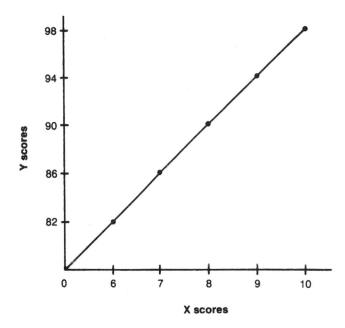

FIGURE 10-4. Graph of scores from Table 10-3, a perfect positive correlation.

cross-products are labeled as $zXzY$ in the table. For subject 2, the cross-product is calculated as $-0.71 \times -0.71 = 0.5$. To take the average of the cross-products, add them and divide by the number of cross-products. Thus, the formula for r is $(\Sigma zXzY)/n$. The sum of the cross-products ($\Sigma zXzY$) is 5; dividing that by 5 (the number of cross-products) results in $r = 1$. The scores are plotted in Figure 10-4. When the dots are joined they form a straight line, which indicates a perfect relationship.

To demonstrate a perfect negative correlation, reverse the scores on the Y variable (Table 10-4). Subject 1 still gets the lowest score on X but now also gets the

TABLE 10-4 *A Perfect Negative Correlation between Two Variables*

Subjects	X	Y	zX	zY	zXzY
1	6	98	−1.42	1.42	−2.0
2	7	94	−0.71	0.71	−0.5
3	8	90	0.00	0.00	0.0
4	9	86	0.71	−0.71	−0.5
5	10	82	1.42	−1.42	−2.0

$\bar{X} = 8$, $sd = 1.41$ $\qquad$ $\bar{Y} = 90$, $sd = 5.66$ $\qquad$ $\Sigma zXzY = -5.00$

$$r = \frac{\Sigma zXzY}{n} = \frac{-5.00}{5} = -1.00$$

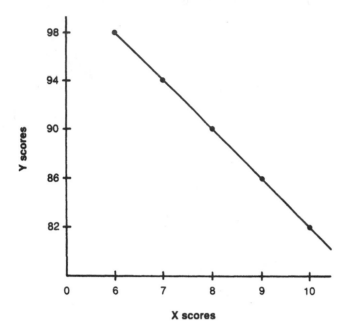

FIGURE 10-5. Graph of scores in Table 10-4, a perfect negative correlation.

highest score on *Y*. Carrying out the same procedure, the sum of the cross-products is −5; thus, $r = -5/5$, or −1, a perfect negative correlation. Figure 10-5 shows the graph of these scores.

In Table 10-5, the *Y* scores are scrambled in such a way that there is no relationship between the *X* and *Y* scores. These scores are plotted in Figure 10-6.

Strength of the Correlation Coefficient

How large should *r* be for it to be useful? As is often the case, it depends. Alternate forms of a test should be measuring the same thing, so the correlation between them

TABLE 10-5 *A Demonstration of No Relationship between Two Variables*					
Subjects	*X*	*Y*	*zX*	*zY*	*zXzY*
1	6	94	−1.42	0.71	−1.0
2	7	82	−0.71	−1.42	1.0
3	8	90	0.00	0.00	0.0
4	9	98	0.71	1.42	1.0
5	10	86	1.42	−0.71	−1.0

$\bar{X} = 8, sd = 1.41$ $\bar{Y} = 90, sd = 5.66$ $\Sigma zXzY = 0.00$

$$y = \frac{\Sigma zXzY}{n} = \frac{0.00}{5} = 0.00$$

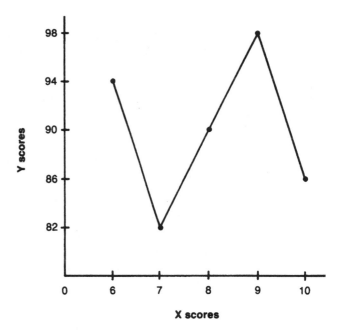

FIGURE 10-6. Graph of scores in Table 10-5.

should be high. With tests (such as the GRE) whose results are used to make important decisions, the correlations between two forms of the same test must be very high, approximately .95. However, when studying the relationships among various aspects of human behavior, we may be happy with a correlation of .50. Some descriptors that can be attached to *r*s of varying strengths are listed below. The direction of the relationship does not affect the strength of the relationship: a correlation of −.90 is just as high, or just as strong, as one of +.90. The following categories apply to positive or negative *r*s:

    .00–.25: little if any
    .26–.49: low
    .50–.69: moderate
    .70–.89: high
    .90–1.00: very high

Significance of the Correlation

If you want to generalize the *r* that you calculate from the sample to the correlation of these two variables in the population, you must determine the level of probability of *r*, that is, the probability that *r* occurred by chance alone. You may use either a one-tailed or a two-tailed test for significance, depending on whether you hypothesized about the relationship. When you use statistical programs for the computer, the exact probability of *r* may be retrieved. When you calculate *r* by hand, you can consult a table, such as that in Appendix E.

The level of statistical significance is greatly affected by the size of the sample, *n*. It makes sense that if *r* is based on a sample of 1,000, there is a much greater likelihood that it represents the *r* of the population than if it were based on a sample of 10. With a two-tailed test and a sample of 100, $r = 0.20$ is statistically significant at the 0.05 level, but with a sample of 10, the correlation must be 0.632 or larger to be significant. With large samples, *r*s that are described as demonstrating "little if any" relationship are statistically significant. To reiterate, the statistical significance implies that the *r* did not occur by chance; the relationship actually is greater than zero. However, a "highly significant" correlation may be quite small. For this reason, many people also speak about the *meaningfulness* of *r*.

Meaningfulness of the Correlation Coefficient

The coefficient of determination, r^2, often is used as a measure of the meaningfulness of *r*. This is a measure of the amount of variance the two variables share. The circle containing *X* represents all the variability or variance of *X*, and the other circle represents the total variance for *Y*. The overlapping area indicates their shared variance. This area can be determined by squaring the correlation coefficient *r*. To determine the meaningfulness of an *r* of .20, square the coefficient: $r^2 = (.20)^2 = .04$, or 4%. You can then say that the variance shared between these two variables equals 4%. When reporting this, researchers usually say that the independent variable, *X*, accounts for 4% of the variance of the dependent variable. Obviously, this is not very much, because another 96% of variance is not accounted for. To account for approximately half of the variance, you would need an *r* of .70 (because $.70^2 = .49$, or 49%).

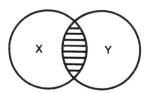

Confidence Intervals

We constructed confidence intervals around mean scores and stated that 95% (or 99%) of the confidence intervals would include the population mean. We also may construct confidence intervals around *r*. This is another way of determining the meaning of the *r* you calculate.

TRANSFORMING *r*-VALUES

Methods for testing differences between means and developing confidence intervals are based on the characteristics of the normal curve. When a distribution is asymmetric, these methods are not appropriate. When the value of *r* in the population exceeds approximately .25, the sampling distribution becomes skewed and becomes more skewed as the value of r increases (Thorndike, 1988). Thus, before rs in different samples can be compared and before confidence intervals can be constructed, the r values must be transformed to values for which distribution will be symmetric. This transformation is known as Fisher's z. Appendix F contains a table that can be used to transform r values into z_r values.

CALCULATION OF CONFIDENCE INTERVALS

To set up the confidence interval around a given r, r must first be transformed into a Fisher's z_r using the table in Appendix F. For example, assume that we had 103 subjects and an r of .9. The first step is to convert r to z_r. In Appendix F, note that an r of .9 equals a z_r of 1.472.

The second step is to determine the standard error. The formula for the standard error is. The third step is to determine the confidence interval to choose. The 95% and 99% levels are commonly used. The formulas are:

95% = z_r ± (1.96) (standard error)
99% = z_r ± (2.58) (standard error)

For our example, they become:

95% = 1.472 ± (1.96) (0.1) = 1.276 and 1.668
99% = 1.472 ± (2.58) (0.1) = 1.214 and 1.730

The fourth step is to transform the z_rs back to rs using Appendix F. When using the table, you will see that not every possible z_r is listed. Select the one closest to the number you calculated.

  a. 95%: z_rs = 1.276 and 1.668; after transformation back to rs, they become 0.855 and 0.930, respectively.
  b. 99%: z_rs = 1.214 and 1.730; after transformation back to rs, they become 0.840 and 0.940, respectively.

The fifth step is to set up the confidence intervals. Note that the confidence intervals are not symmetrical around the r value.

Level	Confidence Interval for r
a. 95%	0.855–0.930
b. 99%	0.840–0.940

OTHER MEASURES OF RELATIONSHIP

There are measures other than the Pearson r for measuring relationships. An overview is given here, but computational formulas are not presented.

Shortcut Versions of *r*

Three "shortcut" versions of *r* are *phi, point-biserial*, and *Spearman rho*. Many researchers assume that shortcut versions of *r* are different from the Pearson *r* and that applying *r* and one of these formulas to a set of data would result in different results. Actually, these measures usually give the same result as *r*. The only advantage of using them is when doing hand calculations. They are really shortcut versions of *r* that can be used with specific types of data.

PHI

When both variables being correlated are dichotomous (ie, each has only two values), a shortcut version of *r* can be used. Examples of dichotomous variables include gender (male and female), a yes or no response choice, and pass or fail. When using the computer to analyze your data, you can use *r* and will get exactly the same result as if you had used phi. See Chapter 4 for a more complete description of phi.

POINT-BISERIAL AND SPEARMAN RHO

When you want to correlate one dichotomous variable with one continuous variable, you can use the point-biserial formula. When you have two sets of ranks, you can use the Spearman rho formula. You might ask two groups to rank a list of stressors from most stressful to least stressful. You could compare the rankings of the two groups by using the Spearman rho formula. Spearman rho is often called a nonparametric test, as though it were distribution free, which is not true. It is better thought of as a shortcut version of *r*.

Nonparametric Measures

KENDALL'S TAU

This measure is a nonparametric measure and is not a shortcut formula for *r*. It was developed as an alternative procedure for Spearman rho. It is sometimes used when measuring the relation between two ranked (ordinal) variables. Kendall's tau might be an alternative if your data seriously violated the assumptions underlying *r*. It can be calculated using most of the major computer packages, such as SAS or SPSS.

CONTINGENCY COEFFICIENT

One nonparametric technique can be used to measure the relationship between two nominal level variables. The variables need not be dichotomous but may have multiple levels. For example, this technique could be used to determine the relationship between ethnicity and political affiliation. To calculate this coefficient, you must use the chi-square statistic, which is discussed in Chapter 4.

Estimating *r*

Two formulas are not shortcut versions of *r* but estimate results that might be obtained using *r*. Nunnally and Bernstein (1994) recommend that these techniques should not be used, but because they are sometimes reported in the literature and are often mentioned in statistics texts, they are outlined here.

BISERIAL

This technique can be used when one variable is dichotomized and the other is continuous. Dichotomized means that the variable has been made dichotomous (cut into two levels from a variable that would have been naturally continuous). For example, scores could be divided into high and low, creating a dichotomized variable. A biserial correlation estimates what the correlation would be if you changed the dichotomized variable into a continuous variable (perhaps by including the entire range of scores). Nunnally and Bernstein (1994) argue against such a use, stating that the resulting coefficient is usually artificially high.

TETRACHORIC

This coefficient estimates *r* from the relationship between two dichotomized variables. If there are serious problems with estimating *r* from one dichotomized variable (biserial), there are obviously even more difficulties with estimating *r* from two dichotomized variables.

"Universal" Measure

We have been discussing the relationship between two variables that have a linear relationship. When we graph these relationships, they suggest a straight line across the graph. Although the relationship may be positive or negative, it is the same across all the scores. An example of a nonlinear relationship can be seen in Figure 10-1*D*. In this case, low scores on the *X* variable are related to low scores on the *Y* variable, but high scores on *X* also are related to low scores on *Y*. Such a relationship is called *curvilinear*. An example might be the possible relationship between anxiety and test scores. In this graph, those with moderate anxiety could perform the best on tests; those with very low or very high anxiety perform poorly. There is a real advantage to having data plotted to determine whether a nonlinear relationship exists, because *r* cannot be used to test such a relationship.

Eta, sometimes called the correlation ratio, can be used to measure a nonlinear relationship. The range of values for eta is 0 to +1. It can be used with all variables, whether nominal or continuous. Eta is closely related to *r* and has been called a "universal" relationship because it can be used regardless of the form of the relationship (Nunnally & Bernstein, 1994). When it is used with two continuous variables that have a linear relationship, it reduces to *r*.

PARTIAL CORRELATION

When discussing research design, we confront the notion of control. How do we control variance that will distract or mislead us? There are several ways. If we are concerned about the impact of a variable, such as age, we might use random assignment of subjects to groups as a method of control, we might select only one age group, or we might match subjects by age before assigning them to groups. There also are statistical measures of control: We can record the age of the subjects and use that as a variable in the study.

One method of statistical control is *partial correlation*. This technique also allows us to describe the relationship between two variables (or more, if you go to multiple partial correlation) after statistically controlling for the influence of some third variable. When studying research design, you learned that the relationship between two variables may be unclear because of the confounding influence of another variable. For example, if you calculate the correlation between mental age and height in children 1 to 10 years of age, you will find a high correlation. Does that mean that height causes intelligence? The key factor is age, not height. Once you control for age, the relationship between height and mental age becomes trivial.

One study was conducted to determine whether the number of hours spent studying was related to grades; the researchers found a negative correlation. This does not mean that studying less results in higher grades. Once they controlled for intelligence, the researchers found a significant positive relation between grades and hours of study. (Although that study indicates that "smarter" people study fewer hours, more recent evidence suggests that in most cases, brighter students study more.)

Partial correlations may be written as $r_{12.3}$. This indicates that you are measuring the correlation between variables 1 and 2 with the effect of variable 3 removed from both the variables being correlated. Consider the example of college grades (variable 1) with hours of study (variable 2) and intelligence (variable 3). If we used partial correlation to study this relationship, the correlation between intelligence and grades (r_{13}) is removed, and the correlation between intelligence and hours of study (r_{23}) also is removed. The confounding influence of intelligence is thus removed statistically, and the relationship between grades and hours of study can be measured accurately. Partial correlation also may be written as $r_{y1.2}$, which would indicate the correlation of an independent variable, 1, with a dependent variable, y, with the effect of variable 2 removed from the independent and dependent variables.

SEMIPARTIAL CORRELATION

This is the correlation of two variables with the effect of a third variable removed from only one of the variables being correlated. It is closely tied to multiple correlation, as is discussed in the next section. Semipartial correlation may be written as $r_{1(2.3)}$ or $r_{y(1.2)}$.

The first way indicates the correlation between variables 1 and 2 with the effect of variable 3 removed from 2 alone; the second way indicates the correlation between the dependent variable, y, and an independent variable, 1, with the effect of variable 2 removed from 1 alone. The following diagram explains further.

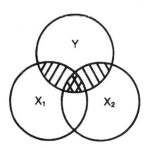

The circles represent the amount of variance of each of the variables. Remember that the variance shared by two variables is measured by r^2. If we take variable X_1 into account first, the variance accounted for in Y equals the variance contributed by X_1 (r_{y1}^2), plus the unique variance accounted for by X_2. That unique variance is the variance shared between Y and X_2 after the effect of X_1 on X_2 has been removed (or after the cross-hatched area has been subtracted). The squared semipartial correlation between X_2 and Y is the unique variance contributed by X_2 ($r_{y(2.1)}^2$). Therefore, in this case, R^2 (the squared multiple correlation, which is explained more fully in the following section) equals the r^2 between X_1 and Y plus the semipartial correlation squared between X_2 and Y, or $R^2 = r_{y1}^2 + r_{y(2.1)}^2$.

MULTIPLE CORRELATION

We have been discussing correlation as measuring the relationship between two variables. This concept can be extended to one in which the relationship is measured between one variable and a combination of other variables. When discussing r, we were talking about one independent variable (X) and one dependent variable (Y). In multiple correlation (R), we are talking about more than one independent variable (X_1, X_2, X_3, and so on) and one dependent variable (Y). It is also possible to have more than one dependent variable (Y_1, Y_2, Y_3, and so on); this is called canonical correlation and is discussed in Chapter 12.

The multiple correlation, R, can go from 0 to 1. There are no negative Rs because the method of least squares is used to calculate R, and squaring numbers eliminates negatives. R^2 is the amount of variance accounted for in the dependent variable by the combination of independent variables. When reporting multiple correlations, R^2 rather than R is often presented.

As we demonstrated in the discussion of semipartial correlation, the calculation of the squared multiple correlation, R^2, may require more than simply adding the squared correlation of each independent variable with the dependent variable. This is because if there were no correlations between the independent variables, the correlations might be as follows:

	X_1	X_2	Y
X_1	1.00	0.00	0.40
X_2	0.00	1.00	0.30

This could be depicted as:

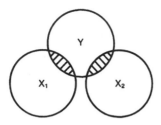

In this case, there is no overlap between variables X_1 and X_2. They are not correlated; thus, each accounts for a different portion of the variance in Y. We could add their squared correlation (r^2s) with Y ($.40^2$s + $.30^2$) and determine that $R^2 = 0.25$.

Usually in behavioral research, however, the independent variables are correlated among themselves, as depicted in the following:

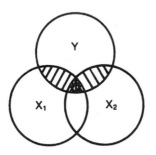

In this case, there is correlation between X_1 and X_2, and if you add the squared correlation of X_1 with Y and the squared correlation of X_2 with Y, you would add in the cross-hatched area twice. The variance accounted for in Y is actually all that is explained by one of the variables plus the additional variance explained by the second variable. The additional variance is measured by the squared semipartial correlation of the second variable with the dependent variable. If X_1 is counted first, it accounts for all of its shared variance with Y, and X_2 adds the variance that it alone contributes (its shared variance with Y minus the cross-hatched area). The first variable gets credit for the first piece of variance accounted for, even though it shares some of that with X_2.

The order of entry of variables into a multiple correlation may be important when understanding the relationships being studied. This is discussed in more detail in Chapter 11. Multiple correlation is a technique for measuring the relationship between a dependent variable and a weighted combination of independent variables.

EXAMPLE FROM THE LITERATURE

Table 10-6 contains a bivariate correlation matrix from an article by Ulrich, Soeken, and Miller (2003). The authors were investigating the ethical conflict of nurse practitioners practicing in a managed care environment. We quote their results in relation to this table to demonstrate how investigators summarize the important features of a table:

> Bivariate analysis revealed a significant positive relationship between ethical concern and ethical conflict in practice. Those with higher ethical concern scores tended to report an increase in ethical conflict ($r = .501, p < .01$). Significant relationships were also found between the perception of the ethical environment, ATGR and ethical conflict. Here, an inverse relationship was noted with respect to the perception of the ethical environment and ethical conflict. The more questionable NPs perceived the environment to be the higher their ethical conflict in practice scores ($r = -.637, p < .01$). Subsequently, the perceived need for governmental regulation of managed care also was associated with higher ethical conflict scores ($r = .225, p < .01$). (Ulrick, Soeken, & Miller, 2003, p. 173)

TABLE 10-6 *Bivariate Correlation Results*

	Variables						
	Ethical Conflict	ATGRS	EEQ	EC	Income	Ethical Relativism	Ethics CEd
ATGRS	.225**	1.0					
EEQ	−.637**	−.210**	1.0				
EC	.501**	.125	−.504**	1.0			
Income	−.131	−.143*	.135*	−.051	1.0		
Ethical Relativism	.091	−.065	.005	.040	.00	1.0	
EthicsCEd	−.107	.020	.037	−.054	.096	−.040	1.0
Percentage Uninsured	.158*	.206**	−.077	.011	−.145*	.033	.054
Medicare	−.093	−.114	.149*	.056	.230**	−.039	−.040
Medicaid	−.011	.172*	−.077	.034	.079	−.143*	−.049
Private	−.095	−.119	.052	−.194**	−.135*	.062	−.001

Note: ATGRS = Attitudes Toward Government Regulations Scale; EEQ = Ethical Environment Questionnaire; EC = Ethical Concern; EthicsCEd = Ethics in Continuing Education.
*$p < .05$.   **$p < .01$.
From Ulrich, C. M., Soeken, K. L., & Miller, N. (2003). Ethical conflict associated with managed care. *Nursing Research 52*(3), p. 173.

SUMMARY

Correlation is a procedure for quantifying the relationship between two or more variables. It measures the strength and indicates the direction of the relationship. Multiple correlation measures the relationship between one variable and a weighted composite of the other variables. Partial correlation is a statistical method for describing the relationship between two variables, with the effect of another confounding variable removed. In semipartial correlation, the influence of a third variable is removed from only one of the variables being correlated.

Application Exercises and Results

Exercises

1. What are the correlations between the following variables: Inventory of Personal Attitudes items 2, 5, 7, and 15?

Results

1. The correlations are contained in Exercise Figure 10-1. Because all the items are taken from the same instrument, and all are related to anxiety and stress, we expect that the correlations will be high and positive. All the correlations are significant at the 0.01 level and range from .337 to .632.

Correlations

Correlations

		Reaction to pressure	Experience anxiety	Fearful	Concentration during stress
Reaction to pressure	Pearson Correlation	1	.409(**)	.337(**)	.548(**)
	Sig. (2 tailed)	.	.000	.000	.000
	N	695	692	690	693
Experience anxiety	Pearson Correlation	.409(**)	1	.632(**)	.391(**)
	Sig. (2 tailed)	.000	.	.000	.000
	N	692	698	694	696
Fearful	Pearson Correlation	.337(**)	.632(**)	1	.397(**)
	Sig. (2 tailed)	.000	.000	.	.000
	N	690	694	696	694
Concentration during stress	Pearson Correlation	.548(**)	.391(**)	.397(**)	1
	Sig. (2 tailed)	.000	.000	.000	.
	N	693	696	694	699

** Correlation is significant at the 0.01 level (2 tailed).

EXERCISE FIGURE 10-1. Correlation coefficients.

CHAPTER
11

Regression

Barbara Hazard Munro

Objectives for Chapter 11

After reading this chapter, you should be able to do the following:

1. Know when it is appropriate to use regression techniques.
2. Understand the statistics generated by the regression procedure.
3. Set up and solve a prediction equation.
4. Explain the difference between testing the significance of R^2 and the significance of a *b*-weight.
5. Code categorical variables.
6. Discuss methods for selecting variables for entry into a regression equation.
7. Interpret the results section of research studies that report these techniques.

RESEARCH QUESTION

We are constantly interested in predicting one thing based on another. We want to predict the weather to plan our weekend. We want to predict how well a student will do in nursing practice. We want to predict how long a patient may remain ill. Countless predictions are necessary for us to move through life. A brilliant statistical invention is regression, which permits us to make predictions from some known evidence about some unknown future events. Only about a century old, regression is the basis of many statistical methods, and in this book there is nothing more important to understand.

Regression makes use of the correlation between variables and the notion of a straight line to develop a prediction equation. Once a relationship has been established between two variables, you can develop an equation that will allow you to predict the score of one of the variables, given the score of the other. In the case of a multiple correlation, regression is used to establish a prediction equation in which the independent variables are each assigned a weight based on their relationship to the dependent variable. For example, in a study of acculturation, resilience, and depression in midlife women from the former Soviet Union, Miller and Chandler (2002) used multiple regression to examine the relationship of predictor variables to acculturation and cultural assimilation. Age, English usage, demands of immigration, and resilience were significant predictors.

Regression is a useful technique that allows us to predict outcomes and explain the interrelationships among variables. The type of data required and the underlying assumptions are the same for regression as for correlation. We repeat them here for your convenience. Information about testing assumptions is provided in Chapter 12 in the discussion of the testing of residuals.

TYPE OF DATA REQUIRED

To calculate r, there must be at least two measures on each subject. It is often assumed that both of these measures must be at the interval level. In most cases, however, valid results also may be obtained with ordinal data. Moreover, we can code categorical variables for use with r and with regression equations. Mathematically, it is possible to use any level of data when calculating r, but factors other than the level of the data must be considered when deciding whether a correlation coefficient is appropriate.

ASSUMPTIONS

Although we can calculate correlations with data at all levels, certain assumptions must be made if we are to generalize beyond the sample statistic; that is, if we are to make inferences about the population itself:

1. The sample must be representative of the population to which the inference will be made.
2. The variables that are being correlated, say X and Y, must each have a normal distribution; that is, the distribution of their scores must approximate the normal curve.
3. For every value of X, the distribution of Y scores must have approximately equal variability. This is called the assumption of homoscedasticity.
4. The relationship between X and Y must be linear; that is, when the two scores for each individual are graphed, they should tend to form a straight line. The points will not all fall on this line, but they should be scattered closely around it.

POWER ANALYSIS

Multiple regression is a useful technique, but there are numerous examples of its misuse. A major problem is including too many variables for the number of subjects.

Computer programs provide an adjusted R^2 as well as the actual R^2. The adjusted R^2 is a more conservative estimate given the number of subjects and variables. It also has been called a shrinkage formula, because it predicts how much the R^2 is likely to shrink. There are several formulas for this adjustment; one is given here (Pedhazur & Schmelkin, 1991, p. 446):

$$\text{Adjusted } R^2 = 1 - (1 - R^2)\frac{n - 1}{n - k - 1}$$

The formula is based on the number in the sample (n) and the number of independent variables (k). The more variables compared to subjects, the greater the shrinkage will be. If you put in the same number of subjects as independent variables, you will get a perfect R^2 (1) no matter which variables you use. (However, the adjusted R^2 will be zero.) Thus, you must always consider the number of subjects and independent variables. Very high and seemingly impressive R^2s may be an artifact of too few subjects. Nunnally and Bernstein (1994) state that one should have at least 10 subjects per predictor "in order to even hope for a stable prediction equation" (p. 201).

Cohen (1987) provides a formula for determining sample size, given an effect size index, which he calls L. He defines a small effect as an R^2 of 0.02, a moderate effect as an R^2 of 0.13, and a large effect as an R^2 of 0.30. The formula is:

$$N = \frac{L(1 - R^2)}{R^2} + u + 1,$$

where N = total sample size
L = effect size index
u = number of independent variables

L can be obtained from a table and is defined by Cohen as a function of power and number of independent variables at a given level of alpha. For our example, we select a power of 0.80, an alpha of 0.05, a moderate effect size, and two different numbers of independent variables to determine appropriate sample sizes.

For three independent variables, the value of L is 10.90, and the formula is:

$$N = \frac{10.90(1 - 0.13)}{0.13} + 3 + 1$$

$$N = 77.$$

For six independent variables, the value of L is 13.62, and the formula is:

$$N = \frac{13.62(1 - 0.13)}{0.13} + 6 + 1$$

$$N = 98$$

Software programs also can calculate sample size. Sample size must be determined before data collection to ensure an adequate sample to conduct the proposed analyses.

It is possible to increase the accuracy of the prediction by adding predictor variables to the equation. The best additional variables to add are highly correlated with the dependent variable but not highly correlated with the other independent variables. Usually four or five predictors are enough. Adding more than that adds little to the R^2 because of intercorrelations among the predictors.

Because the analysis uses error variance and true variance, the multiple correlation is usually inflated by such error variance. In addition to the shrinkage formula, another way to evaluate the R^2 is to calculate it with a second sample. This is called *cross-validation*. A weakness of multiple regression is a tendency to throw variables into the equation. There should be some rationale for each variable included.

SIMPLE LINEAR REGRESSION

We begin by explaining simple regression. A correlation between two variables is used to develop a prediction equation. The techniques described in this chapter are for predictions based on a linear relationship between variables. If the relationship is curvilinear, other techniques, such as trend analysis, must be used.

If the correlation between two variables were perfect ($+1$ or -1), we would be able to make a perfect prediction about the score on one variable, given the score on the other variable. We never get perfect correlations, so we are never able to make perfect predictions. The higher the correlation, the more accurate the prediction. If there were no correlation between two variables, knowing the score of one would not help in estimating the score on the other. When you have no information to aid you in predicting a score, your best guess for any subject would be the mean, because that is the center of the data.

To be able to make predictions, the relationship between two variables, the independent (X) and the dependent (Y), must be measured. If there is a correlation, a regression equation can be developed that will allow prediction of Y given X. For example, in the study previously mentioned, Miller and Chandler (2002) regressed scores on a measure of acculturation and cultural assimilation (CES-D) on four variables: age, English usage, score on the demands of Immigration scale (DI), and resilience. All of these measures contributed significantly to the regression equation. Combined, they explained 33% of the variation in CES-D.

Understanding Regression through the Use of Standardized Scores

In previous chapters, standardized scores (*z*-scores) were used to explain the concepts of standard deviation and correlation. Remember that once scores have been converted to *z*-scores, they have a mean of 0 and a standard deviation of 1 (Fig. 11-1). Direct comparisons between sets of *z*-scores can be made because they are measured on the same scale. Given *z*-scores, the formula for a prediction (regression) equation is simple. It is $Y' = rX$, where Y' is the predicted score and X is the "known" or predictor variable. Given a perfect positive correlation, $Y' = X$. For

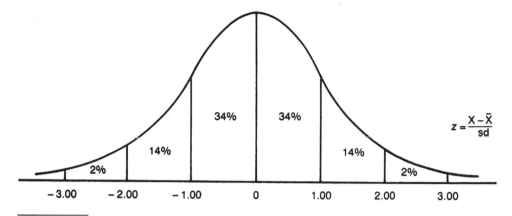

FIGURE 11-1. Normal curve with standardiized scores.

example, someone with a z-score of $+2$ on X would also score $+2$ on Y.

$$Y' = (1)(2)$$

In Chapter 10 we demonstrated that with a perfect positive correlation ($r = +1$), everyone receives exactly the same z-score on Y as on X. With a perfect negative correlation ($r = -1$), each subject receives exactly the opposite z-score on Y as on X. For example, someone with a -3 on X would get a $+3$ on Y'.

$$Y' = (-1)(-3) = +3$$

As previously mentioned, if there is no correlation between the variables, no prediction can be made, and our best guess for Y' is the mean. Using the formula for Y', with $r = 0$ and $X = +3$, we calculate Y' as $(0)(3) = 0$. Zero is, of course, the mean of a z-score distribution. These extreme cases, perfect correlations and zero correlations, however, are uncommon in the world of research. Therefore, consider what happens with more reasonable correlations. Suppose an individual, Jill, scored $+2$ on X. Given the following rs, what Y score would you predict for Jill? Work these equations before continuing.

$r = -.20$
$r = .60$
$r = .20$
$r = -.60$

For $r = -.20$, our equation would be $Y' = (-.20)(2)$, or $-.40$. The other answers are, respectively, 1.20, .40, and -1.20. If you predicted each Y score correctly, you have mastered this simplest type of prediction, for which you have only the standard scores and the correlation coefficient.

Regression literally means a falling back toward the mean. With perfect correlations, there is no falling back; the predicted score is the same as the predictor. With less-than-perfect correlations, there is some error in the measurement, and we would expect that in the case of a person who received an extremely high score, chance may have been working in her favor; therefore, on a second measure, her score would be somewhat less—it would have fallen back toward the mean. In the same way, a person with an extremely low score perhaps had all the fates against her and on a second measure would do better, thus moving her score closer to the mean.

Each prediction regresses toward the mean, depending on the strength of the correlation. If there is no correlation ($r = 0$), $Y' = 0$ (the mean). As the correlation rises toward 1, Y' moves proportionately outward from the mean, toward the position of the X predictor. The correlation coefficient tells us exactly what percentage of this distance Y' moves. Figure 11-2 shows predictions based on an r of .50. Note on the figure that all the predicted scores (Y's) are halfway between the mean and the X score. This is because the correlation is 0.5. (If the correlation had been 0.7, the Y'

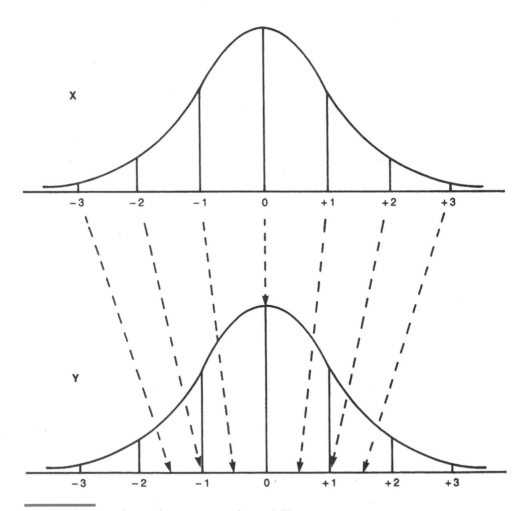

FIGURE 11-2. Predicting from X to Y with $r = 0.50$.

scores would have moved 0.7 times the distance between the mean and X.) If the X score is above the mean, the predicted score will be lower than the X score and closer to the mean. With an r of .5 and an X score of $+2$, $Y' = (.5)(2) = 1$. With a correlation of .5, a person who was 2 standard deviations above the mean would be predicted to be 1 standard deviation above the mean on Y.

If the X score is below the mean, the predicted score is higher and closer to the mean. An X score of -3 would result in a predicted score of $(.5)(-3) = -1.5$. Remember that these are predictions based on a correlation of .5, so you would not be able to predict perfectly an individual's score. The person's actual score will differ from the predicted score. This discrepancy between predicted and actual scores reflects the error in the prediction and is discussed more fully in the next section of this chapter. Because most measures will not be in z-scores, we now present the more general regression equation.

Regression Equation

The regression equation is the equation for a straight line and is written as:

$$Y' = a + bX$$

Y' is the *predicted score*.

Given data on X and Y from a sample of subjects called the *regression sample*, a and b can be calculated. With these two measures, Y can be predicted, given X. The letter a is called the *intercept constant* and is the value of Y when $X = 0$. It is the point at which the regression line intercepts the Y axis. The letter b is called the *regression coefficient* and is the rate of change in Y with a unit change in X. It is a measure of the slope of the regression line.

An example is given in Figure 11-3. The intercept constant, a, is equal to 3; you can see that is the value of Y when $X = 0$. It is the point at which the regression line connects with the Y axis. The regression coefficient, b, is .5. This means that the value of Y goes up .5 of a point for every 1-point change in X. When $X = 0$, $Y = 3$, and when X goes up to 1, Y goes up to 3.5. As you will see when we are calculating a and b, a is based on the means of the two variables and b is based on the correlation between them. The regression line is the "line of best fit" and is formed by a technique called the *method of least squares*. The concept of least squares was presented in Chapter 2 with a discussion of characteristics of the mean. Because the mean is (in one sense) the center of the data, the sum of the deviations of the scores around the mean, $\Sigma(X - X)$, is 0. Also, if you square these deviations and add them, that number will be smaller than the sum of the squared deviations around any other measure of central tendency. In the same way, the regression line passes through the exact center of the data in the scatter diagram. Therefore, it is the "line of best fit." There are deviations around the regression line, just as there are deviations around the mean. The regression line represents the predicted scores (Y's), but because a prediction is not perfect, the actual scores (Ys) would deviate somewhat from the predicted scores. Because the regression line passes through the center of the pairs of scores, if you add the deviations from the regression line $\Sigma(Y - Y')$, they

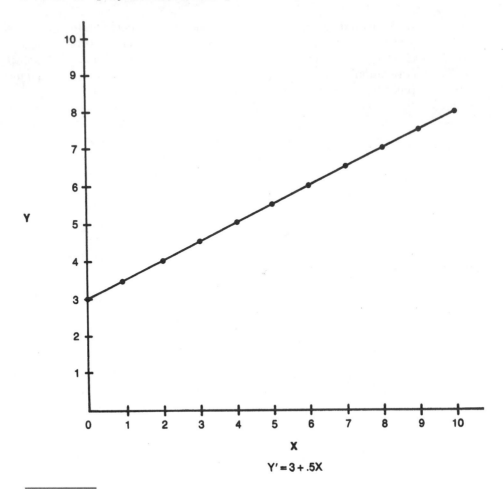

FIGURE 11-3. The regression line.

will equal 0. Also, if you square those deviations and add them, the sum of the squared deviations around the regression line is smaller than the sum of the squared deviations around any other line drawn through the scatter diagram.

If Miller and Chandler (2002) applied their prediction equation to the midlife women in their sample, they would find that the women's actual scores on acculturation (Y) would vary from their predicted (Y') score. Because the correlations between the predictors and the outcome measure were not perfect, there is error in the prediction. Even using the sample on which the prediction equation was calculated, there will be differences between Y and Y'. $Y - Y'$ equals the deviations from the predicted scores, just as $X - \bar{X}$ equals the deviations around the mean. The regression equation minimizes the squared differences of the predicted score from the actual score.

Given a regression equation of $Y' = 4 + 0.2X$ and three individuals with scores on X of 5, 10, and 20, respectively, the predicted scores for the three would be calculated as follows:

$$a + bX = Y'$$

1. $4 + (0.2)(5) = 5$
2. $4 + (0.2)(10) = 6$
3. $4 + (0.2)(20) = 8$

Confidence Intervals

Because there is error in predictions, we need to know how accurate a prediction is. The standard error of estimate can be used to construct confidence intervals around predicted scores. The standard error of estimate is the standard deviation of the errors of prediction. We use that in the same way that we use the standard errors of the mean and the correlation coefficient to construct confidence intervals. Given a predicted score, we can then say that 95% or 99% of the confidence intervals will capture the actual score.

MULTIPLE REGRESSION

Multiple regression is possible when there is a measurable multiple correlation between a group of predictor variables and one dependent variable. The prediction equation is:

$$Y' = a + b_1X_1 + b_2X_2 + b_3X_3 + \cdots b_kX_k$$

There is still one intercept constant, a, but each independent variable (eg, X_1, X_2, X_3) has a separate b-weight. Given a prediction equation of:

$$Y' = 2 + 0.5X_1 + 0.2X_2 + 0.4X_3$$

and three individuals with the following scores:

	X_1	X_2	X_3
1.	8	4	7
2.	12	3	5
3.	10	6	9

their predicted scores would be calculated as:

1. $2 + (0.5)(8) + (0.2)(4) + (0.4)(7) = 9.6$
2. $2 + (0.5)(12) + (0.2)(3) + (0.4)(5) = 10.6$
3. $2 + (0.5)(10) + (0.2)(6) + (0.4)(9) = 11.8$

If adding extra variables increases the amount of variance accounted for in the dependent variable, that will also increase the accuracy of our prediction. Multiple regression simply extends the multiple correlation into the computation of the regression equation.

SIGNIFICANCE TESTING

When doing a simple linear regression, the correlation between the two variables is tested for significance, and r^2 represents meaningfulness. With multiple correlation, we are interested not only in the significance of the overall R and the amount of variance accounted for (R^2), but also in the significance of each of the independent variables. Just because R^2 is significant does not mean that all the independent variables are contributing significantly to the explained variance. In multiple regression, the multiple correlation is tested for significance, and each of the b-weights also is tested for significance. Testing the b-weight tells us whether the independent variable associated with it is contributing significantly to the variance accounted for in the dependent variable.

The F-distribution is used for testing the significance of the R^2s, and either the F- or t-distribution is used to test the significance of the bs. See Appendix D for the F-distribution. When using computer programs, the Fs or ts and associated probabilities are printed out. The F-distribution is used for demonstration here.

When testing for the significance of R^2s, the degrees of freedom (df) are calculated as $k/(n - k - 1)$. In other words, there are two dfs; a numerator, k; and a denominator, $(n - k - 1)$. The k stands for the number of independent variables, and n stands for the number of subjects. When testing the significance of a b-weight, the $df = 1/(n - k - 1)$.

We start with examples of testing the Fs associated with R^2s for significance. If we had two independent variables and a sample size of 63, the df would be $2/(63 - 2 - 1)$, or $2/60$. In Appendix D, the dfs for the numerator are listed across the top of the page. The numerator also is known as the greater mean square. The dfs for the denominator are listed down the left side of the page. The denominator also is called the lesser mean square. In our example, there are 2 dfs in the numerator and 60 dfs in the denominator. The tabled values for 2/60 df, which must be equaled or exceeded, are 3.15 at the 0.05 level and 4.98 at the 0.01 level. Note that the 0.05 level is in light print, and the 0.01 level is in dark print. An F of 4.50 would be significant at the 0.05 level but not at the 0.01 level. Two additional examples follow:

F	k	n	df	p
4.05	3	129	3/125	<0.01
2.00	6	207	6/200	ns

To test the *b*-weights, the procedure is the same except that the numerator of the *df* is always 1. Some examples for testing *b*-weights follow:

F	k	n	df	p
5.25	2	68	1/65	<0.05
8.00	3	154	1/150	<0.01

COMPUTER ANALYSIS

The question to be addressed is whether a measure of mental competence can be predicted by age; education (highest grade completed); feeling full of pep (from 0 = none of the time to 5 = all of the time); and ability to walk more than a mile (from 1 = limited a lot to 3 = not limited). The measure of mental competence is count-ing backward from 100 by subtracting 7. The interviewer stops at five answers. The score is the number of correct answers before the first mistake and ranges from 0 to 5. The data come from Wood's (1997) study. Figure 11-4 contains the correlations among the variables. Note the correlations between each of the four variables and counting backward. The correlations range from a high of .497 to a low of .133. Age is negatively related to ability to count backward. All correlations are significant (*p* = .000 to .003). Because we can see that all of the variables are significantly related to each other, we will use multiple regression to determine how well the combination of independent variables explains the variance in the counting back-wards score. The research question is, "What is the multiple correlation between a set of four predictors (age, education, pep, and walking) and the outcome, mental status?" To answer this question, the counting backward score is regressed on the four predictor variables.

The output from this analysis is contained in Figure 11-5. There are five tables produced by SPSS for Windows. The first simply indicates which variables were entered into the equation. We entered education and age in the first "model" (often called block), and pep and walking in the second model. The method, "enter," indi-cates that all variables within a model (or block) were entered together. In Model Summary, we see that values for each model (block). Entering education and age in the first model resulted in $R = .497$, R^2 is .247, and the adjusted R^2 is .244; thus, at this point the analysis accounted for 24.7% of the variance. The R Square Change is the difference between one model and the next. In the first model, it is the differ-ence between 0 and the R square, or 24.7%. This is significant at $p = .000$. Adding the predictors of pep and walking into the second model, raised the R square from 24.7% to 26.7% an increase of 2% (R Square Change = .019, difference between 1.9 and 2% is due to rounding). This addition is significant at the .004 level.

(text continues on page 273)

		Count backward from 100 by subtracting 7. Interviewer stops at 5 answers. Score # correct answers before 1st mistake.	Age	What is the highest grade or year of school that you completed?	Did you feel full of pep	Walking more than a mile
Pearson Corre-lation	Count backward from 100 by subtracting 7. Interviewer stops at 5 answers. Score # correct answers before 1st mistake.	1.000	−.145	.497	.133	.184
	Age	−.145	1.000	−.306	.016	−.119
	What is the highest grade or year of school that you completed?	.497	−.306	1.000	.087	.103
	Did you feel full of pep	.133	.016	.087	1.000	.405
	Walking more than a mile	.184	−.119	.103	.405	1.000
Sig. (1 tailed)	Count backward from 100 by subtracting 7. Interviewer stops at 5 answers. Score # correct answers before 1st mistake.	.	.001	.000	.003	.000
	Age	.001	.	.000	.372	.007
	What is the highest grade or year of school that you completed?	.000	.000	.	.035	.017
	Did you feel full of pep	.003	.372	.035	.	.000
	Walking more than a mile	.000	.007	.017	.000	
N	Count backward from 100 by subtracting 7. Interviewer stops at 5 answers. Score # correct answers before 1st mistake.	437	435	430	435	427
	Age	435	437	430	435	427
	What is the highest grade or year of school that you completed?	430	430	432	430	422
	Did you feel full of pep	435	435	430	437	427
	Walking more than a mile	427	427	422	427	429

FIGURE 11-4. Correlations from Wood's data set.

Regression

Variables Entered/Removed (b)

Model	Variables Entered	Variables Removed	Method
1	What is the highest grade or year of school that you completed?, Age (a)	.	Enter
2	Did you feel full of pep, walking more than a mile(a)	.	Enter

a All requested variables entered.
b Dependent Variable: Count backward from 100 by subtracting 7. Interviewer stops at 5 answers. Score # correct answers before 1st mistake.

Model Summary

Model	R	R Square	Adjusted R Square	Std. Error of the Estimate	Change Statistics				
					R Square Change	F Change	df1	df2	Sig. F Change
1	.497(a)	.247	.244	1.856	.247	68.887	2	419	.000
2	.517(b)	.267	.260	1.836	.019	5.532	2	417	.004

a Predictors: (Constant), what is the highest grade or year of school that you completed?, age.
b Predictors: (Constant), what is the highest grade or year of school that you completed?, age, did you feel full of pep, walking more than a mile.

AUTHOR COMMENTS
The analysis accounted for 26.7% of the variance in the dependent variable.

FIGURE 11-5. Computer output, multiple regression.

ANOVA (c)

Model		Sum of Squares	df	Mean Square	F	Sig.
1	Regression	474.696	2	237.348	68.887	.000(a)
	Residual	1443.654	419	3.445		
	Total	1918.350	421			
2	Regression	512.013	4	128.003	37.955	.000(b)
	Residual	1406.338	417	3.373		
	Total	1918.350	421			

a Predictors: (Constant), what is the highest grade or year of school that you completed?, age.
b Predictors: (Constant), what is the highest grade or year of school that you completed?, age, did you feel full of pep, walking more than a mile.
c Dependent Variable: Count backward from 100 by subtracting 7. Interviewer stops at 5 answers. Score # correct answers before 1st mistake.

AUTHOR COMMENTS
The overall analysis was significant, p = .000.

Coefficients (a)

Model		Unstandardized Coefficients		Standardized Coefficients	t	Sig.
		B	Std. Error	Beta		
1	(Constant)	−.210	.905		−.232	.816
	Age	.002	.011	.008	.171	.864
	What is the highest grade or year of school that you completed?	.246	.022	.500	11.227	.000
2	(Constant)	−1.067	.932		−1.145	.253
	Age	.004	.011	.017	.382	.703
	What is the highest grade or year of school that you completed?	.240	.022	.487	10.993	.000
	Did you feel full of pep	.067	.073	.042	.917	.360
	walking more than a mile	.278	.109	.118	2.551	.011

a Dependent Variable: Count backward from 100 by subtracting 7. Interviewer stops at 5 answers. Score # correct answers before 1st mistake.

FIGURE 11-5. (*Continued*)

AUTHOR COMMENTS
Two of the independent variables (highest grade in school and walking) contributed significantly to the analysis. The other two independent variables, age and pep, were not significantly related to the outcome measure.

Excluded Variables (b)

| Model | | Beta In | t | Sig. | Partial Correlation | Collinearity Statistics |
						Tolerance
1	Did you feel full of pep	.090(a)	2.121	.035	.103	.990
	walking more than a mile	.135(a)	3.198	.001	.155	.981

a Predictors in the Model: (Constant), what is the highest grade or year of school that you completed?, age.
b Dependent Variable: Count backward from 100 by subtracting 7. Interviewer stops at 5 answers. Score # correct answers before 1st mistake.

FIGURE 11-5. (*Continued*)

The analysis of variance (ANOVA) table is next, and there we see that the overall analysis is significant at the .000 level for both models. Note that rather than sum of squares for between and within, we see sum of squares for regression and residual.

The coefficients are presented in the fourth table. The unstandardized coefficients (*b*-weights) are presented first, then the standardized or beta coefficients. Because the *b*-weight reflects the actual measure with its associated mean and standard deviation, it is not directly interpretable. The standard error is a measure of the difference between predicted and actual scores and can be used to construct confidence intervals around the *b*-weights.

Beta reflects the weight associated with standardized scores (*z*-scores) on the variables. It is a partial correlation coefficient, a measure of the relationship between an independent and a dependent variable with the influence of the other independent variables held constant. In model two, two of the four predictors contribute significantly to the variance in counting backwards: education ($p = .000$) and walking more than a mile ($p = .011$).

Although age and pep had significant zero-order correlations with counting backward (see Fig. 11-4), they do not contribute significantly to the regression equation. Why is this so? Both age and pep are significantly correlated to education and walking thus, beyond what they share with those variables, they do not account for any significant additional variance in counting backward. The final table is Excluded Variables. In the first model, two variables were not entered. We see that each of them was significantly related to the outcome measure. These variables are entered in the second model.

For this analysis, we would report that the hierarchical regression of mental status (counting backward) on four predictor variables, entered in two blocks accounted for 26.7% of the variance and was significant at the .000 level. Education and age were entered in the first block and accounted for 24.7 % of the variance ($p = .000$). Pep and walking were added in the second block and accounted for an additional 1.9% of the variance ($p = .004$). In the final model, education and walking were significantly related to mental status. The positive relationships indicated that people who completed more years of education and who were better able to walk a mile, scored higher on the mental status exam. Confidence intervals may be requested for each b value, but to save space we left them off this table.

The prediction equation based on this table is:

$$\text{Predicted total score on counting} = -1.067 + .004(\text{age}) + .240(\text{education})$$
$$+ .067(\text{pep}) + .278(\text{walking}).$$

CODING

Nominal-level variables can be included in a regression analysis, but they must be coded to allow proper interpretation. You might collect information on the marital status of your subjects, and when entering the information into the computer, you decide on some arbitrary code numbers, such as single = 1, married = 2, and divorced = 3. If you entered that variable into a regression equation, it would be treated as though the numbers really meant something, that 2 was twice as big as 1, and so on. Such coding is not recommended. Instead, coding methods have been developed to allow us to enter such variables; three of these techniques, *dummy*, *effect*, and *orthogonal*, are presented here.

In all the coding methods, variables are coded into vectors, and the rule is that $n - 1$ vectors are used to describe the categories. If the variable has two categories, such as gender, one vector ($2 - 1 = 1$) is enough. If there were four categories, three vectors would be required, and so on.

Dummy Coding

This system uses 1s and 0s. If gender is a variable, you could code all males as 1 and all females as 0 (or vice versa). Correlational techniques applied to such a variable would tell you whether the gender of the subject was related to some measure. The 1 and 0 indicate that you belong to the chosen group or you do not. There is no distinction among members of a group; that is, all the 1s are considered equally male and all the 0s equally female. Suppose you had three groups, experimental group 1, experimental group 2, and a control group. You would need $n - 1$ ($3 - 1$) vectors to describe those categories (Table 11-1). To code those groups, start with the first vector, which we label $X1$. All the subjects in the first experimental group get a 1 on that vector, and all others get a 0. On the second vector, $X2$, all subjects in the

TABLE 11-1 *Dummy Coding*

	Vectors	
Groups	X1	X2
Experimental 1	1	0
Experimental 2	0	1
Control	0	0

second experimental group get a 1, and all the other subjects get a 0. The control group has received 0s on both vectors. On these two vectors, each group has a different pattern; that is, the first experimental group has 1,0; the second experimental group has 0,1; and the control group has 0,0.

This form could be extended for any number of categories. When the regression is run, the vectors $X1$ and $X2$ are entered to represent group membership. When such dummy coding is used, the intercept constant, a, in the prediction equation equals the mean of the dependent variable for the group that is assigned 0s throughout. In our example, that would be the control group. Therefore, in this form of analysis, we are testing the means of the other groups against the mean of a control group. In addition to a, the prediction equation would contain a b-weight for each of the vectors; that is, the prediction equation would look like:

$$Y' = a + b_1 X_1 + b_2 X_2$$

The regression weight, b_1, represents the difference between the group assigned 1s on $X1$ and the group assigned 0s throughout. In our example, testing b_1 for significance would be testing to see whether there is a significant difference between the first experimental group and the control group on some dependent variable, Y. Testing b_2 for significance tells us whether there is a significant difference between the second experimental group and the control group. Although it is most clear when used with a control group, dummy coding may be used to code categorical variables, whether or not a control group exists. You can use dummy coding for ethnicity, marital status, and so on, but you must understand what testing the b-weights means. In addition to comparing a group with the control group, you may want to compare it with some other group. In our example, you may want to compare experimental group 1 with experimental group 2. To do that, you would need to use a method that allows you to make multiple comparisons between means.

Effect Coding

Effect coding looks like dummy coding except that the last group gets -1s throughout instead of 0s (Table 11-2). Five categories of marital status are coded into four vectors. We proceed in the same way as with dummy coding, but we give the last

	Vectors			
Marital Status	X1	X2	X3	X4
Single	1	0	0	0
Married	0	1	0	0
Divorced	0	0	1	0
Widowed	0	0	0	1
Separated	−1	−1	−1	−1

TABLE 11-2 *Efffect Coding*

group −1 on each vector. Vectors $X1$ through $X4$ would then be entered into the regression equation to represent marital status.

When using effect coding, the a in the prediction equation represents the mean of the dependent variable. It is not the mean of one particular group on the dependent variable, but the overall mean for all the subjects in the analysis. This is called the *grand mean*. What you are testing with this type of coding is how each group's mean differs from the grand mean.

In our example, the regression equation would be:

$$Y' = a + b_1X_1 + b_2X_2 + b_3X_3 + b_4X_4$$

If you tested b_1 for significance, you would be testing to see whether the mean score on the dependent variable for single people differed from the overall or grand mean. We could compare the means for single, married, divorced, and widowed against the grand mean, but what about the separated group? There is no b-weight to represent the fifth group. That b-weight can be calculated easily when you know that all the b-weights add up to zero; in the example, this is $b_1 + b_2 + b_3 + b_4 + b_5 = 0$. Given the b-weights for the first four categories from the regression, the fifth b-weight can be obtained by subtracting the sum of the first four from zero. For example, if the b-weights were $b_1 = 1$, $b_2 = 3$, $b_3 = -2$, $b_4 = 2$, then $1 + 3 + (-2) + 2 = 4$, and $0 - 4 = -4$. Thus, the b-weight for the "separated" category would be -4. To compare specific pairs of means, a test for multiple comparisons between means must be applied.

Orthogonal Coding

When you hypothesize ahead of time, you can use more powerful statistical tests. Orthogonal coding allows you to code your hypotheses so they can be tested. To use this technique, you must have hypothesized a priori (ie, before the data were collected). Here, orthogonal means that the comparisons that you want to test are independent of each other; that is, knowing the answer to one does not give you the answer to the other.

	Vectors	
TABLE 11-3 *Orthogonal Coding*		
Groups	*X1*	*X2*
Experimental 1	-1	1
Experimental 2	-1	-1
Control	2	0

To have comparisons that are independent, only $n - 1$ comparisons can be made; that is, if there were three groups (experimental 1, experimental 2, and control), there could be only two orthogonal contrasts. Suppose you were trying to decrease the number of postoperative complications, and you had three groups. Subjects in experimental group 1 were given special preoperative instruction by a nurse and a booklet to which they could refer later. Experimental group 2 received instruction only, and the control group just received the usual care. You would want to know whether the special instructions reduced postoperative complications and whether providing a booklet and instruction was better than instruction alone. We could compare the mean for experimental groups 1 and 2 with the mean of the control group to see whether there was a difference between experimental and control groups. We also could compare the means of the two experimental groups to see whether the booklet made a difference.

Table 11-3 contains the vectors necessary to code such a contrast. On vector $X1$, subjects in both experimental groups receive a -1, and the control group subjects receive a 2. That contrast tests the difference between the mean number of postoperative complications for all the experimental subjects and the mean for the control group subjects. Testing b_1 for significance would tell you whether that difference was statistically significant. The second contrast is given in vector $X2$. The first experimental group is compared with the second. Testing b_2 for significance would tell you whether there was a significant difference in the mean number of postoperative complications between those in the experimental group who received the booklet and those who did not. To ensure that hypothesized contrasts are orthogonal, three tests must be applied:

1. There must be only $n - 1$ contrasts.
2. The sum of each vector must equal zero. In the example, the sum of $X1$ is $(-1) + (-1) + 2 = 0$, and the sum of $X2$ is $1 + (-1) + 0 = 0$.
3. The sum of the cross-products must equal zero. In the example, $(-1 \times 1) + (-1 \times -1) + (2 \times 0) = 0$.

Table 11-4 shows some other examples of possible contrasts, given three groups. Are they all orthogonal? The vectors $X1$ and $X2$ reflect an orthogonal contrast, as do the vectors $Y1$ and $Y2$. Vectors $Z1$ and $Z2$ do not reflect an orthogonal contrast;

	TABLE 11-4 *Contrasts*					

	Pairs of Vectors					
Groups	*X1*	*X2*	*Y1*	*Y2*	*Z1*	*Z2*
1	2	0	−1	1	−1	1
2	−1	1	2	0	0	−1
3	−1	−1	−1	−1	1	0

group 1 is compared to group 2 and to group 3. The sum of the cross-products does not equal zero, $(-1 \times 1) + (0 \times -1) + (1 \times 0) = -1$.

In the regression equation with orthogonal coding, a is the grand mean of the dependent variable and each b represents a hypothesized contrast.

Coding Interactions

As pointed out in Chapter 7, you can study the interaction among variables. Interactions among variables may be coded and entered into the regression equation. Suppose you had two categorical variables to code: group membership and gender. Dummy coding will be used in this example, but any of the coding methods could be used. Figure 11-6 shows the basic design of the study. There are six mutually exclusive groups. We can now look at the effects of group membership, the effects of gender, and whether there is any interaction between group and gender. For example, does the booklet reduce postoperative complications for women but not for men? Coding of an interaction is demonstrated in Table 11-5. (M and F are used for male and female.) The six groups formed by the design are listed. First, we code group membership. To do that, ignore the gender variable. We need two group vectors and will call them $G1$ and $G2$. All EG1 subjects will be assigned 1 on $G1$; all

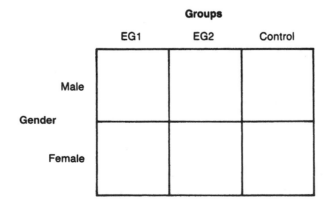

FIGURE 11-6. Design of study.

TABLE 11-5 *Coding Interactions*					
			Vectors		
Groups	G1	G2	S1	I1	I2
EG1, M	1	0	1	1	0
EG1, F	1	0	0	0	0
EG2, M	0	1	1	0	1
EG2, F	0	1	0	0	0
Control, M	0	0	1	0	0
Control, F	0	0	0	0	0

other subjects will be assigned 0. All EG2 subjects will receive a 1 on $G2$, all other subjects will receive a 0. Only one vector ($S1$) is needed to code gender. Males are assigned 1s; females are assigned 0s.

In this example, there are two vectors for group and one for gender, so there must be two (2 × 1) vectors to code the interaction between these two variables. These vectors are labeled $I1$ and $I2$. For $I1$, multiply $G1$ by $S1$, and for $I2$, multiply $G2$ by $S1$.

Summary of Coding

As shown in these examples, coding is the way categorical variables and interactions are entered into the regression equation. Regardless of the method of coding used, the overall R^2 will remain the same, and so will its significance. Predictions based on the resulting prediction equations will be identical. The differences lie in the meaning attached to testing the b-weights for significance. With dummy coding, the b-weight represents the difference between the mean of the group represented by that b and the group assigned 0s throughout. In effect coding, the bs represent the difference between the mean of the group associated with that b-weight and the grand mean. With orthogonal coding, the b-weight measures the difference between two means specified in a hypothesized contrast.

MULTIPLE COMPARISONS AMONG MEANS

None of the coding methods allows us to make all the comparisons among mean scores that we might like. If we have three groups, A, B, and C, and use dummy coding, we can compare the means of A and B with the mean of the control group C to see whether they are statistically different; however, we cannot compare the means of A and B by testing the b-weights. With effect coding, we could compare the means of each of the three groups with the grand mean, but we could not compare

A with B, A with C, and so on. With orthogonal coding, we are restricted to $n - 1$ orthogonal hypothesized contrasts. As discussed in Chapter 6, some contrasts can be measured after the fact, that is, after the overall F is found to be significant. Using these posthoc tests, we can then compare each group with every other group or compare two groups with one group, and so on. Given our two experimental groups (preoperative teaching plus booklet and preoperative teaching alone) and a control group, we could compare each experimental group with the control group, the two experimental groups, the two experimental groups together with the control group, and so forth. Measures for multiple comparisons among means allow us to explore all interesting differences in our data once we have an overall F that is significant. These can be done using ANOVA techniques in SPSS for Windows.

SELECTING VARIABLES FOR REGRESSION

Because there is so much intercorrelation among variables used in behavioral research, we may want to select a subset of variables that does the best job of predicting a particular outcome. Usually, we want to find the smallest group of variables that will account for the greatest proportion of variance in the dependent variable. Using such information, we can make practical decisions. If two predictors are equally good, we will probably decide to use the one that is easiest to administer, most economical, and so forth. Outlined here are some of the commonly used methods for selecting variables, including standard, hierarchical, and stepwise.

Standard

All the independent variables are entered at once. In SPSS it is called ENTER. In the example in this chapter, variables within each model were entered together. All variables are evaluated in relation to the dependent variable and the other independent variables through the use of partial correlation coefficients.

Hierarchical

The researcher may want to force the order of entry of variables into the equation. Suppose you want to know whether a particular intervention would improve pregnancy outcomes. You already have some givens, such as age, socioeconomic status, and nutritional status, and you would like to know whether your intervention makes a difference over and above factors that you cannot change. You might then enter the givens first and add your intervention last. In this chapter, we entered the variables in two blocks. As is shown in Chapter 16, this technique is used in developing path models. The variables may be entered one at a time or in subsets, but there should always be a theoretical rationale for the order of entry. Within each subset, variables may be entered as a group, or in a stepwise fashion. An example of hierarchical regression is a study of the determinants of Medicare home health care service use (Henton et al., 2002). To examine Medicare home health care expenditures, the investigators entered the predictor variables in three blocks: predisposing characteristics (age, sex, marital status, education, and race/ethnicity), enabling resources (income and place of residence), and need (perceived health status, perceived mental health status, cognitive limitation, functional limitation, vision impairment, and hearing impairment). The predisposing characteristics accounted for 16% of the variance, enabling resources added only .8%, and need added an additional 9%.

Stepwise

FORWARD SOLUTION

The independent variable that has the highest correlation with the dependent variable is entered first. The second variable entered is the one that will increase the R^2 the most over and above what the first variable contributed. We have four independent variables, and we calculated the correlations between each independent variable and the dependent variable and found the highest correlation to be 0.50. That independent variable enters the equation and accounts for 0.50^2 or 25%, of the variance. Now we want to know which of the three remaining variables will add the most to the 25% that is already explained. The computer cannot simply select the one with the next-highest correlation with the dependent variable because there is intercorrelation among the independent variables. Therefore, partial correlations are calculated between each of the three remaining independent variables and the dependent variable. Thus, the effect of the first variable is removed from the correlation. The variable that has the highest partial correlation with the dependent variable enters next. Then the partials between the two remaining independent variables and the dependent variable, taking out the effects of the first two variables in the equation, are calculated. The one with the highest partial correlation is entered next. Various criteria may be set for entry into the regression equation. The 0.05 level of significance is often used. In that case, a variable has to contribute a significant ($p < 0.05$) amount of variance to be included in the analysis. Once none of the remaining independent variables can contribute significantly to the R^2, the analysis is ended.

BACKWARD SOLUTION

In this method, we start with the overall R^2 generated by putting all of our independent variables in the equation. Then each variable is deleted one at a time to see whether the R^2 drops significantly. Each variable is tested to see what would happen if it were the last one entered into the equation. With four independent variables, the following differences would be tested:

$R^2y.1234 - R^2y.234$ tests for variable 1
$R^2y.1234 - R^2y.134$ tests for variable 2
$R^2y.1234 - R^2y.124$ tests for variable 3
$R^2y.1234 - R^2y.123$ tests for variable 4

If for any of these variables there is a significant drop in R^2, that variable is contributing significantly and will not be removed. If all the variables contribute significantly, the analysis would end with all four variables remaining in the equation. If one is not significant, there would be three variables left in the equation. Then, each of those three variables would be tested to see whether it would contribute significantly if entered last. The analysis continues until all variables in the equation contribute significantly if entered last.

STEPWISE SOLUTION

The stepwise solution combines the forward solution with the backward solution and therefore overcomes difficulties associated with each. With the forward solution, once a variable is in the equation, it is not removed. No attempt is made to reassess the contribution of a variable once other variables have been added. The backward solution remedies that problem, but the order of entry is not clear (ie, which variable enters first and contributes most to the explained variance?). With the stepwise solution, variables are entered in the method outlined for the forward solution and are assessed at each step using the backward method to determine whether their contribution is still significant, given the effect of other variables in the equation.

Summary of Methods of Entry

Selecting a method for entering variables into the equation is an important decision, because the results will differ depending on the method selected. Stepwise methods were in vogue in the 1970s, but they are less popular today. Because the order of entry is based on a statistical rather than a theoretical rationale, the technique is criticized for capitalizing on chance. This is because the entry is based on the correlations among the variables, and these correlations are not stable with time because error is involved in their measurement. This becomes more of a problem when dealing with variables with low reliability.

Nunnally and Bernstein (1994) state that stepwise solutions are particularly problematic when testing hypotheses. The possibility of making a type I error expands dramatically with increased numbers of predictors. They believe it is preferable to combine stepwise and hierarchical approaches. Variables are not to be "dumped" into an analysis and "large samples are an absolute necessity" (p. 195). They urge a ratio of 50 subjects to 1 variable if you want to use as many as 10 variables. They stress the need to examine the beta weights and R and to cross-validate results.

EXAMPLE FROM THE LITERATURE

Table 11-6 contains results of the Henton and colleagues (2002) study described under the section on hierarchical regression. You can see the variables entered in

TABLE 11-6 *Hierarchical Regression of Personal Annual Medicare Home Health Care Expenditures on Population Characteristics (N = 239)*

Population characteristics	R^2	R^2 change
Predisposing	.159	.159
Age		
Sex		
Marital status		
Education		
Race/ethnicity		
Enabing resources	0.167	0.008
Income		
Place of residence		
Need	0.259	0.093
Perceived health status		
Perceived mental health status		
Cognitive limitation		
Functional limitation		
Vision impairment		
Hearing impairment		

Note. Adjusted R^2 = .212.
From Henton, F. E., Hays, B. J., Walker, S. N., & Atwood, J. R. (2002). Determinants of Medicare home healthcare service use among Medicare recipients. *Nursing Research, 51*(6), p. 360.

each group and their contribution to the overall model. The predisposing characteristics were entered first and accounted for the largest portion of the variance, 15.9%. Only two of the variables, age (p = .001) and race/ethnicity (p = .008), made significant contributions. None of the enabling resources made significant contributions, and only one of the need variables, functional limitation (p = .012), made a significant contribution.

SUMMARY

Multiple regression may be used for explanation and prediction. It is a flexible technique that allows the use of categorical and continuous variables. Overall, this is one of the most powerful techniques in our field; if used wisely, it can be of great assistance in studying many problems related to human behavior and the health professions.

Application Exercises and Results

Exercises

1. What is the multiple correlation of three sets of predictors and overall state of health? The first set of predictors contains age and years of education. The second set contains confidence and life satisfaction. The third set contains smoking history and satisfaction with current weight.

Results

1. A hierarchical multiple regression was run to answer the question. The results are contained in Exercise Figure 11-1. The variables were entered in three blocks (models). Education and age were entered in the first model and accounted for 4.1% of the variance ($p = .000$). Confidence and life purpose were entered in the second model and accounted for an additional 22.8% of the variance ($R^2 = .269, p = .000$). Satisfaction with current weight and smoking history were entered in the third model and accounted for an additional 6.5% of the variance ($p = .000$). The three models accounted for 33.4% of the variance in overall state of health. In the final model, age, education in years, life satisfaction, smoking history, and satisfaction with current weight accounted for significant portions of the variance. Being younger, having more education and higher life satisfaction, smoking less, and being more satisfied with current weight were associated with greater health. Self-confidence was not significantly related to overall health. (Note that these variables are not all normally distributed and, therefore, the results should be interpreted with caution.)

Regression

Variables Entered/Removed (b)

Model	Variables Entered	Variables Removed	Method
1	Education in years, subject's age(a)	.	Enter
2	CONFID, LIFE(a)	.	Enter
3	Smoking history, satisfaction with current weight(a)	.	Enter

a All requested variables entered.
b Dependent Variable: Overall state of health.

EXERCISE FIGURE 11-1. Regression analysis.

Model Summary

Model	R	R Square	Adjusted R Square	Std. Error of the Estimate	Change Statistics				
					R Square Change	F Change	df1	df2	Sig. F Change
1	.202(a)	.041	.038	1.706	.041	13.792	2	646	.000
2	.519(b)	.269	.264	1.492	.228	100.469	2	644	.000
3	.578(c)	.334	.327	1.427	.065	31.072	2	642	.000

a Predictors: (Constant), education in years, subject's age.
b Predictors: (Constant), education in years, subject's age, CONFID, LIFE.
c Predictors: (Constant), education in years, subject's age, CONFID, LIFE, Smoking History, satisfaction with current weight.

ANOVA (d)

Model		Sum of Squares	df	Mean Square	F	Sig.
1	Regression	80.329	2	40.164	13.792	.000(a)
	Residual	1881.237	646	2.912		
	Total	1961.566	648			
2	Regression	527.713	4	131.928	59.254	.000(b)
	Residual	1433.853	644	2.226		
	Total	1961.566	648			
3	Regression	654.259	6	109.043	53.550	.000(c)
	Residual	1307.307	642	2.036		
	Total	1961.566	648			

a Predictors: (Constant), education in years, subject's age.
b Predictors: (Constant), education in years, subject's age, CONFID, LIFE.
c Predictors: (Constant), education in years, subject's age, CONFID, LIFE, Smoking history, satisfaction with current weight.
d Dependent Variable: overall state of health.

EXERCISE FIGURE 11-1. (*Continued*)

Coefficients (a)

Model		Unstandardized Coefficients		Standardized Coefficients		
		B	Std. Error	Beta	t	Sig.
1	(Constant),	7.124	.373		19.123	.000
	subject's age,	−.017	.005	−.128	−3.321	.001
	education in years	.083	.019	.165	4.280	.000
2	(Constant),	3.336	.424		7.876	.000
	subject's age,	−.018	.005	−.136	−4.026	.000
	education in years,	.041	.017	.081	2.348	.019
	CONFID,	.011	.007	.084	1.638	.102
	LIFE	.043	.005	.419	8.072	.000
3	(Constant),	3.075	.422		7.291	.000
	subject's age,	−.013	.004	−.093	−2.825	.005
	education in years,	.035	.017	.069	2.084	.038
	CONFID,	.009	.007	.068	1.372	.170
	LIFE,	.036	.005	.354	6.971	.000
	Smoking history,	−.219	.085	-.087	−2.586	.010
	satisfaction with current weight	.163	.022	.252	7.479	.000

a Dependent Variable: overall state of health.

Excluded Variables (c)

Model		Beta In	t	Sig.	Partial Correlation	Collinearity Statistics Tolerance
1	CONFID,	.396(a)	11.113	.000	.401	.983
	LIFE,	.482(a)	14.062	.000	.484	.967
	Smoking history,	−.148(a)	−3.793	.000	−.148	.953
	satisfaction with current weight	.358(a)	9.887	.000	.363	.985
2	Smoking history,	−.084(b)	−2.391	.017	−.094	.920
	satisfaction with current weight	.251(b)	7.414	.000	.281	.917

a Predictors in the Model: (Constant), education in years, subject's age.
b Predictors in the Model: (Constant), education in years, subject's age, CONFID, LIFE.
c Dependent Variable: overall state of health.

EXERCISE FIGURE 11-1. (*Continued*)

Regression Diagnostics and Canonical Correlation

Barbara Hazard Munro

Objectives for Chapter 12

After reading this chapter, you should be able to do the following:

1. Test the assumptions underlying regression.
2. Understand the statistics generated by a canonical correlation.
3. Interpret the results section of research studies reporting canonical correlation.

TESTING REGRESSION ASSUMPTIONS

Before the Analysis

As with all analyses, there are steps to be taken before conducting an analysis. Checking for outliers and being sure that variables are normally distributed are important whenever parametric techniques are being used. In addition, when linear regression is being used, one should check the bivariate relationships to be sure they are linear. Scatter diagrams can be used to visualize the relationship between each pair of variables. A problem for behavioral researchers is the interrelatedness of the independent variables. This is called *multicollinearity*.

Multicollinearity

Because variables collected in behavioral research often provide very similar information, they are often highly correlated with each other. Such high interrelatedness makes evaluation of results problematic. Schroeder (1990) and Fox (1997) provide details on diagnosing and dealing with multicollinearity. Indications of the problem include high correlations between variables (>0.85); substantial R^2 but statistically insignificant coefficients; unstable regression coefficients (ie, weights that change dramatically when variables are added or dropped from the equation); unexpected size of coefficients (much larger or smaller than expected); and signs (positive or negative) that are unexpected.

The *tolerance* of a variable is used as a measure of collinearity. It is the proportion of the variance in a variable that is not accounted for by the other independent variables (SPSS, 1999c). To obtain measures of tolerance, each independent variable is treated as a dependent variable and is regressed on the other independent variables. A high multiple correlation indicates that the variable is closely related to the other independent variables. If the R^2 were 1, then the independent variable would be completely related to the others. Tolerance is simply $1 - R^2$; therefore, a tolerance of 0 $(1 - 1 = 0)$ indicates perfect collinearity. The variable is a perfect linear combination of the other variables. Tolerances may be requested as part of the output in the regression procedure. By default, tolerances are set as criteria for entry into regression equations. These values may be changed by the investigator.

The *variance inflation factor* is the reciprocal of tolerance (SPSS, 1999c). Therefore, variables with high tolerances have small variance inflation factors, and vice versa.

In Chapter 11, we used regression to predict mental status (see Fig. 11-5). In Figure 12-1, we have added the collinearity statistics to the coefficients that were presented in that analysis. The tolerance values go from a low of .820 to a high of .906. Because the tolerance equals $1 - R^2$, a tolerance of .820 for walking more than a mile means that 18% $(1 - .820 = .18)$ of the variance in this variable is shared with the other predictors. Because the other values for tolerance are even higher, multicollinearity is not a problem in this analysis.

Coefficients (a)

Model		Unstandardized Coefficients		Standardized Coefficients	t	Sig.	Collinearity Statistics	
		B	Std. Error	Beta			Tolerance	VIF
1.	(Constant),	−.210	.905		−.232	.816		
	what is the highest grade or year of school that you completed?	.246	.022	.500	11.227	.000	.906	1.103
	age	.002	.011	.008	.171	.864	.906	1.103
2	(Constant),	−1.067	.932		−1.145	.253		
	what is the highest grade or year of school that you completed?	.240	.022	.487	10.993	.000	.897	1.115
	age,	.004	.011	.017	.382	.703	.892	1.121
	did you feel full of pep	.067	.073	.042	.917	.360	.827	1.208
	walking more than a mile	.278	.109	.118	2.551	.011	.820	1.220

a Dependent Variable: Count backward from 100 by subtracting 7. Interviewer stops at 5 answers. Score # correct answers before 1st mistake.

FIGURE 12-1. Collinearity statistics.

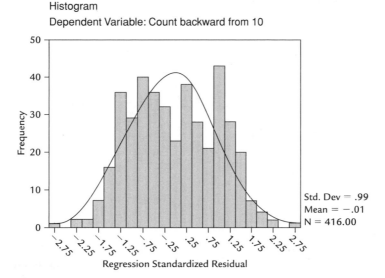

FIGURE 12-2. Histogram of residuals.

TESTING ASSUMPTIONS BY ANALYZING RESIDUALS

Another important tool for checking the assumptions is residual analysis. Verran and Ferketich (1987) present an overview of the use of residual analysis to test linear model assumptions. The residual is the difference between the actual and the predicted score. If the analysis were perfect, there would be no residuals; they would be zero.

NORMAL DISTRIBUTION

If the relationships are linear and the dependent variable is normally distributed for each value of the independent variable, then the distribution of the residuals should be approximately normal (SPSS, 1999c). This can be assessed by using a histogram of the standardized residuals (Fig. 12-2). The normal curve is interposed on the standardized residuals. On the counting backward from 100 by 7s score, the residuals are fairly normally distributed, but there are peaks at 1.25 and .75 standard deviations below the mean and at 1.0 standard deviation above the mean. It is possible to transform the data mathematically if residual analysis indicates violation of the assumption of normality.

HOMOSCEDASTICITY

To check this assumption, the residuals can be plotted against the predicted values and against the independent variables. When standardized predicted values are plotted against observed values, the data would form a straight line from the lower-left corner to the upper-right corner, if the model fit the data exactly. Although the

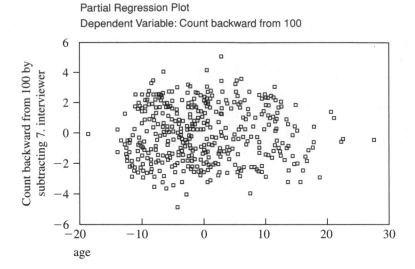

FIGURE 12-3. Plot of residuals against independent variable.

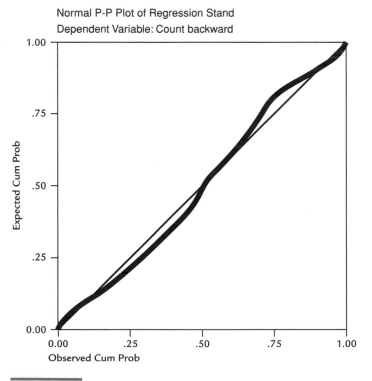

FIGURE 12-4. Normal probability plot.

regression line is not drawn, if you took a ruler and drew a line from the lower-left to the upper-right corner, you would have it. In Figure 12-3, we demonstrate plotting residuals against one of our independent variables, age. Note that the actual scores vary around the prediction line. When the residuals are from a normal distribution, the plotted values fall close to the line in the normal probability plot (SPSS, 1999c). Figure 12-4 is an example from our analysis. Basically, this is a different look at what we saw in the histogram. There are peaks above and below the mean.

Summary of Assessing Assumptions in Regression Analysis

It is important, as always, to check data before it is entered into an analysis for normality, linear relationships, and so forth. In addition, we can request collinearity statistics and analyses of residuals as part of our computer analysis. It is very important to check these assumptions; otherwise, the results may be very questionable, and future analyses may show quite different results.

CANONICAL CORRELATION

Research Question

When calculating a multiple correlation, you have more than one independent variable but only one dependent variable. Often, however, we are interested in more than one dependent variable. We could run separate regressions for each dependent variable, but that would not allow us to explore all the variation in the data. A method that takes all the information into account, thus giving a better understanding of all the relationships, is *canonical correlation*. This technique measures the relationship between a set of independent variables and a set of dependent variables. For example, Bournaki (1997) studied the responses of school-aged children to venipuncture. The independent variables included the age of the child, medical fears, distractibility, and sensory threshold. There were three outcome measures: pain quality, behavioral responses, and magnitude in heart rate change. She used canonical correlation to examine the relationships between the independent and dependent variables. The method of least squares is used to give two composites, one for the independent variables (sometimes called the variables on the left) and one for the dependent variables (variables on the right). Because of the complexity of the analysis, this technique was rarely used until sophisticated computer software became available. Use of the technique is increasing, and overviews of the method have been presented in the literature. For example, Wikoff and Miller (1991) discussed the use of canonical analysis in a "Methodology Corner" in *Nursing Research*. Although the variables are weighted through the procedure of canonical correlation, the main emphasis of this technique is on assessing relationships, rather than on prediction.

Type of Data Required

To calculate a correlation coefficient, r, there must be at least two measures on each subject. It is often assumed that both of these measures must be at the interval level.

In most cases, however, valid results also may be obtained with ordinal data. More-over, we can code categorical variables for use with r and with canonical correlation equations. Mathematically, it is possible to use any level of data when calculating r, but factors other than the level of the data must be considered when deciding whether a correlation coefficient is appropriate.

Assumptions

Although we can calculate correlations with data at all levels, certain assumptions must be made if we are to generalize beyond the sample statistic; that is, if we are to make inferences about the population itself:

1. The sample must be representative of the population to which the inference will be made.
2. The variables that are being correlated, say X and Y, must each have a normal distribution; that is, the distribution of their scores must approximate the normal curve.
3. For every value of X, the distribution of Y scores must have approximately equal variability. This is called the assumption of homoscedasticity.
4. The relationship between X and Y must be linear; that is, when the two scores for each individual are graphed, they should tend to form a straight line. The points will not all fall on this line, but they should be scattered closely around it.

Power Analysis

As with multiple regression, there must be adequate numbers of subjects per inde-pendent variable or the results will be distorted. The calculations are fairly complex for determining sample size and power, but one can use computer programs for this determination.

Results of Canonical Correlation

More than one canonical correlation coefficient can be generated from a single analysis, because each coefficient represents the relationship between one factor in one of the groups of variables and a related factor in the other group. In this way, canonical correlation is like factor analysis. As is demonstrated in Chapter 14, there may be several factors in a group of variables. If there are three factors in one set of variables and three related factors in the second group of variables, three canonical correlation coefficients might emerge, one for each pair of factors. There cannot be more canonical correlation coefficients (Rcs) than there are variables in the smaller set. For example, Bournaki (1997) had four independent variables and three dependent variables; thus, the most Rcs that could be calculated is three. The vari-ance accounted for by each Rc is unique. The first canonical correlation accounts for the largest amount of variance, the second accounts for the second-largest amount, and so on. The procedure ends when no significant Rcs are left.

Canonical Correlation Terminology

A *canonical variate* is a weighted composite of the variables in a set. It is a "new" variable or construct derived from the original variables. *Canonical weights*, which are in standard score form, are generated for each variable. Like standardized regression coefficients (betas), they are used more for explanation than for prediction. Because they are in standard score form, they indicate the relative importance of the variable with which they are associated. They must be interpreted with caution, however. Canonical weights, like the betas in regression equations, may be unstable because they may vary a great deal from one analysis to another. Because of this, many researchers prefer to interpret loadings called *structure coefficients*. These loadings represent the correlation between the canonical variates and the real (or original) variables. If there is a high correlation between the new variable (canonical variate) and the original variables, the canonical variate represents what the original variables were measuring. Loadings or structure coefficients of 0.30 or higher are treated as meaningful (Pedhazur, 1982). They are interpreted like the loadings in factor analysis. The higher loadings give meaning to the canonical correlation and are used to name it. The square of a loading is the proportion of variance accounted for, so you can say how much of the variance is accounted for by an *Rc*.

To test the significance of a canonical correlation, *Wilks' lambda* is used. Lambda varies from 0 to 1 and stands for the error variance, the variance not accounted for by the independent variables. Thus, it is interpreted in an opposite way to the squared multiple correlation, R^2. A 1 means that the independent variables are not accounting for any of the variance in the dependent variable, and a 0 means that the independent variables are accounting for all of the variance. The smaller the lambda, the greater the variance accounted for. One minus lambda would be equivalent to R^2. A chi-square statistic (called Bartlett's test) is used to test the significance of lambda.

The *redundancy* of the variables is often mentioned when canonical correlation results are presented. The higher the redundancy, or correlation, among a group of variables, the better the ability to predict from one group to another.

Computer Analysis

We extend the example used earlier in this chapter and in Chapter 11 for the regression analysis. There we used Wood's (1997) data with a measure of mental status (counting backward) as the dependent variable. In this analysis, we add a measure of the subjects' knowledge of breast self-examination (TOTKNOW) as a second dependent variable. The independent variables: age, years of education (HIGHED), feeling full of pep (FEEL1), and the ability to walk a mile (ADL7) remain the same. Figure 12-5 contains the printout produced by using the macro for canonical correlation in SPSS for Windows (SPSS, 1999b, pp. 396–397).

Two canonical correlations are produced, equal to the number of variables in the smaller set (two dependent variables). The first canonical correlation equals .546. Squaring that (Rc^2), equals .298, which indicates that it explains 29.8% of

(text continues on page 296)

Run MATRIX procedure:

Correlations for Set-1

	AGE	HIGHED	FEEL1	ADL7
AGE	1.0000	−.2963	.0195	−.1094
HIGHED	−.2963	1.0000	.0926	.0963
FEEL1	.0195	.0926	1.0000	.4019
ADL7	−.1094	.0963	.4019	1.0000

Correlations for Set-2

	COUNT	TOTKNOW
COUNT	1.0000	.1364
TOTKNOW	.1364	1.0000

Correlations Between Set-1 and Set-2

	COUNT	TOTKNOW
AGE	−.1397	−.1294
HIGHED	.4984	.2483
FEEL1	.1491	.0037
ADL7	.1860	.0077

Canonical Correlations

1	.546
2	.108

Test that remaining correlations are zero:

	Wilk's	Chi-SQ	DF	Sig.
1	.694	150.233	8.000	.000
2	.988	4.805	3.000	.187

AUTHOR COMMENTS
Only the first canonical correlation is significant.

Standardized Canonical Coefficients for Set-1

	1	2
AGE	.008	−.622
HIGHED	−.943	.091
FEEL1	−.088	−.314
ADL7	−.187	−.639

AUTHOR COMMENTS
Standardized coefficients are like betas in regression.

Raw Canonical Coefficients for Set-1

	1	2
AGE	.001	−.073
HIGHED	−.216	.021
FEEL1	−.065	−.231
ADL7	−.206	−.703

AUTHOR COMMENTS
Raw coefficients are like b-weights in regression.

FIGURE 12-5. Computer output of canonical correlation.

Standardized Canonical Coefficients for Set-2

	1	2
COUNT	−.909	−.438
TOTKNOW	−.310	.961

> **AUTHOR COMMENTS**
> *The canonical loadings (structure coefficients) are usually interpreted.*

Raw Canonical Coefficients for Set-2

	1	2
COUNT	−.427	−.206
TOTKNOW	−.015	.047

Canonical Loadings for Set-1

	1	2
AGE	.306	−.585
HIGHED	−.972	.185
FEEL1	−.251	−.574
ADL7	−.314	−.688

Canonical Loadings for Set-2

	1	2
COUNT	−.952	−.307
TOTKNOW	−.434	.901

Redundancy Analysis:

Proportion of Variance of Set-1 Explained by Its Own Can. Var.

	Prop Var
CV1-1	.300
CV1-2	.295

Proportion of Variance of Set-1 Explained by Opposite Can.Var.

	Prop Var
CV2-1	.089
CV2-2	.003

Proportion of Variance of Set-2 Explained by Its Own Can. Var.

	Prop Var
CV2-1	.547
CV2-2	.453

Proportion of Variance of Set-2 Explained by Opposite Can. Var.

	Prop Var
CV1-1	.163
CV1-2	.005

——— END MATRIX ———

FIGURE 12-5. (*Continued*)

the variance. The second canonical correlation (.108) explains about 1.2% of the variance. Only the first canonical correlations is significant ($ps = .000$ and .187). Next, two sets of coefficients associated with the independent variables (Set 1) are presented. The standardized canonical coefficients are like the beta weights in regression. They are based on the standard scores of the variables and indicate the relative importance of each variable. The raw canonical coefficients are equivalent to the *b*-weights in regression and can be used to calculate predicted scores based on subject's actual scores. Next, the standardized and raw canonical coefficients for the dependent variables (Set 2) are presented. Finally, the canonical loadings for each set are presented. These are what are generally interpreted. They represent the correlations between the dependent and canonical variables and are also called structure coefficients. Values greater than .30 are treated as meaningful.

Using the rule that coefficients greater than .30 are meaningful, and paying attention to the signs associated with the loadings, we can say that the first canonical variate indicates that having lower mental ability and less knowledge of breast self-examination are related to being older having less education and having less ability to walk a mile. Feeling full of pep is not meaningful in this analysis. Because the second canonical correlation is not significant. It is not interpreted.

Example from the Literature

Table 12-1 contains a table from the Bournaki (1997) study described earlier. What was the maximum number of canonical variates possible? The answer is three, because there were three variables in the smaller set (the dependent variables). Only two of the three were significant, however. Now try to interpret the two variates. The author has helped by putting an "a" next to loadings greater than or equal to 0.30. As always, it is important to know how a variable is scored to interpret the sign associated with the relationship. In this study, for example, a higher score indicates higher distractibility but lower sensory threshold. On the first variate, we see that older children with a higher sensory threshold have lower quality of pain, fewer behavioral changes, and a lower magnitude of heart rate change. The second variate indicates that younger children who have fewer fears and are less distractible have higher pain quality and a higher magnitude of heart rate changes. The author reports that it is children with more fears who have higher pain quality, and that makes sense, so there may be a typographical error in the table in relation to the loading -0.582 associated with medical fears on the second variate. The variable is scored so that a higher score indicates higher fear. Thus, the negative relationship indicates lower fears with higher pain.

SUMMARY

Canonical correlation is an extension of multiple regression that enables the researcher to include more than one dependent variable in the analysis. It is a powerful technique that helps us study the complex relationships that exist in health care research.

TABLE 12-1 *Canonical Correlation Analysis Summary Table between Age, Distractibility, Threshold, and Medical Fears (Set 1) and Pain Quality, Behavioral Responses, and Heart Rate Magnitude (Set 2)*

Variables Sets	Canonical Variates	
	1	2
Set 1: independent variables		
Age of child	0.884[a]	−0.328[a]
Medical fears	−0.146	−0.582[a]
Distractibility	−0.251	−0.793[a]
Threshold	−0.572[a]	−0.504[a]
Set 2: dependent variables		
Pain quality	−0.463[a]	0.414[a]
Behavioral responses	−0.994[a]	0.055
Magnitude in heart rate change	−0.308[a]	0.912[a]
Canonical correlations	0.526	0.411
	$p < 0.001$	$p = 0.014$
Variance explained	12.0%	5.7%
Total variance explained	17.7%	

[a]Structure coefficients $\geq$ 0.30.
From Bournaki, M. C. (1997). Correlates of pain-related responses to venipunctures in school-age children. *Nursing Research, 46*(3), 152.

Application Exercises and Results

Exercises

1. The following is the same analysis requested in the exercise for Chapter 11, but now we ask you to request the collinearity statistics and a histogram of the residuals. What is the multiple correlation of three sets of predictors and overall state of health? The first set of predictors contains age and years of education. The second set contains confidence and life satisfaction. The third set contains smoking history and satisfaction with current weight.

2. What is the canonical correlation between the following two sets of variables: the predictor set (age, education, smoking history, depressed state of mind, exercise, and current quality of life) and the outcome set (positive psychological attitudes and overall state of health).

Results

1. The results are the same as those reported for the exercise in Chapter 11. Here we will concentrate on the multicollinearity statistics and the histogram of the residuals (Exercise

Fig. 12-1). An examination of the tolerances in model 3 indicates that two of the variables, confidence and life satisfaction, have low tolerances, indicating multicollinearity. Because tolerance is equal to $1 - R^2$, the tolerance for self-confidence indicates that 58% of the variance is shared with other variables. For life satisfaction, 60% of the variance is shared. Because these are two subscales from one instrument, it is not surprising that they are highly correlated. Thus, it would be better to use one or the other of these variables or to use the total IPPA score rather than the two subscale scores. The histogram of the residuals indicates more scores at the positive side of the mean. The variable is health, and because these data were drawn from friends of doctoral students, it is no wonder that most of the subjects were healthy. Obviously, students would be unlikely to ask a sick friend to complete their questionaire.

Regression

Coefficients (a)

Model		Unstandardized Coefficients		Standardized Coefficients	t	Sig.	Collinearity Statistics	
		B	Std. Error	Beta			Tolerance	VIF
1	(Constant),	7.124	.373		19.123	.000		
	subject's age,	−.017	.005	−.128	−3.321	.001	.996	1.004
	education in years	.083	.019	.165	4.280	.000	.996	1.004
2	(Constant),	3.336	.424		7.876	.000		
	subject's age,	−.018	.005	−.136	−4.026	.000	.988	1.013
	education in years,	.041	.017	.081	2.348	.019	.962	1.040
	CONFID,	.011	.007	.084	1.638	.102	.429	2.331
	LIFE	.043	.005	.419	8.072	.000	.422	2.368
3	(Constant),	3.075	.422		7.291	.000		
	subject's age,	−.013	.004	−.093	−2.825	.005	.953	1.050
	education in years,	.035	.017	.069	2.084	.038	.942	1.061
	CONFID,	.009	.007	.068	1.372	.170	.421	2.374
	LIFE,	.036	.005	.354	6.971	.000	.403	2.480
	Smoking history,	−.219	.085	−.087	−2.586	.010	.920	1.087
	satisfaction with current weight	.163	.022	.252	7.479	.000	.916	1.091

a Dependent Variable: overall state of health.

EXERCISE FIGURE 12-1. Regression diagnostics. Collinearity statistics.

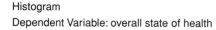

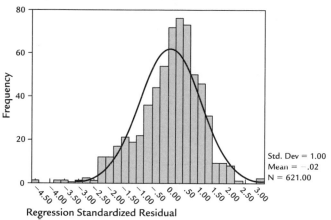

Histogram
Dependent Variable: overall state of health

Std. Dev = 1.00
Mean = −.02
N = 621.00

Regression Standardized Residual

EXERCISE FIGURE 12-1. (*Continued*)

2. The results of the canonical correlation are contained in Exercise Figure 12-2. Both canonical correlations are significant. The first accounts for 55% of the variance, the second 9%. We have included just the canonical loadings because they are what is usually interpreted. We would interpret the first canonical variate as indicating that positive psychological attitudes and good health are associated with being less depressed, exercising more, and reporting a higher current quality of life. The second canonical variate indicates that people who are younger, smoke less, and exercise more are healthier.

Run MATRIX procedure:

Canonical Correlations

1   .740
2   .306

Test that remaining correlations are zero:

	Wilk's	Chi-SQ	DF	Sig.
1	.410	547.670	12.000	.000
2	.907	60.233	5.000	.000

Canonical Loadings for Set-1

	1	2
AGE	.034	−.613
EDUC	.251	.173
SMOKE	−.225	−.357
DEPRESS	−.855	.234
EXER	.481	.670
QOLCUR	.794	−.016

Canonical Loadings for Set-2

	1	2
TOTAL	.965	−.263
HEALTH	.697	.717

———— END MATRIX ————

EXERCISE FIGURE 12-2. Canonical correlation, Exercise 2.

Logistic Regression

Barbara Hazard Munro

As described in Chapter 11, multiple regression is used extensively by researchers. It allows us to find the best fitting and most parsimonious model to describe the relationship between the dependent variable and a set of independent or predictor variables.

Although the independent variables can be of differing levels of measurement (nominal to ratio), the dependent variable is supposed to be continuous and meet the assumptions underlying the technique. Suppose, however, the outcome measure is categorical. For example, in medical and epidemiologic studies, outcomes may be occurrence or nonoccurrence, mortality (dead or alive), and so forth. It is possible to code a dichotomous outcome variable as 1 or 0 and run a regression. In that case, the statistics generated will be the same as if you ran a *discriminant function analysis*. With more than two outcome categories, multiple regression cannot be used. Although discriminant function analysis may be used, logistic regression is more often the technique of choice. People who have studied the methods report that logistic regression is better suited to the data, and the results include *odds ratios* that lend interpretability to the data.

The odds of an outcome being present as a measure of association has found wide use, especially in epidemiology, because it approximates how much more likely (or unlikely) it is for the outcome to be present given certain conditions. For example, when looking at lung cancer in smokers and nonsmokers, an odds ratio of 2 indicates that smokers had twice the incidence of lung cancer in the study population. The odds ratio approximates another indicator called *relative risk*. Before describing logistic regression, we present a brief overview of discriminant function analysis, because it is still reported in the literature.

DISCRIMINANT FUNCTION ANALYSIS

Research Question

Discriminant function analysis allows us to distinguish among groups based on some predictor variables. The mathematical function that combines information from predictor variables to obtain the maximum discrimination among groups is called the *discriminant function*. With two groups, the results are the same as using multiple regression with a dummy-coded dependent variable.

Type of Data Required

This technique tells us which set of predictors will most clearly distinguish among these groups. When we use this technique, we are interested in explanation and prediction. We want to know which factors are most related to these groups and how well they can predict group membership. The aim of the procedure is to find a way to maximize the discrimination among groups. As with canonical correlation, more than one statistic may be derived. The most discriminant functions that can be derived are one less than the number of categories in the dependent variable or the number of independent variables, whichever is smaller. The first discriminant function derived from the data explains most of the between-group variance, the second discriminant function explains the next largest piece of variance, and so on. These functions are not correlated with each other. All the variables may be entered at once, or a stepwise procedure may be used to select the most discriminating variables. Eigenvalues and their associated canonical correlations are used to judge the most discriminating variables. Eigenvalues represent the amount of variance explained by a discriminant function.

As with multiple regression, each variable is weighted, and these weights may be used to calculate a discriminant score for each subject. The mean of the discriminant scores for a given group is called the *centroid*.

The discriminant functions are calculated by a method similar to factor analysis. Principal components analysis is used on a matrix of indices of discrimination between and within groups. This type of analysis discriminates among subjects, rather than among variables. Rotation may be used to increase the interpretability of the functions.

Wilks' lambda (L) is used to measure the association between the independent and dependent variables. Using the discriminant function scores, the members of the known groups are classified to see how well the system works. We want to know what percentage are classified correctly and what percentage are classified incorrectly.

The analysis produces *raw coefficients* (like *b*s in multiple regression), *standardized coefficients* (like betas), and *structure coefficients* (like those in canonical correlation). The raw coefficients are commonly used to calculate scores for each individual. The standardized coefficients represent the relative importance of the independent variables with which they are associated. Like betas, they should be interpreted with caution, however, because they tend to be unstable.

The correlations between the discriminant score for each individual and the scores on the original variables are called *structure coefficients*, or *loadings*. The square of that coefficient is the proportion of variance in a particular variable explained by the discriminant functions. Structure coefficients of 0.30 or greater are considered meaningful (Pedhazur, 1982). These coefficients are used to interpret the discriminant functions.

Assumptions

When studying this method of analysis, the general conclusion is that discriminant function estimators are sensitive to the assumption of normality. In particular, the estimators of the coefficients for nonnormally distributed variables are biased away from zero. The practical implication for dichotomous independent variables is that the discriminant function estimators will overestimate the magnitude of the association (Hosmer & Lemeshow, 1989).

When the dependent variable has only two values—either the event occurs or it does not—the assumptions underlying regression analysis are violated because the distribution of errors is not normal but binomial (because the outcome is either 1 or 0) (SPSS, 1999d). Discriminant analysis does allow direct prediction of group membership, but the assumption of multivariate normality of the independent variables and equal variance–covariance matrices in the two groups are required for the prediction rule to be optimal. "Logistic regression requires far fewer assumptions than discriminant analysis; and even when the assumptions required for discriminant analysis are satisfied, logistic regression still performs well" (SPSS, 1999d, p. 35). In logistic regression, estimates of the probability of an event are given. This provides information not obtainable from regression weights. The method of least squares is used in regression. The coefficients minimize the squared distances between the observed and predicted scores. In logistic regression, the *maximum likelihood method* is used. This means that the coefficients make our observed results most likely. The logistic model is nonlinear; when graphed, the data assume an S-shaped curve. Therefore, an iterative algorithm is necessary for parameter estimation. This technique is used more often now that the computer software is available.

ODDS RATIOS VERSUS RELATIVE RISK

Before giving an example of logistic regression, we need to explain some of the terms used with this analysis. An *odds ratio* is defined as the probability of occurrence over the probability of nonoccurrence. Table 13-1 contains data from a study on the abuse

TABLE 13-1 *The Relationship between Smoking During Pregnancy and Low Birth Weight*

Count

| | | Low birth weight | | Total |
		no	yes	
smoking	no	2165	144	2309
	yes	670	76	746
Total		2835	220	3055

From: Hawkins, J. W., Pearce, C. W., Kearney, M. H., Munro, B. H., Haggerty, L. A., Dwyer, J., Higgins, L. P., Aber, C. S., & Mahony, D. (1996). *Abuse, women's self-care, and pregnancy outcomes.* Funded by the National Institute for Nursing Research, National Institutes of Health AREA grant 1 R15 NRO4246-01.

of pregnant women (Hawkins et al. 1996) to demonstrate calculations of an odds ratio. Data were collected from 3,055 women. Of those, 220 had a baby that weighed less than 2,500 grams (LBW), and 2,835 did not. Seven hundred and forty-six of the women reported smoking during their pregnancy, and 2,309 did not.

Table 13-2 contains probabilities based on the data in Table 13-1. The probability of having a normal weight infant when the mother does not smoke during pregnancy is calculated as the number of normal weight infants in the group with

TABLE 13-2 *Probabilities*

Probability of Normal Birth Weight with No Smoking

$$\frac{\text{Normal weight}}{\text{No smoking}} \quad \frac{2165}{2309} = 0.94$$

Probability of Low Birth Weight (LBW) with No Smoking

$$\frac{\text{LBW}}{\text{No smoking}} \quad \frac{144}{2309} = 0.06$$

Probability of Normal Birth Weight with Smoking

$$\frac{\text{Normal weight}}{\text{smoking}} \quad \frac{670}{746} = 0.90$$

Probability of LBW with Smoking

$$\frac{\text{LBW}}{\text{smoking}} \quad \frac{76}{746} = 0.10$$

TABLE 13-3 *Odds*

Odds of low birth weight (LBW) infant, when No Smoking:

$$\frac{\text{Probability of occurrence}}{\text{Probability of nonoccurrence}} = \frac{.06}{.94} = .06$$

Odds of LBW infant, with Smoking:

$$\frac{\text{Probability of occurrence}}{\text{Probability of nonoccurrence}} = \frac{.10}{.90} = .11$$

nonsmoking mothers over the total number who did not smoke during pregnancy (2,165/2,309). The resulting probability is 0.94. In the same way, the probability of a low birth weight (LBW) baby with a nonsmoking mother is the number of LBW babies (144) over the total number of nonsmoking mothers (2,309). Therefore, for nonsmoking women, the probability of having a normal weight baby is 0.94 and that of having an LBW infant is 0.06. For the smoking mothers, the probabilities are 0.90 for normal weight and 0.10 for LBW.

The odds of an event are the probability of occurrence over the probability of nonoccurrence. The odds of these events are presented in Table 13-3. The odds of having an LBW infant for nonsmoking mothers is 0.06 and for smoking mothers is 0.11. The odds ratio, which is the ratio of one probability to the other, is calculated as 1.85 in Table 13-4. We can say that the odds of having an LBW infant are almost two times greater when the woman smokes than when she doesn't.

Odds ratios are used to estimate what epidemiologists call *relative risk*. A risk is the number of occurrences out of the total. Relative risk is the risk given one condition versus the risk given another condition. Table 13-5 contains the calculation of the risks of LBW with and without smoking. Table 13-6 contains a calculation of the relative risk. The relative risk of LBW is 1.67 times higher for women who smoke. The odds ratio is at least equal to relative risk but often overestimates it, especially if the occurrence of the event is not rare. Here the odds ratio was 1.85, and the relative risk was 1.67. Because odds ratios are generated by the logistic regression procedure, it is important to understand what they are and not confuse them with actual measures of relative risk.

TABLE 13-4 *Odds Ratio*

Ratio of one probability to the other:

$$\frac{.11}{.06} = 1.85$$

TABLE 13-5 *Risks of Low Birth Weight*

Without Smoking:

$$\frac{144}{2309} = .06$$

With Smoking:

$$\frac{76}{746} = .10$$

LOGISTIC REGRESSION

Research Question

Logistic regression is used to determine which variables affect the probability of a particular outcome. For example, McCullagh, Lusk, and Ronis (2002) studied the factors influencing the use of hearing protection among farmers. Interpersonal support, barriers, and situational influences were significantly related to the decision to use hearing protection. For every 1 point increase on the measure of interpersonal support (a 3-point scale), the odds of using hearing protection went up 7 times. The sensitivity (users correctly classified) was 72%, and specificity (nonusers correctly classified) was 85%.

Type of Data Required

In logistic regression, the independent variables may be at any level of measurement from nominal to ratio. Nominal-level variables must be coded before entry, as discussed in Chapter 11 on multiple regression. The dependent variable is categorical, and until recently most statistical software programs handled only dichotomous dependent variables. SPSS Regression Models 9.0 (1999d) provides two procedures for logistic regression. The first, called *binary*, is used when the outcome variable has only two values. The second procedure, called *multinomial logistic regression* (also referred to as *polychotomous logistic regression*), can be used for outcome variables with two or more values. In this chapter, we will confine ourselves to describing the binary model.

TABLE 13-6 *Relative Risk*

$$\frac{.10}{.06} = 1.67$$

Issues Related to Power

Computer software and books such as Cohen (1987) do not cover logistic regression. As more people use the technique, it is reasonable that authors will add calculations of effect and sample sizes to their materials.

Computer Analysis

The data in this example come from the study of abuse of pregnant women (Hawkins et al., 1996). Almost 3,000 women were included in the sample. The outcome variable is dichotomous with two groups: those who had a LBW (less than 2,500 grams) infant and those who did not. The predictor variables are:

1. GAINRISK—A dichotomous variable where those who gained less that 15 pounds = 1, and those who gained more = 0.
2. HTNRISK—risk of hypertension = 1, no risk = 0.
3. NUMPNC—number of prenatal visits. Ranged from 0 to 39.

Figure 13-1 contains an edited version of the printout. The dependent variable, LBW, was entered as 0 = normal weight baby, and 1 = LBW baby. This is appropriate coding for the logistic regression procedure, so the original (value given by the investigator) and internal (value assigned by the computer) are the same. If the data had been entered as LBW = 1 and normal weight = 2, for example, the variable would have been recoded.

CODING

Just as in multiple regression, categorical independent variables are coded. You can use dummy- (indicator), effect (deviation), or orthogonal coding. The computer program will produce the dummy or effect coefficients for you. You name the variable and tell it what type of coding you want. You also can specify orthogonal contrasts.

Interaction terms also may be entered into the equation. This is especially important when considering risk factors. Does smoking and low weight gain increase the odds of LBW more than adding up the odds of each taken separately?

−2 LOG LIKELIHOOD

"The probability of the observed results, given the parameter estimates, is known as the *likelihood*. Since the likelihood is a small number, less than 1, it is customary to use −2 times the log of the likelihood (−2 LL) as a measure of how well the estimated model fits the data" (SPSS, 1999d, p. 45). In regression, we evaluate models with and without particular variables to determine whether they are making a significant contribution to the explanatory power. In logistic regression, comparison of observed to predicted values is based on the log likelihood (LL) function. A good model is one that results in a high likelihood of the observed results. This means a small value for −2 LL. (If the model fit perfectly, −2 LL would equal 0.) In our example, for the logistic regression model containing only the constant, −2 LL equals 1481.285.

(text continues on page 310)

Logistic Regression

Dependent Variable Encoding

Original Value	Internal Value
no	0
yes	1

Block 0: Beginning Block

a Constant is included in the model.
b Initial -2 Log Likelihood: 1481.285.
c Estimation terminated at iteration number 5 because parameter estimates changed by less than .001.

Classification Table (a,b)

			Predicted		
			Low birth weight		Percentage Correct
	Observed		no	yes	
Step 0	birth weight <2500g	no	2694	0	100.0
		yes	205	0	.0
	Overall Percentage				92.9

a Constant is included in the model.
b The cut value is .500.

Block 1: Method = Enter

Omnibus Tests of Model Coefficients

		Chi-square	df	Sig.
Step 1	Step	64.796	2	.000
	Block	64.796	2	.000
	Model	64.796	2	.000

AUTHOR COMMENTS
Step—*If variables within block are entered in steps, tests each step, ie, each variable separately. Because variables in this example were entered as a group within the block, step = block.*
Block—*Test of variables entered in this block.*
Model—*Test of overall model at this point.*

FIGURE 13-1. Computer output, logistic regression.

Model Summary

Step	-2 Log likelihood	Cox & Snell R Square	Nagelkerke R Square
1	1416.489	.022	.055

AUTHOR COMMENTS
Cox & Snell and Nagelkerke are estimates of the variance accounted for in the analysis. Here they indicate that 2.2% to 5.5% of the variance has been accounted for.

Hosmer and Lemeshow Test

Step	Chi-square	df	Sig.
1	.001	1	.977

AUTHOR COMMENTS
The nonsignificant goodness of fit test (p = .977) indicates that the data fit the model.

Classification Table (a)

	Observed		Predicted		
			Low birth weight		Percentage
			no	yes	Correct
Step 1	birth weight <2500g	no	2694	0	100.0
		yes	205	0	.0
	Overall Percentage				92.9

a The cut value is .500.

Variables in the Equation

		B	S.E.	Wald	df	Sig.	Exp(B)
Step 1(a)	GAINRISK	1.094	.192	32.357	1	.000	2.986
	HTNRISK	1.229	.190	41.938	1	.000	3.418
	Constant	-2.875	.088	1059.521	1	.000	.056

a Variable(s) entered on step 1: GAINRISK, HTNRISK.

AUTHOR COMMENTS
Exp (B) = odds ratio

Block 2: Method = Enter
Omnibus Tests of Model Coefficients

		Chi-square	df	Sig.
Step 1	Step	90.776	1	.000
	Block	90.776	1	.000
	Model	155.572	3	.000

FIGURE 13-1. (*Continued*)

Model Summary

Step	−2 Log likelihood	Cox & Snell R Square	Nagelkerke R Square
1	1325.713	.052	.131

Hosmer and Lemeshow Test

Step	Chi-square	df	Sig.
1	17.005	8	.030

Classification Table (a)

			Predicted		
			Low birth weight		Percentage
	Observed		no	yes	Correct
Step 1	birth weight <2500g	no	2692	2	99.9
		yes	200	5	2.4
	Overall Percentage				93.0

a The cut value is .500.

Variables in the Equation

		B	S.E.	Wald	df	Sig.	Exp(B)
Step 1(a)	GAINRISK	.997	.199	25.110	1	.000	2.710
	HTNRISK	1.278	.198	41.738	1	.000	3.588
	NUMPNC	−.174	.019	84.474	1	.000	.840
	Constant	−.968	.207	21.880	1	.000	.380

a Variable(s) entered on step 1: NUMPNC.

FIGURE 13-1. (*Continued*)

CLASSIFICATION TABLE

At this point, no variables are in the equation and the best that can be done is simply predict that each individual will fall into the larger category. In this case, far more subjects had normal weight babies, so everyone is predicted as falling into that category. So for the actual 2,694 normal weight infants, the prediction is correct (specificity), but for all the LBW infants (205) the prediction (sensitivity) is incorrect.

The method is enter, which means that all the variables were entered together in each step, not in a stepwise fashion. Two variables, weight gain risk, and hypertension risk, were entered in the first block; the third variable, number of prenatal visits, was entered in block 2.

OMNIBUS TESTS OF MODEL COEFFICIENTS

The chi-square is based on the difference between successive -2 LLs. In other words, does adding our predictors do anything for the model? It tests the null hypothesis that the coefficients for the independent variables equal 0. This is comparable to the overall F in regression. As you can see in the table, there are three chi-squares, one for Step, one for Block, and one for Model. In this analysis, the variables were entered together in each block, so the values for Step and Block are the same throughout. If we had entered the variables in a stepwise fashion within each block, those values would vary. In the first Block, there is also no difference between the values for Block and Model, as the model at that point only includes those variables entered in the first block.

Two variables were entered in the first block, the risks of low weight gain and of hypertension. -2 LL changed from the initial value of 1481.285 to the current value of 1416.489. The difference between those two values is 64.796, which, as you can see is the chi-square value. It is the difference between -2 LL for the model with only a constant and -2 LL for the complete model. The result is significant ($p = .000$). The null hypothesis is rejected, indicating that the two variables add to the model. In the model summary table there are values for Cox & Snell and Nagelkerke R Squares. The variance explained thus far is only 2.2% to 5.5%. The Nagelkerke is a modification of the Cox & Snell, which cannot equal 1 (SPSS, 1999d).

GOODNESS OF FIT STATISTIC

This statistic compares the observed probabilities to those predicted by the model (like regression, in which you compare the scores that would be predicted for each subject given the prediction equation with the scores they actually received). In other words, it examines the residuals. When the significance is large for the test of -2 LL or the goodness of fit statistic, you do not reject the null hypothesis that the model fits. In other words, a nonsignificant result indicates that the model fits; a significant result indicates that it does not fit. The goodness of fit statistic is tested by the Hosmer-Lemeshow Test. We see that the chi-square is .001 with 1 df, and the p value is .977. This indicates that the model does fit the data.

CLASSIFICATION TABLE

In our example, we see that 205 subjects were misclassified (all of the low birth weight infants). At this block, the model has no value in terms of specificity (0%). It is still simply placing all subjects in the normal birth weight category.

VARIABLES IN THE EQUATION

The b-weights associated with each independent variable and the constant term are given in the first column. The b-weights in multiple regression are used to create a prediction equation; that is, knowing a person's score on each variable, we can use the weights and the constant term to predict the individual's score on some outcome measure. In logistic regression, these weights are used to determine the probability of a subject doing one thing or the other. In our example, this is the probability of having a low birth weight infant or not. Instead of a score, as with the continuous variables used as dependent variables in regression, we get a probability from 0 to 1. Because this variable was coded as LBW = 1, and no LBW = 0, if the probability is greater than 0.5, the prediction would be for a LBW infant; if less than 0.5, the infant would be predicted to be normal weight. We demonstrate the formula for these calculations after explaining the other columns in this section. The signs associated with the *b*-weights indicate the direction of the relationship. Looking at the signs, both of which are positive, we would predict that those with low weight gain and risk of hypertension would be more likely to have a LBW infant.

The next column contains the standard errors for the predictors and the constant. In general, a statistic is divided by its standard error to give the value that is tested for significance. For large sample sizes, the test that a *b* coefficient is equal to 0 can be based on the Wald statistic, which has a chi-square distribution. When a variable has 1 *df*, the Wald statistic is simply the square of the result of dividing the *b* value by its standard error. For example, the coefficient for GAINRISK is 1.094. Dividing that by the standard error of .192 and then squaring the result equals the Wald value of 32.357. (For categorical variables, the Wald statistic has *df*s equal to one less than the number of categories.) The value is significant at the .000 level. The Wald statistic has an undesirable property: When the absolute value of the regression coefficient becomes large, the estimated standard error is too large. This produces a Wald statistic that is too small, leading to nonsignificant results, even when the null hypothesis should be rejected. When you have a large coefficient, you should not rely on the Wald statistic for hypothesis testing. Instead, you should build a model with and without that variable and base your hypothesis test on the difference between the two likelihood-ratio chi-squares (SPSS, 1999d).

Exp (B) is the odds ratio. Mathematically, this is *e* (the base of the natural logarithm, 2.718) raised to the power of *b*. In this example, 2.718 raised to the power of 1.094 (*b* for GAINRISK) is 2.986. Remember that the odds ratio is the ratio of one probability to the other. In this example, it is the probability of having a LBW infant over the probability of having a normal weight infant. In linear regression, *b* indicates the amount of change in the dependent variable for a one-unit change in the independent variable with the other variables held constant. To understand logistic coefficients, we need to think in terms of the odds of an event occurring. The logistic coefficient (*b*) is the change in the log odds associated with a one-unit change in the independent variable with the other variables held constant. Thus, if GAINRISK went up 1 point, the log odds would go up 2.986. The confidence intervals around the odds ratios can be requested. The odds ratio does not fall in the middle of the confidence interval the way mean scores do. This is due to the J-shaped distribution of the data used in maximum likelihood analyses.

DIAGRAM OF OBSERVED GROUPS AND PREDICTED PROBABILITIES

The predicted classification is based on the probabilities, that is, greater than or less than 0.5. As you can see, all the subjects were had probabilities lower than .5 and were, therefore, predicted to have normal weight infants.

We entered one more variable in block 2. Now -2 LL = 1325.713. The difference between the original -2 LL of 1481.285 and 1325.713 equals 155.572, the figure given for the Model; and the difference between -2 LL at the first block (1416.489) and -2 LL at the second block (1325.713) equals 90.776, listed for the Block. What this means is that testing "Model" means that you are testing the overall model at this point in the analysis, whereas testing "Block" is a test of what this block of variables added to the model. Because there was only one variable entered in this Block, Block and Step are the same. We would say that the overall model is significant ($p = .000$), and the variables entered in this block (number of prenatal visits) made a significant contribution ($p = .000$).

The amount of variance accounted for ranges from 5.2% (Cox & Snell) to 13.1% (Nagelkerke). The Hosmer and Lemeshow goodness of fit test is significant ($p = .030$), indicating that the data do not fit the model well. Looking at the classification table, we see that the model still is unable to specify accurately those who will have a LBW infant and those who will not. Because the model is so poor, we could not draw conclusions from it, but to complete the analysis for the sake of pedagogy, we look at the variables. All made significant contributions, but did not account for enough of the variance in the outcome variable to provide a useful prediction. The odds ratios indicate that having low weight gain increases the odds of having a LBW infant 2.7 times. Hypertension increases the odds of having a LBW infant 3.6 times. For every 1-point increase on the measure of number of prenatal visits, the odds of a LBW infant go up .840.

The clearest use of the odds ratio is when the independent variable is categorical. Because this variable is not categorical, its interpretation is much less clear. The number of prenatal visits varied from zero to 39. A one-visit increase in that scale is not of any practical interest. You can calculate the odds for some more meaningful change by multiplying the b value by the change you want and then performing an exponentiation on that number. For NUMPNC, if 10 visits were of interest, $-.174 \times 10 = 1.74$. Raising 2.718 to the power of 1.74 = 5.70 so for every decrease (due to negative sign) of 10 visits NUMPNC, the odds go up 5.70 times of having a LBW infant.

Because the odds ratio is usually the parameter of interest in a logistic regression because of its ease of interpretation, be aware that as a point estimate, the distribution is skewed, because it is bounded away from zero. If the sample size is large enough, this is not a problem. Confidence intervals often are used to demonstrate more clearly the odds ratio. These interval estimates are provided in some software packages. (An exponentiation is performed on the usual formula; that is, you raise 2.718 to a power derived from the b-weight $\pm$ 1.96 $\times$ the standard error.)

Example

The following example helps clarify the relationships expressed in this table of variables in the equation. The probability of an event is determined by the following formula:

$1/1 + e^{-z}$
e = base of the natural logarithm, 2.718
z = constant + $b_1X_1 + b_2X_2 + b_3X_3 + \cdots$

In our example:

$$z = -.968 + .997(\text{GAINRISK}) + 1.278(\text{HTNRISK}) - .174(\text{NUMPNC})$$

Ratings of two individuals:

	Angeleen	*Wilaiporn*
Low weight gain	1	1
Hypertension	1	0
Number of prenatal visits	10	10

Our two students (these are the names of actual students in my class, but their scores are fictional) have identical scores except that Angeleen had hypertension and Wilaiporn did not. What is the probability of each of these having an LBW infant, given the data collected?

First, the z-scores for each individual are calculated as:

Angeleen: $z = -.968 + .997(1) + 1.278(1) - .174(10) = -.433$
Wilaiporn: $z = -.968 + .997(1) + 1.278(0) - .174(10) = -1.711$

The formulas for determining the estimated probabilities of these individuals having an LBW infant are:

$$\text{Angeleen } \frac{1}{1 + 2.718^{-(-.433)}}$$

$$\text{Wilaiporn } \frac{1}{1 + 2.718^{-(1.711)}}$$

$$\text{Angeleen } \frac{1}{1.6486} = .6066$$

$$\text{Wilaiporn } \frac{1}{1.1807} = .8470$$

Because both probabilities are more than 0.5, we would predict that both of these women would have an LBW infant. As we pointed out, the odds of an event are the probability of occurrence over the probability of nonoccurrence. Thus, for our subjects, the odds of falling into the depressed group are:

$$\text{Angeleen } \frac{.6066}{1 - .6066} = 1.54$$

$$\text{Wilaiporn } \frac{.8470}{1 - .8470} = 5.54$$

and the odds ratio is: $\dfrac{5.54}{1.54}$

We would say that the odds for Angeleen having an LBW infant are 3.59 times higher than for Wilaiporn. The only difference in their scores on the three predictor variables was that Angeleen had hypertension and Wilaiporn did not. Look again at the odds ratio for HTNRISK. It is 3.588, the same as the odds ratio for Angeleen and Wilaiporn. What we have demonstrated is that a 1-point increase on a variable results in an increase in odds as listed in Exp(B), the odds ratio.

Example from the Literature

Table 13-7 contains a table from the McCullagh, Lusk, and Ronis (2002) article that was mentioned in the beginning of this chapter. They studied the factors associated with the use of hearing protection among farmers. As you can see in the table, all three variables were significantly related to the use of hearing protection. For every 1-point increase on the 3-point interpersonal scale, the odds of using hearing protection goes up seven times. Situational influences was measured on a 6-point scale. A 1-point increase is associated with an odds ratio of 1.82. You can calculate other point increases as previously described. For example, if you were interested in a 3-point change, you would multiply the *b*-weight by the desired change (.61 × 3 = 1.83), and then raise 2.1718 to the power of 1.83 (6.23). Then, you could say that for every 3-point increase in situational influences, the odds of using hearing protection go up six times.

TABLE 13-7 *Logistic Regression of Selected Model Variables on HPD*

Variable	b	SE	Likelihood Ratio Statistic	p	Odds Ratio	CI
Barriers	−1.76	.38	31.82	<.005	.18	.08–.36
Interpersonal support	1.93	.60	11.89	<.005	7.12	2.12–22.45
Situational influences	.61	.24	6.93	<.025	1.82	1.16–2.82
Constant	.56	1.48				

Note: HPD = hearing protection device.
Chi-square = 67.39, df = 3.
*p < .0001.
From: McCullagh, M., Lusk, Sally L., & Ronis, D. L. (2002). Factors influencing use of hearing protection among farmers. *Nursing Research, 51*(1), p. 37.

SUMMARY

Logistic regression is now more commonly reported when the outcome measure is categorical. As with all methods of regression, it is of utmost importance to select variables for inclusion in the model based on a clear scientific rationale. You can use a stepwise method (forward or backward) in which variables are selected strictly on statistical criteria. An alternative selection method is best subsets. Stepwise, best subsets, and other mechanical selection procedures have been criticized because they are based solely on correlations derived from variables measured with some error. Following the fit of the model, the importance of each variable included in the model should be verified (SPSS, 1999d). This should include the examination of the Wald statistic for each variable and a comparison of each estimated coefficient with the coefficient from the univariate model containing only that variable. Variables that do not contribute to the model based on these criteria should be eliminated and a new model fit. The new model should be compared with the old model through the likelihood ratio test. Once you have obtained a model that you believe contains the essential variables, you should consider whether to add interaction terms.

As with regression, residuals may be examined to evaluate the model. The residuals in logistic regression are the differences between the observed and predicted probabilities of an event. They should be normally distributed with a mean of 0 and a standard deviation of 1.

Deviance compares the predicted probability of being in the correct group based on the model to the perfect prediction of 1. It can be viewed as a component of $-2\ LL$, which compares a model to the perfect model. Large values for deviance indicate that the model does not fit the case well.

Logistic regression programs are available with most of the software packages for the personal computer; they manage model building with a dichotomous outcome variable very well and provide the additional benefit of odds ratios, which lend interpretability to the data. Programs for managing outcomes with more than two categories are also available.

Application Exercises and Results

Exercises

1. Calculate the odds, odds ratio, risks, and relative risk of smoking when not on a sports team.

	Smokes	
On a Sports Team	*Yes*	*No*
No	270	500
Yes	50	430

2. Recode the depressed state of mind variable into a dichotomous variable with two groups: those who rated themselves as rarely depressed are scored 0, and those who rated themselves as sometimes to routinely depressed are scored 1. Using the new variable as the outcome measure, determine which of the following variables increase the odds of being depressed:

   1. Smoking history: recoded into currently smoking = 1, and not currently smoking = 0.

   2. Gender: male = 0; female = 1.

   3. Quality of life in the past month: recoded so that values 1 to 3 (sometimes to very unhappy) become 0, and 4 to 6 (sometimes to extremely happy) become 1.

   4. Total score on the Inventory of Positive Psychological Attitudes scale (IPPA) (Kass et al., 1991). Enter recoded smoking history and gender in the first block and recoded quality of life and total IPPA score in the second block.

Results

1.

On a Sports Team	Smokes		Row Totals
	Yes	No	
No	270	500	770
Yes	50	430	480
	320	930	1,250

Probabilities:

Of smoking when not on team	270/770 = 0.35
Of not smoking when not on team	500/770 = 0.65
Of smoking when on team	50/480 = 0.10
Of not smoking when on team	430/480 = 0.90

Odds:

Of smoking when not on team	0.35/0.65 = 0.54
Of smoking when on team	0.10/0.90 = 0.11
Odds ratio:	0.54/0.11 = 4.91

Risks:

Of smoking when not on team	270/770 = 0.35
Of smoking when on team	50/408 = 0.10
Relative risk:	0.35/0.10 = 3.5

The odds of smoking when not on a team are almost 5 times higher than when on a team. The relative risk of smoking when not on a team is 3.5 times higher.

2. A logistic regression was run to answer the research question (n = 653). The results are contained in Exercise Figure 13-1. The variables were entered in two blocks. Smoking status and gender were entered in block 1, which was significant (p = .003), and

accounted for 1.8 to 2.4% of the variance. The Hosmer and Lemshow Test indicated a good fit ($p = .808$). Only smoking made a significant contribution ($p = .001$). Quality of life and total IPPA score were entered in block 2, which was significant ($p = .000$). The total model was significant ($p = .000$), and accounted for 34.3 to 45.7% of the variance. The model was a good fit (Hosmer and Lemeshow, chi-square $= 4.068$, df $= 8$, $p = .851$). The sensitivity of the model in predicting depression was 72.3%. The specificity in predicting those who were not depressed was 80. Three of the variables, smoking status ($p = .032$), quality of life ($p = .000$), and total IPPA score ($p = .000$) were significant predictors. The odds of being depressed were 2 times higher for those who smoked. Higher quality of life was related to lower probability of depression. The IPPA scale is scored from 30 to 210, therefore, a 1-point increase in that score would be of no practical interest. To calculate the effect of a 30-point change in IPPA, multiply the *b*-weight for TOTAL times 30 and raise 2.1718 to that power ($.057 \times 30 = 1.71$), raising 2.1718 to the power of 1.71 $= 5.53$. So, for every 30-point increase in the IPPA score the odds of being depressed go down (negative *b*-weight) 5.5 times.

Logistic Regression

Dependent Variable Encoding

Original Value	Internal Value
Rarely	0
Sometimes to routinely	1

Block 1: Method = Enter

Omnibus Tests of Model Coefficients

		Chi-square	df	Sig.
Step 1	Step	11.848	2	.003
	Block	11.848	2	.003
	Model	11.848	2	.003

Model Summary

Step	−2 Log likelihood	Cox & Snell R Square	Nagelkerke R Square
1	892.445	.018	.024

Hosmer and Lemeshow Test

Step	Chi-square	df	Sig.
1	.059	1	.808

Variables in the Equation

		B	S.E.	Wald	df	Sig.	Exp(B)
Step 1(a)	SMOKEREC	.903	.273	10.978	1	.001	2.468
	GENDER	.169	.166	1.037	1	.309	1.184
	Constant	−.275	.137	4.039	1	.044	.759

a Variable(s) entered on step 1: SMOKEREC, GENDER.

Block 2: Method = Enter

Omnibus Tests of Model Coefficients

		Chi-square	df	Sig.
Step 1	Step	262.275	2	.000
	Block	262.275	2	.000
	Model	274.123	4	.000

EXERCISE FIGURE 13-1. Logistic regression results.

Model Summary

Step	−2 Log likelihood	Cox & Snell R Square	Nagelkerke R Square
1	630.170	.343	.457

Hosmer and Lemeshow Test

Step	Chi-square	df	Sig.
1	4.068	8	.851

Classification Table (a)

	Observed		Predicted		Percentage Correct
			Depression recoded		
			rarely	sometimes to routinely	
Step 1	Depression recoded	Rarely	273	66	80.5
		Sometimes to routinely	87	227	72.3
	Overall Percentage				76.6

a The cut value is .500.

Variables in the Equation

		B	S.E.	Wald	df	Sig.	Exp(B)
Step 1(a)	SMOKEREC	.771	.359	4.621	1	.032	2.162
	GENDER	.225	.206	1.187	1	.276	1.252
	QOLREC	−1.066	.292	13.320	1	.000	.344
	TOTAL	−.057	.005	117.961	1	.000	.944
	Constant	9.433	.832	128.681	1	.000	12499.450

a Variable(s) entered on step 1: QOLREC, TOTAL.

EXERCISE FIGURE 13-1. (*Continued*)

Exploratory Factor Analysis

Jane Karpe Dixon

Objectives for Chapter 14

After reading this chapter, you should be able to do the following:

1. Identify research situations in which factor analysis would be appropriate.
2. Describe the steps involved in carrying out a factor analysis procedure.
3. Interpret factor analysis results from a computer printout or published study.

FACTOR ANALYSIS

Researchers in the health care fields often focus their attention on multiple variables. This is a direct result of the nature of the problems under study, which are complex in the real world of patient care. For example, with regard to major causes of illness and death in the developed world (eg, cancer, heart disease, stroke, diabetes, accidents), we have learned to speak of risk factors rather than one single cause. In some cases, a particular disease may exist only in the presence of a particular agent (eg, clinical mononucleosis with the Epstein-Barr virus). Even then, however, variables describing personal and environmental characteristics are crucial in influencing the course of the illness or even whether symptoms occur. Also, multiple issues affect such nursing concerns as recuperation following surgery and self-management of chronic disease. In other chapters of this book, we discuss how multivariate strategies can be used to understand the way multiple causes may lead to a single event. Factor analysis is often an early step in the process of achieving a multivariate perspective on a clinical research problem.

This chapter addresses the understanding of concepts. Often when labeling variables, a single word or phrase is used to represent a phenomenon with multiple parts. Our language may be overly general, blending together the multiple aspects of the phenomenon of interest. Consider, for example, the term *satisfaction with care*. Superficially, it seems logical to measure this with a single rating. ("Rate your satisfaction with the care you received.") However, such a rating might involve opinions on a variety of matters, such as perceived competence of caregivers, convenience, and pleasantness of the environment. (As an exercise, think of at least two other aspects of satisfaction with care.) It is hard to know which of these influences are reflected in a subject's satisfaction rating and what such a rating really means. Instead of a global rating, should the various aspects be measured separately? There are so many potential variables, we may be unable to decide which should be measured and which should not. Factor analysis can help us make such decisions.

The amount of information on which our minds can focus simultaneously is limited. As a convenience, we may concentrate on variables thought to be primary. This will reduce the data burden. In some research endeavors, however, such simplicity of questionnaire may not be necessary, because we have techniques for organizing multivariate data—data on many variables. Factor analysis is one of these techniques. Factor analysis can serve the purpose of data reduction. In factor analysis, many variables are "reduced" (grouped) into a smaller number of factors. This is analogous to univariate approaches in which a mean, variance, or correlation coefficient is calculated to reduce individual scores on one or two values. In this chapter, the purposes of factor analysis are explained, and the steps used to carry out a factor analysis are introduced. Because factor analysis is a complex technique, and it is carried out by computer, this chapter emphasizes interpretation rather than calculation. Confirmatory factor analysis, an advanced form of factor analysis, is presented in Chapter 15.

RESEARCH QUESTIONS

To explicate the types of research questions that can be answered using factor analysis, a hypothetical example of a factor analysis situation may be helpful. Suppose a researcher measures six variables within a sample of adult female participants in a health maintenance organization. Three of these variables are aspects of body size: height, arm length, and leg length. Three are derived from a health history in which the subject is asked to report the number of specific episodes occurring in the last year. These variables are number of sore throats, number of headaches, and number of earaches. A researcher may want to see how these variables group—which ones go together and which ones do not? How strongly does each variable go with its group? Altogether, how many dimensions are needed to explain relationships among the variables (Nunnally & Bernstein, 1994)? You may begin to explore answers to these questions through careful examination of the patterns of correlations among these variables. In the matrix of correlations for these six variables, we will probably see that the three size variables have high intercorrelations and that

TABLE 14-1 *Six × Six Correlation Matrix: Size and History Variables*

	Height	Arm Length	Leg Length	Number of Sore Throats	Number of Headaches	Number of Earaches
Height	—	Hi	Hi	Lo	Lo	Lo
Arm Length		—	Hi	Lo	Lo	Lo
Leg Length			—	Lo	Lo	Lo
Number of Sore Throats				—	Hi	Hi
Number of Headaches					—	Hi
Number of Earaches						—

"Hi" means correlation of high magnitude, regardless of direction (approaching 1.00 or approaching −1.00).
"Lo" means correlation of low magnitude (near zero).

the three history variables also have high intercorrelations; that is, a woman with longer than average legs also may have longer than average arms. She is also likely to be taller than average. A person reporting frequent sore throats also may report other discomforts. On the other hand, it would be surprising if the size variables and the history variables were highly related.

A simplified representation of a correlation matrix is shown in Table 14-1. If such a matrix is factor analyzed, a factor matrix defining the two groups of variables would be derived, as shown in Table 14-2. Each column in this table reflects one of the variable groupings or factors. The size variables have high values in one column, and the history variables have high values in the other column. This table, indicating the

TABLE 14-2 *Abbreviated Factor Matrix: Size and History Variables*

	Factors	
	I	*II*
Height	Hi	Lo
Arm Length	Hi	Lo
Leg Length	Hi	Lo
Number of Sore Throats	Lo	Hi
Number of Headaches	Lo	Hi
Number of Earaches	Lo	Hi

"Hi" Means above 0.40 or below −0.40 (especially approaching 1.00 or −1.00).
"Lo" means between 0.40 and −0.40 (especially near zero).

presence of two distinct groups of variables—two factors—summarizes the information contained in the larger correlation matrix. It reduces the data. Thus, we see that much of the information from a 6 × 6 correlation matrix is also conveyed in a 6 × 2 factor matrix.

You may object that the groupings derived were already easily apparent from the correlation table and that an advanced statistical technique is not needed to show what is obvious. This is true, but in the usual case, factor analysis does help us know what we would not otherwise know. Suppose that we had a 20 × 20 correlation matrix with widely ranging correlation coefficients, and the groupings among the variables were subtle. The variables would appear in random order, rather than neatly arranged according to grouping. Then patterns would not be obvious. Factor analysis is a tool through which we may uncover groupings of variables that are not obvious.

USE OF FACTOR ANALYSIS

Factor analysis is a statistical tool for analyzing scores on large numbers of variables to determine whether there are any identifiable dimensions that can be used to describe many of the variables under study. Sometimes researchers assume that observed covariation between variables is due to some underlying common factors. The collection of intercorrelations is treated mathematically in such a way that underlying traits are identified.

Factor analysis may be exploratory or confirmatory. This chapter concerns exploratory factor analysis, which is used to summarize data by grouping together variables that are intercorrelated. Most often, this occurs in the early stages of research. Chapter 15 concerns confirmatory factor analysis, which tests hypotheses about structure of variables. Confirmatory factor analysis may follow an exploratory factor analysis, or it may come directly from theory. Exploratory factor analysis and confirmatory factor analysis are complementary techniques that are often used together in a single study or coordinated program of research.

The direct purpose of exploratory factor analysis is to reduce a set of data so that it may be described and used easily. This usually occurs in the context of instrument development. Theory construction work may also be involved.

Instrument Development

In the research literature of nursing and other health care professions, factor analysis is most often used as a part of the instrument development process. Factor analysis may be a vital step in creation of a new measurement tool. It is a method for organizing the items into factors. A factor is a group of items that may be said to belong together. A person who scores high on one item of a particular factor is likely to score above average on other items of the factor and vice versa. Such an item has high correlations with other items of the same factor and not so high correlations with items of different factors. This principle provides the mathematical basis for assignment of items to factors through the statistical technique of factor analysis.

Factor analysis is often used to test the validity of ideas about items in order to decide how items should be grouped together into subscales and which items should be dropped from the instrument entirely. The method helps to provide justification for our use of summated scales (sets of items summed into scale scores). For example, a researcher may start with 18 items and based on factor analysis decide that these should be organized into two subscales: For each subject, two scores will be calculated. It is also common for some items to be dropped from a scale based on factor analysis results. Factor analysis is an important statistical tool for providing validity evidence concerning the structure of our instruments. In most cases, this is followed by computation of Cronbach's alpha coefficient, which is a measure of internal consistency reliability. Such reliability is an alternative way of looking at the extent to which items go together, similar to the factor analysis itself; however, in computation of reliability, only one set of items is dealt with at a time. Also, reliability computations are useful for further identifying weak items that may be omitted in subsequent analysis. In any case, items that form a strong factor in factor analysis generally yield acceptable alpha coefficients when grouped together in a scale, thus providing evidence of internal consistency reliability, as well as supporting beginning evidence of construct validity for a developing scale.

Theory Development

The building of theory is a principal purpose of research, and factor analysis may support such efforts in a variety of ways: by describing clinical phenomena, exploring relationships, identifying constructs that unite a set of elements, creating units of classification for systems construction, and testing hypotheses. All of these are theory-building functions. Ideally, development of theory and of instruments are closely related endeavors.

It is in relation to the theory development purpose of factor analysis that the distinction between exploratory and confirmatory goals is of most importance. In a truly exploratory approach, a researcher uses factor analysis to discover a structure that can be meaningfully interpreted. The researcher begins without preconceived expectations about the nature of the structure that will emerge; rather, the structure is allowed to unfold from the data. In a truly confirmatory approach, a hypothesis is developed, and variables relevant to that hypothesis are then identified and (once data are collected) submitted to factor analysis. The researcher asks whether the data fit the hypothesized model better than they fit alternative models. More details on this approach appear in the Chapter 15.

Data Reduction for Subsequent Analysis

Sometimes factor analysis is used solely for data reduction, simply because such reduction may be needed for subsequent analysis. One goal of scientific inquiry is parsimony, simplicity of explanation; that is, it is preferable to use one variable, rather than many, to explain a phenomenon. Factor analysis provides a means for creating a single composite variable out of many variables. Often it is used to identify several composite variables, which taken together, summarize the sources of variance contained in all (or most) variables included in a study (or at least of those variables of a particular type). These composite variables are mathematically constructed through a combination of the measured variables. The several composite variables, rather than the larger number of measured variables, are then used in subsequent data analysis. Data reduction of this sort may serve a highly pragmatic function. The researcher may collect a large amount of data, reduce the data through factor analysis, and conduct other analyses (such as regression or analysis of variance) on the reduced data. In these subsequent analyses, the number of variables relative to the number of subjects is kept within reasonable bounds, reliability is augmented, and provided that the meanings of factors are clearly defined and communicated, interpretation of the analysis may be simplified. Often, this is combined with instrument development or theory development.

TYPE OF DATA REQUIRED

Most often, the factor analysis process begins with raw data of subjects by variables and the calculation of Pearson product-moment correlations between these variables. However, you may also carry out a factor analysis based simply on a correlation matrix, even without access to the raw data by subjects. Whatever the actual starting point, the correlation matrix is submitted to factor analysis.

You are already familiar with the correlation matrix, the beginnings of many of our statistical treatments. In such a matrix, the two halves are identical; that is, the correlation of X with Y is the same as the correlation of Y with X. We call such a matrix symmetrical. Factor analysis may be performed on any symmetrical matrix of correlations.

In the development of a new instrument, however, it is common for some items to be eliminated from consideration prior to conducting factor analysis. This is based on the univariate and multivariate characteristics of each item. This systematic evaluation of individual items is called *item analysis*. For example, Fleury (1998) created the Index of Self-Regulation to measure self-regulation in the maintenance of health behavior change. From a sample of cardiac rehabilitation patients, data were collected on 37 Likert-type items, but only 16 of these were included in the factor analysis. Others were omitted through the item analysis process. Criteria for inclusion of an item included consideration of item variance of each item. Another criterion was moderate correlations with other items (between .30 and .70). In factor analyzing the 16 items, Fleury obtained three factors that she named cognitive reconditioning, stimulus control and behavioral monitoring.

Criteria used to select some items for factor analysis and eliminate others vary from one study to another; however, they are largely based on understanding of the assumptions and meaning of correlation and the role of factor analysis in summarizing or reducing a correlation matrix.

ASSUMPTIONS

Factor analysis is based on a matrix of correlations between variables, so all data assumptions applicable to calculation and interpretation of correlations apply to factor analysis as well. Data should be interval level or data that the researcher has specifically decided to treat as interval, as typically occurs with Likert-type self-report data. Data should be approximately normally distributed. It is customary to base factor analysis on variables that are measured on a common metric or response format.

A curvilinear relationship between two variables cannot be detected using the Pearson product-moment correlation. Therefore, such a relationship will not be reflected in factor analysis results either.

In general, for meaningful results to be obtained in a factor analysis, correlations between variables should be substantial so that each variable included correlates highly with at least one other variable. It is common to look for correlations with other variables between .30 and .70, as did Fleury (1998) whose work is described earlier. Nunnally and Bernstein (1994) recommend inclusion of marker variables with known properties to increase the likelihood of obtaining substantial correlations. Also, all variables included must be reliably measured, and subjects must show some variation in their responses.

SAMPLE SIZE CONSIDERATIONS AND "POWER"

For statistical tests treated earlier in this book, there is a direct relationship between sample size and power of the test to identify statistically significant differences between groups (or relationships between variables), when such differences (or relationships) exist in the population from which the sample is drawn. With a larger sample size, the ability to generalize from the sample to the population is increased. In exploratory models of factor analysis, statistical significance is not tested, and strictly speaking, the concept of "power" does not apply. However, the value of observed sample data in reflecting reality as it exists in the larger population is a major concern in most factor analytic studies, as in most research generally. It is desirable that our results be generalizable beyond the sample from which the data is obtained.

In factor analysis, the number of subjects needed is usually assessed in relation to the number of variables being measured. Although factor analysis is especially appropriate when working with a large amount of data, the number of variables that may be included in a factor analysis procedure is limited. It is tied to sample size. Certainly, the number of cases should always exceed the number of variables. A ratio of at least 10 subjects for each variable is desirable to generalize from the sample to a wider population. With smaller ratios, the influence of relationships based on random patterns within the data becomes more pronounced. However, Knapp and Brown (1995) note that ratios as low as three subjects per variable are sometimes acceptable. Another perspective on sample size is that because it is based on correlation, 100 to 200 subjects are enough for most purposes. In any case, sample

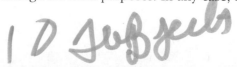

size may be problematic, and the need for replication of factor studies is increasingly apparent. If two different datasets yield similar factor structures, this would greatly increase our confidence that the factor structures obtained may be generalized to other samples not yet studied.

SIX MATRICES

The mathematics of factor analysis is complex. It is based on matrix algebra—the branch of mathematics that deals with the manipulation of matrices. However, matrix algebra is beyond the scope of this book, and you do not need an understanding of matrix algebra to conduct a factor analysis. All mathematics can be done by computer.

The process of conducting a factor analysis, as experienced by the clinical researcher working within the structure of a statistical computer program, is now presented. This process may involve as many as six matrices with each matrix derived from a previous one.

Raw Data Matrix

These are the data that the researcher collects about the study subjects and enters into the computer. Each line contains information about one subject. Each column represents a variable. You are familiar with this sort of matrix; it is the beginning of any data analysis. A raw data matrix to be factor analyzed would contain many variables with data on each variable from many subjects.

Correlation Matrix

You are also familiar with the correlation matrix. When fully depicted, the correlation matrix is a square, symmetrical matrix in which the number of rows and the number of columns each equals the number of variables. Because the correlation matrix is symmetrical (therefore, containing much duplication), it is often depicted in one of several abbreviated forms. The correlation matrix summarizes information in the raw data matrix. It is smaller, with fewer rows and fewer elements than the raw data matrix. This is the beginning of the data-reduction process. In some situations, the correlation matrix is altered prior to conducting the factor analysis. This alteration concerns the diagonal that extends from the upper-left corner to the lower-right corner—the correlation of each variable with itself. Each variable correlates perfectly with itself, so the conventional correlation matrix contains "1.0" as every element in this diagonal. However, in a correlation matrix to be used for a factor analysis, this may not be maintained. Depending on decisions about the factor analysis model to be used, these 1s are sometimes replaced by a number smaller than 1.0 and selected to be specific for each variable, such as an estimate of the common variance with other variables or the reliability of measurement. This is explained later.

Factor Matrix, Unrotated

Based on the correlation matrix, the first of two (or more) factor matrices are calculated. In a factor matrix (Table 14-3), each row represents one variable included in the factor analysis. There are fewer columns, each column representing one factor. In the unrotated factor matrix, the elements within the matrix are the unrotated factor loadings—numbers ranging between -1 and $+1$, which are like correlations of the variable with the factor. The square of a factor loading represents the proportion of variance that the item and factor have in common; in other words, this is the proportion of item variance explained by the factor. For example, in Table 14-3, illustrating an unrotated factor matrix, the first variable (1) has a loading of .85 on factor I; approximately 72% of variance is accounted for by this loading ($[.85]^2 = .7225$). Adding the squared loadings across a row, you arrive at the item communality (h^2). This is the portion of item variance accounted for by the various factors. For variable 1 in Table 14-3, the squared factor loadings are totaled as follows: $.85^2 + .22^2 + .03^2 = .77$. The item communality is .77; that is, 77% of item variance is "explained" by the three factors.

Likewise, if you add the squared loadings contained in a single column, you will obtain the eigenvalue for the factor. The eigenvalue represents the total amount of variance explained by a factor. The average of the squared loadings in a column is obtained by dividing the eigenvalue by the number of items in the column (eigenvalue/n). This average represents the percent of interitem variance accounted for by the factor. For the first factor in Table 14-3, the eigenvalue is calculated as follows: $.85^2 + .15^2 + .51^2 + .83^2 + .26^2 = 1.76$. This eigenvalue of 1.76 is divided by 5 (because there are five variables), yielding .352. Thus, approximately 35% of total item variance is accounted for by the first factor. Adding the percent of variance accounted for by each factor tells us how much variance is explained by all the factors.

Factor eigenvalues and variance accounted for are the most important figures contained in the unrotated factor matrix. You may be especially interested in how

TABLE 14-3 *Factor Loading Matrix*

		Factors			
		I	*II*	*III*	h^2
	1	0.85	0.22	0.03	0.77
	2	0.15	•	•	•
Variables	**3**	0.51	•	•	•
	4	0.83	•	•	•
	5	0.26	•	•	•
Eigenvalues		1.76			
% of variance		0.35			

much variance is accounted for altogether by the important factors; this is simply the sum of variance accounted for by individual factors. Either factor eigenvalues or the variance accounted for by factors may be used to determine the number of potentially interpretable factors contained in the data. Typically, researchers want to interpret the number of factors that each account for at least 5% of variance or the number of factors for which the eigenvalue is 1 or greater. Determination of the appropriate number of factors paves the way for the next matrix of the factor analysis process. However, before moving on to this next matrix, a diversion is needed.

A NOTE ON EXTRACTION MODELS

For the ambitious reader, further explanation is provided here concerning the choices facing the researcher who is conducting a factor analysis. (If you are a less-ambitious reader, you may want to skip this section.) The unrotated factor matrix is obtained through use of an extraction method, and the statistical software packages that are generally used offer a choice of extraction methods. Basically, two general approaches are based on two different assumptions about the data (Ferketich & Muller, 1990).

The distinction has to do with the nature of the variance in the data. One possible assumption is that all measurement error is random. In this case, the mean of deviations (representing the error) is zero. Based on this assumption, a researcher chooses to use the extraction method known as principal components. Using this method of extraction, new variables are exact mathematical transformations of the original data. When this method of extraction is used, all variance in the observed variables contributes to the solution. Because each variable correlates perfectly with itself, the 1s (unities) in the diagonal of the correlation matrix are a part of the variance that is analyzed. Using the principal components method, the goal is to convert a set of variables into a new set of variables that is an exact mathematical transformation of the original data.

The other possible assumption to be made is that measurement error consists of a systematic component and a unique component. The systematic component may reflect common variance due to factors that are not directly measured (Ferketich & Muller, 1990). These are called *latent factors*. Based on this assumption, a researcher chooses to use any of a class of extraction methods categorized as "common factor analysis." This includes methods named *principal axis, image, alpha, generalized least squares*, and *unweighted least squares*. Because the researcher making this assumption wants to focus on the common variance, it is not appropriate to use the full correlation matrix. Instead, the diagonals are altered so that instead of consisting of unities (1s), an estimate of the communalities (h^2) is used. Such modification of a matrix may seem surprising to someone new to factor analysis. In common factor analyses, the matrix analyzed does not reflect the full variance in the data; rather, the covariance is analyzed.

Although some research methodologists place strong emphasis on the distinction between principal components and common factor analysis (Ferketich & Muller, 1990), Nunnally and Bernstein (1994) argue that in a well-designed study involving a sufficient number of subjects, choice of extraction model makes little practical difference in the results obtained. They do note, however, that the principal component method will lead to elements of the matrix being a bit larger. This is because approaches to common factor analysis always involve replacing the "ones" in the diagonal of the correlation matrix with numbers that are less than 1. Thus, the factor loadings that emerge are a bit smaller. We have seen that eigenvalues, variance accounted for by factor, and item communalities are all a direct function of the magnitude of the loadings, so it follows that these are smaller also. Thus, the factor solution may appear to be less good, but this is simply an artifact of the methods decision. Nunnally and Bernstein (1994) also note that the principal components method is more reliable because with this method, you always obtain a factor solution. In common factor analysis, obtaining a solution may not be a sure thing.

Given the potential for differences between extraction methods, some researchers routinely run multiple factor analyses of the same dataset with varying methods. This enables the researcher to gauge the importance of these distinctions and other decision points in the factor analytic process as these affect the specific data under study.

Later in this chapter, we return to the problem of choosing a specific extraction model. Now, we return to discussion of the fourth of six matrices.

Factor Matrix, Rotated

The unrotated factors are created (based on the correlations between variables) so that the amount of variance accounted for by each successive factor is maximized. This means that factors may (in geometric terms) run between independent groups of related variables, rather than accurately reflect the meaning of a group of variables. The consequence of this is that unrotated factors rarely can be meaningfully interpreted. However, just as you may alter an algebraic equation by performing the same operation on both sides, you may transform or "rotate" a factor matrix into any one of an infinite number of mathematically equivalent matrices. If factor rotation is conducted according to the criterion of simple structure as described by Thurstone in 1947, the result is a set of factors that are distinct from one another and that, in most situations, can be meaningfully and creatively interpreted by the researcher. In simple structure, factors are set to maximize the number of loadings of great magnitude (near −1 and +1) and loadings of small magnitude (near 0.00) for each factor; that is, a distinct pattern emerges in the factor matrix so that each factor has certain variables that go with it, while other variables do not. Likewise, as simple structure is approached, each variable is identified with only one factor. According to Thurstone (1947), the following occur in a factor matrix:

1. Each row should have at least one loading close to zero.
2. Each column should have at least as many variables with near-zero loadings as there are factors.
3. For pairs of columns (factors), several variables should load on one and not on the other.

The essence of interpreting factor analytic results is the process of identifying, from the rotated factor matrix, which variables go with a factor and then naming the factor based on whatever meanings these variables with high loadings have in common. The criterion for considering a loading high varies from study to study, with some researchers using cutoff points as low as 0.30; others use cutoff points as high as 0.55. In the example given previously, Fleury (1998) used .40 for her criterion in determining whether or not a particular item loaded substantially on a factor. She also looked for a difference of at least .20 between the highest loading of an item and its next highest loading.

When naming and describing factors, the researcher uses not only knowledge of the statistical technique and how it works, but also an understanding of the subject matter under study, especially an ability to construct new understandings of that subject matter. By facilitating the organization of individual variables into variable groupings, factor analysis opens the door to new conceptualizations and new ways of thinking, provided that the researcher is ready to discover these in the data. More than any other statistical technique, factor analysis requires the full exercise of creative potential.

Factor Score Matrix

Based on the rotated factor matrix, a score for each subject on each factor may be computed. To calculate such factor scores, an individual's score on each variable included in a factor is multiplied by the factor loading for the particular variable. The sum of these products is the individual's factor score.

Factor scores can be calculated automatically within factor analysis procedures in statistical packages for the computer. Consider an individual included in the data of Table 14-3 who received scores as follows:

Variable	Scores
1	2
2	4
3	1
4	5
5	2

This person's factor score on factor 1 would be calculated as follows:

$$(.85)(2) + (.15)(4) + (.51)(1) + (.83)(5) + (.26)(2)$$
$$= 1.7 + .6 + .51 + 4.15 + .52 = 7.48.$$

This factor score, based on the strength of the correlation of each variable with the factor, could be used instead of the individual's unweighted (ie, summative) score on the factor. The factor score is based on the relative "importance" of each variable to the factor as indicated by that correlation. It is conventional among researchers to use factor scores when conducting further analysis on the same dataset. This operationalizes the data reduction purpose of factor analysis.

		Factors			
		I	*II*	•	•
Subjects	1	7.48	•	•	•
	2	•	•		
	•	•	•		
	•	•	•		
	•	•	•		
	n	•	•		

TABLE 14-4 *Factor Score Matrix*

In contrast, when factor analysis is used primarily for the purpose of instrument development, it is conventional to derive an approach for creation of unweighted scores from the factor results obtained. These are the summative scales (usually subscales) that become a part of the protocol for how the instrument is to be scored and interpreted in future usage. This individual's unweighted score would be simply the sum of the scores on the three variables with substantial loadings on the factor (2 + 1 + 5 = 8). This is a much more user-friendly approach for other researchers who will utilize the instrument in future studies.

The factor score matrix has as many rows as subjects, with each column representing one factor. The structure of such a matrix is illustrated in Table 14-4. The factor score matrix is smaller than the raw data matrix because there are fewer factors than variables. The data have been reduced.

Factor Correlation Matrix

Factor rotation is often orthogonal, with resulting factors uncorrelated with each other. This is usually desirable for instrument development, in which the researcher seeks to create subscales that are independent of one another. Alternatively, factor rotation also may be oblique, with factors that are not totally unrelated to each other. Advocates of oblique rotation assert that in the real world, important factors are likely to be correlated; thus, searching for unrelated factors is unrealistic. Novice factor analysts should probably plan to use an orthogonal, rather than oblique, rotation because it is easier to interpret. The Varimax (variance maximized) method, is available on widely used computer packages. This tends to produce factors that have low loadings with some variables and high loadings with other variables. Other alternatives are Quartimax, which is likely to yield a first, very general factor with many high loadings, and Equamax, which combines characteristics of Quartimax and Varimax, balancing the advantages and disadvantages of each.

With orthogonal rotation, one factor loading matrix is produced. It represents regression weights (called a *pattern matrix*) and correlation coefficients (called a *structure matrix*). Because the solution is orthogonal, the regression weights are

TABLE 14-5 *Factor Correlation Matrix*			
	Factor 1	**Factor 2**	**Factor 3**
Factor 1	1.00	0.65	0.30
Factor 2		1.00	0.45
Factor 3			1.00

equal to the correlation coefficients. The loadings are interpreted as were those in the unrotated factor matrix. A squared loading represents the variance accounted for in a variable by a particular factor. The squared loadings may be added across a row to determine total variance accounted for in a variable by all the factors and so on.

Because with oblique rotation there is correlation among the factors, the factor pattern matrix (the regression weights) and the factor structure matrix (containing correlation coefficients) are not the same. The two matrices are produced and interpreted differently. The pattern matrix is generally considered preferable as a basis for interpreting the meanings of factors. The square of a loading in a factor pattern matrix represents the variance accounted for by a particular variable, but because other factors may share some of this variance (due to intercorrelation among factors in an oblique solution), the total variance in an item accounted for by all the factors cannot be determined by adding the squared loadings in a row (h^2).

In oblique rotation, a matrix displaying the correlation of each factor with every other factor is displayed in a factor correlation matrix. The structure of such a matrix is shown in Table 14-5.

STEPS OF A FACTOR ANALYTIC STUDY

The steps of a factor analytic study are as follows:

1. Formulate a research question or hypothesis. If factor analysis is the appropriate statistical technique for answering research questions or testing the hypothesis, proceed with the following steps.
2. Collect data of interest.
3. Calculate and examine univariate data on a variable-by-variable basis, identifying variables that should not be included in the factor analysis because of failure to meet initial assumptions or criteria.
4. Calculate and examine bivariate relationship data—again with an eye toward identifying variables and relationships that should not be included in the factor analysis.
5. "Run" the factor analysis. Unless you have a good reason to do otherwise, use an orthogonal rotation. If you have predicted certain factors, specify in the computer program how many factors you expect; otherwise, let the computer determine the number of factors in the course of the factor analysis, based on eigenvalues

in the unrotated factor matrix. Note the total proportion of interitem variance accounted for by the factor solution and the number of factors involved.

6. Name and interpret factors from the rotated factor loading matrix. (Sometimes researchers experiment with several factor solutions to choose the one that can be most meaningfully interpreted.)

7. If subsequent analyses are planned, use factor analysis results to decide how to combine variables; calculate these new or combined variables for each subject. (Usually, factor scores can be easily calculated on the computer.) Consider the reliabilities of the derived scores. Then conduct the subsequent analyses.

8. Relate findings to the existing literature, and disseminate results through presentation and publication. If appropriate, repeat the analysis with other available populations.

COMBINING FACTOR ANALYSIS WITH OTHER APPROACHES

Factor analysis is often used as an early stage of a multistage analysis, as indicated by steps 7 and 8. Subsequent analyses may be conducted as part of an instrument development and validation process or because of substantive interest. For example, after Lenoci et al., (2002) identified three factors of their Chronic Illness Assessment Interview for Sickle Cell Disease (CIAI-SCD) and determined internal consistency of these as subscales (as well as test-retest reliability), they asessed construct validity by performing a multiple regression analysis using the factors scores to predict self-care behaviors. Scores on *Personal Satisfaction and Perceived Control* factor and *Feeling Concerned and Worried* factor were both positive predictors of self-care behaviors. In another analysis, scores on the *Feeling Supported* factor were related to satisfaction with services received from staff and physicians. The authors note that these findings are consistent with prior studies and with their expectations. These data were taken as evidence of the potential usefulness of the new instrument for adults with Sickle cell disease.

Such findings may have important substantive and instrument development implications. Generally, factor analysis tends to be most useful when combined with other analyses within a single study.

EXAMPLE OF A COMPUTER PRINTOUT

As an example, an edited computer printout of a principal components analysis is shown in Figure 14-1. The data analyzed are from the Inventory of Personal Attitudes (IPA). The dataset, which is provided with this text, includes 30 items. These items are the variables of the factor analysis. Items are shown in Appendix G. Full data on each of the variables was provided by 661 subjects. Thus, there are 22 subjects per variable—well above the 10 to 1 ratio that is recommended. This data was analyzed by principal components extraction method with Varimax rotation using the SPSS computer package.

KMO and Bartlett's Test

Kaiser-Meyer-Olkin (KMO) Measure of Sampling Adequacy.		.964
Bartlett's Test of Sphericity	Approx. Chi-Square	10608.051
	df	435
	Sig.	.000

AUTHOR'S COMMENTS

In this section, KMO Measure of Sampling Adequacy and Bartlett's Test of Sphericity are shown. These results meet criteria and support use of factor analysis for this data.

FIGURE 14-1. Computer printout of a principal component analysis.

The first table shows two approaches that are used to examine the strength of the relationships among the variables as a part of deciding whether factor analysis is appropriate (Norusis, 1993). Bartlett's Test of Sphericity is used to evaluate whether a correlation matrix is suitable for factor analysis by testing the hypothesis that the matrix is an identity matrix—a matrix in which all coefficients not in the diagonal are zeroes. If a low probability is obtained and the hypothesis of an identity matrix is rejected, this supports the use of factor analysis as an appropriate procedure. In this analysis, the probability reported is .000.

The Kaiser-Meyer-Olkin (KMO) measure is based on the principle that if variables share common factors, then partial correlations between pairs of variables should be small when the effects of other variables are controlled. The KMO measure provides an approach to comparing the zero-order correlations to the partial correlations. The KMO measure may vary between zero and one with larger numbers indicating a greater difference between the zero-order correlations and the partial correlations. If a KMO measure in the .80s or .90s is achieved, this supports the use of factor analysis for the data. In this analysis the KMO measure of sampling adequacy is .964. These calculations provide support for preceding with the analysis.

The next table shows communalities for each of the items. The column labeled "initial" presents 1.000 for each of the 30 variables. This simply indicates that the number 1.000 was kept in the diagonal of the correlation matrix that was analyzed—always the case when using the extraction method of principal components. In the column labeled "extraction" there is listing of communalities as calculated for each item, based on the four-factor solution. The communality for the first item may be rounded to .49, indicating that, for that item, $.49^2$ or 24% of variance is accounted for by the four factors.

The next table contains information needed relative to general characteristics of the factors, both before and after rotation. Note that some information ("initial eigenvalues") is provided for 30 potential factors. This is because the number of unrotated factors obtainable equals the number of variables included in a principal components analysis. The purpose of this part of the analysis is, however, to determine how many of the 30 potential factors should be rotated for conceptual interpretation. Three

(text continues on page 339)

Communalities

	Initial	Extraction
energy level	1.000	.492
reaction to pressure	1.000	.651
characterization of life as a whole	1.000	.617
daily activities	1.000	.553
experience anxiety	1.000	.630
expectations of every day	1.000	.566
fearful	1.000	.581
think deeply about life	1.000	.508
productivity of life	1.000	.585
making mistakes	1.000	.525
value of work	1.000	.516
wishing I was different	1.000	.645
defined goals for life	1.000	.517
worrying that bad things will happen	1.000	.622
concentration during stress	1.000	.649
standing up for myself	1.000	.492
adequacy in most situations	1.000	.556
frustration to problems	1.000	.548
sad things	1.000	.514
worthwhile life	1.000	.646
satisfaction of present life	1.000	.629
respond positively in difficult situations	1.000	.595
joy in heart	1.000	.623
when relaxing	1.000	.492
trapped by life	1.000	.615
panic in frightening situations	1.000	.672
thinking about past	1.000	.427
feeling loved	1.000	.612
worry about future	1.000	.474
thinking about problems	1.000	.596

Extraction Method: Principal component analysis.

AUTHOR'S COMMENTS
This table shows initial "communalities" of correlation matrix, as well as communalities derived through the analysis.

FIGURE 14-1. (*Continued*)

Total Variance Explained

Component	Initial Eigenvalues			Extraction Sums of Squared Loadings			Rotation Sums of Squared Loadings		
	Total	% of Variance	Cumulative %	Total	% of Variance	Cumulative %	Total	% of Variance	Cumulative %
1	12.633	42.110	42.110	12.633	42.110	42.110	5.874	19.579	19.579
2	2.107	7.023	49.133	2.107	7.023	49.133	4.422	14.740	34.319
3	1.233	4.111	53.243	1.233	4.111	53.243	3.469	11.563	45.883
4	1.176	3.921	57.164	1.176	3.921	57.164	3.384	11.281	57.164
5	.947	3.158	60.322						
6	.843	2.811	63.134						
7	.777	2.592	65.725						
8	.714	2.379	68.104						
9	.674	2.246	70.350						
10	.648	2.159	72.509						
11	.630	2.101	74.610						
12	.573	1.909	76.519						
13	.536	1.788	78.307						
14	.534	1.780	80.086						
15	.513	1.710	81.796						
16	.475	1.582	83.378						
17	.450	1.500	84.878						
18	.446	1.486	86.364						
19	.425	1.417	87.781						
20	.406	1.354	89.134						
21	.396	1.321	90.456						
22	.376	1.254	91.709						
23	.373	1.242	92.952						
24	.342	1.142	94.093						
25	.335	1.116	95.210						
26	.323	1.077	96.287						
27	.295	.982	97.269						
28	.293	.977	98.246						
29	.273	.909	99.155						
30	.254	.845	100.000						

Extraction Method: Principal component analysis.

AUTHOR'S COMMENTS
In this table, variance accounted for by factors before rotation and after rotation is shown. "Total" refers to total variance accounted for by the factor. This is the eigenvalue. Four factors have eigenvalues greater than one. Only these factors are rotated. "Cumulative %" refers to percent of variance accounted for cumulatively by previous factors and this factor. Thus, the first four factors account for 57.164% of variance—rounded to 57.2%. After rotation, the cumulative % of the four-factor solution remains the same at 57.2%. However, after rotation, variance is more evenly distributed between factors. Printout of this table is pasted together to duplicate how it appears on screen. It prints as two separate tables.

FIGURE 14-1. (*Continued*)

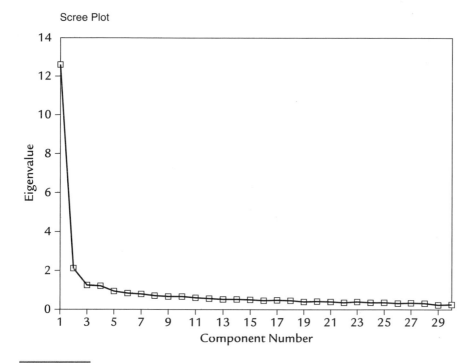

Scree Plot

FIGURE 14-1. (*Continued*)

types of information are given about each potential factor: This includes the total eigenvalue, percent of variance accounted for by this factor, and the cumulative percent of variance accounted for by all factors so far (indicated as "Cumulative %"). The first four factors each have an eigenvalue greater than 1. Variance accounted by these factors (as rounded) is 42%, 7%, 4%, and 4%, respectively. Together, these factors account for 57.2% of the overall variance between items. Based on the criterion that the minimum eigenvalue (for rotated factors) is one, the first four factors are rotated. The second set of three columns simply repeats information already provided for these first four factors. The third set of three columns (under the heading "Rotation Sums of Squared Loadings") provides equivalent information for the factors after rotation. Note that numbers listed under "total" are now considerably closer to each other in value than were the original eigenvalues of the unrotated factors, indicating that the variance is now more equally distributed between the factors. However, both sets account for 57.2% of variance. The total variance accounted for by the four factors has not changed.

In this printout, a plot of eigenvalues was requested. This is called the Scree Plot. It provides a graphic representation of the relative values of eigenvalues. Because eigenvalues often are the key criteria for determining number of factors to be rotated, this can be useful as it provides a basis for identifying a logical breaking point between eigenvalues. This visual representation of eigenvalues may help the researcher to determine the number of factors in the data.

(*text continues on page 342*)

Component Matrix (a)

	Component			
	1	2	3	4
thinking about problems	.764			
joy in heart	.752	−.211		−.118
respond positively in difficult situations	.737			.227
satisfaction of present life	.734	−.280		
worthwhile life	.732	−.265	−.177	
trapped by life	.722	−.178		−.233
wishing I was different	.720		−.327	−.129
characterization of life as a whole	.709	−.240	.235	
sad things	.693	.172		
feeling loved	.690	−.238	−.227	−.165
frustration to problems	.663	.301		.133
productivity of life	.662	−.304	−.206	.113
when relaxing	.659		.136	−.171
adequacy in most situations	.655	.154	−.316	
value of work	.646	−.303		
defined goals for life	.637	−.304		.137
think deeply about life	.634	−.314		
daily activities	.622	−.287	.285	
thinking about past	.613		−.154	−.165
fearful	.611	.338	.116	−.284
panic in frightening situations	.610	.471		.279
experience anxiety	.609	.390	.174	−.279
concentration during stress	.607	.380		.368
making mistakes	.602	.228	−.329	
energy level	.593		.305	.214
standing up for myself	.573	.203	−.348	
worry about future	.549	.112	.197	−.349
reaction to pressure	.524	.450		.404
expectations of every day	.522	−.214	.470	.164
worrying that bad things will happen	.512	.406	.245	−.368

Extraction Method: Principal component analysis.
(a) Four components extracted.

AUTHOR'S COMMENTS
This is the unrotated matrix. You do not use this to interpret the meanings of the factors. Loadings that are near zero are not printed. This helps to make the matrix easier to read.

FIGURE 14-1. (*Continued*)

Rotated Component Matrix (a)

	Component			
	1	2	3	4
daily activities	.695	.111	.124	.205
characterization of life as a whole	.694	.198	.173	.256
expectations of every day	.688	−.121	.209	.186
satisfaction of present life	.647	.363		.268
defined goals for life	.611	.341	.160	
value of work	.592	.381	.123	
think deeply about life	.590	.379	.115	
joy in heart	.575	.434		.309
worthwhile life	.561	.541	.186	
energy level	.560		.374	.195
trapped by life	.548	.366		.424
productivity of life	.534	.528	.145	
respond positively in difficult situations	.507	.328	.453	.159
wishing I was different	.309	.678	.164	.251
feeling loved	.446	.604		.218
adequacy in most situations	.159	.602	.316	.262
making mistakes		.576	.344	.263
standing up for myself		.562	.376	.168
thinking about problems	.468	.483	.260	.275
thinking about past	.274	.480	.139	.319
reaction to pressure	.156		.769	.168
concentration during stress	.216	.194	.731	.172
panic in frightening situations	.114	.255	.728	.252
frustration to problems	.239	.302	.548	.315
sad things	.330	.335	.432	.326
worrying that bad things will happen			.234	.742
experience anxiety	.144	.191	.319	.686
fearful	.153	.246	.281	.646
worry about future	.280	.180		.598
when relaxing	.368	.258	.223	.490

Extraction Method: Principal component analysis. Rotation Method: Varimax with Kaiser Normalization.
(a) Rotation converged in 13 iterations.

AUTHOR'S COMMENTS
This is the rotated matrix. Use this one to interpret meanings of the factors.

FIGURE 14-1. (*Continued*)

The next table, labeled "Component Matrix," is analogous to the unrotated factor matrix. Because the extraction method was principal components analysis, SPSS refers to components rather than factors, but we will continue use of the term *factors* here. This table presents loadings for the four factors extracted. As usual, the first factor is a generalized factor on which all variables load. The other factors have only a few loadings in the moderate range and none above .5. Typically, no attempt is made to derive conceptual interpretations of these unrotated factors.

Next, the four factors with eigenvalues greater than 1 are rotated, and the final solution is derived. The last table, "Rotated Component Matrix," represents the culmination of this effort. These rotated factors are to be conceptually interpreted. Note that the items are listed by strength of loading. In SPSS this is done by checking "sort by size" under Options.

After inspecting the items that load on a factor and their respective loadings, the investigator gives each factor an appropriate name as a way of capturing its meaning. Note that, in contrast to the unrotated matrix previously displayed, this analysis results in a distribution of highest loadings among the four factors. In the naming process, the researcher gives most emphasis to the three or four variables with the highest loadings. Remember that items with negative wordings were reversed as they were coded. In this analysis, the factors may be named Life Satisfaction, Self-Love, Reactivity, and Pessimistic Worry. The researcher should not expect that all items loading on a factor will seem to fit conceptually or that factor names selected will perfectly reflect the meanings of all items. In any case one could calculate a score for each subject on each factor, and these could be used for further analysis.

Other Options

A factor analysis may be considerably more complicated than the one shown here. Rather than principal components analysis, any of a variety of extraction methods representing common factor analysis may be used. Principal axis factoring differs from principal components mainly in that the correlation matrix diagonals are squared multiple correlations, rather than 1s, in the first step. Following this initial step, communalities are estimated from the factor matrix, and factoring is repeated with these communalities in the diagonal. Each such step is one iteration. This is repeated until the estimated communalities and calculated communalities are approximately the same.

Another important method of extraction within the class of common factor analysis is alpha factoring, which is designed to maximize the alpha reliability of the factors. It is assumed that the particular variables measured are a sample of the universe of variables represented by the factor. You want to generalize not to the population of cases from which research subjects were drawn, but to the universe of variables from which the measured variables were sampled. Ferketich and Muller (1990) point out that this method is highly appropriate for instrument development efforts, particularly the early stages.

Other extraction methods available in the common statistical packages are image factoring, unweighted least squares, and generalized least squares. However, these may be less important to the sort of applications discussed here. Finally, the maximum likelihood method of extraction is an available option. This method provides a form of confirmatory factor analysis.

PRESENTATION IN THE LITERATURE

Parshall (2002) employed factor analysis as part of the process of developing an instrument to measure sensory qualities of dyspnea among persons with exacerbated chronic obstructive pulmonary disease (COPD). The researcher notes that dyspnea is the most common symptom of COPD patients in the emergency department (ED). In this study 104 patients who presented to the ED with exacerbated COPD were asked to rate the intensity of the 16 dyspnea sensory quality descriptors, as experienced at 2 points in time—when the person made the decision to come to ED, and 1 week earlier. Intensity ratings could vary from 0 to 10. Factor analysis was reported in detail for the data describing the time point of the decision to come to the ED.

One item ("*I felt that I was breathing more.*") was eliminated prior to the analysis. The researcher reported that this item was confusing to subjects, and the frequency of use by subjects was low. The remaining 15 items were included in a exploratory factor analysis using principal axis factor analysis (PAF) with Varimax rotation. With 104 subjects and 15 items, there is a ratio of 6.9 subjects per item.

Another item was omitted based on the initial factor analysis results. The item ("*My breath did not go all the way in.*") had weak loadings on multiple factors, rather than being strongly associated with a single factor. Thus, the item did not meet the threshold loading used in this study. Nor was the item consistent with simple structure. After this item was eliminated, multiple runs of factor analysis were conducted, varying the number of factors. The researcher found that the five factor solution was best at yielding a clear pattern of loadings. This solution accounted for almost 63% of the total variance between items. This factor solution from the article is reproduced here in Table 14-6. In a footnote to the table, Parshall indicates the names that he assigned to the factors—*Work/Effort; Suffocating/Smothering; Heavy/Rapid; Tight/ Constricted;* and *Shallow/Not Enough.*

Parshall constructs the table so that loadings above .45 are indicated in bold type, other loadings of magnitude greater than .2 are indicated in type which is not bold, and lower loadings are simply omitted leaving some blank space in the published table. This approach to presenting a factor table in publication is intended to be reader-friendly, by emphasizing the information which is most important, and omitting information of lesser importance. The connection between item wordings and factors names is, thus, made clear, even to readers who may not be familiar with the details of factor analysis, but who may be very interested in the content of the research. The table also includes supplementary information about item and factors. Item communalities are shown in a column to the right of the factors. For each factor, information is provided concerning the initial eigenvalues (before rotation), variance accounted for after rotation (rotation sum of squares), percentage of variance explained (also after rotation), and internal consistency reliability as indicated by Cronbach's alpha of the items loading on the factor.

TABLE 14-6 *Rotated Factor Matrix for "Descriptive" Solution (14 Descriptors) at Decision (n = 98)*

Descriptor	Factor[a] 1	2	3	4	5	$h^{2\,b}$
EFFORT	**.79**		.29	.25		.81
WORK	**.70**	.29	.30			.72
OUT OF BREATH	**.54**	.33			.26	.52
SUFFOCATING	.22	**.87**		.27		.94
SMOTHERING	.22	**.63**	.40		.30	.72
COULDN'T BREATHE	.39	**.53**			.25	.52
HUNGER FOR AIR	.44	**.48**	.30		.28	.62
HEAVY	.28	.21	**.61**			.52
NOT OUT ALL THE WAY			**.59**			.40
RAPID	.22	.33	**.46**			.41
CONSTRICTED	.40			**.83**		.89
TIGHT		.37		**.58**		.52
NOT ENOUGH	.41	.22			**.71**	.73
SHALLOW			.26		**.58**	.46
Initial Eigenvalues[c]	6.56	1.14	1.03	0.98	0.88	
Rotation sums of squares	2.32	2.27	1.54	1.35	1.30	
Percentage of variance explained	16.6%	16.2%	11.0%	9.6%	9.3%	
Cronbach's α^{d}	.84	.87	.67	.74	.67	

Bold type indicates primary factor loading for each item.
[a]Factor 1 = Work/Effort; Factor 2 = Suffocating/Smothering; Factor 3 = Heavy/Rapid; Factor 4 = Tight/Constricted; Factor 5 = Shallow/Not enough. Factor loadings <.20 not shown.
[b]h^2 = extraction (final) communalities (row sums of squared loadings).
[c]Eigenvalues = prerotation column sums of squared loadings.
[d]Cronbach's α reported for primary loadings (bold type).
From Parshall, M. B. (2002). Psychometric characteristics of dyspnea descriptor ratings in Emergency Department patients with exacerbated Chronic Obstructive Pulmonary Disease. *Research in Nursing and Health, 25,* p. 339.

Parshall (2002) notes that two of the five factors had low internal consistency reliability, as indicated by Cronbach's alpha below .70. He suggests that this argues "against retention" of these factors. The researcher proceeded to eliminate items one at a time, rerunning the analysis at each step. The optimal solution consisted of seven items and three factors. Factors were named as follows: *Smothering/ Suffocating/Hunger for air, Effort/Work, Tight/Constricted.* This reduced factor solution from the article is shown in Table 14-7. This solution accounted for almost 74% of the variance between items. Parshall (2002) observed that the item referring to *Hunger for air* had a clearer primary loading in the reduced analysis. Further, the

TABLE 14-7 *Rotated Factor Matrix for Reduced Solution at Decision (n = 98)*

Descriptor	Factor[a]			$h^{2\,b}$
	1	2	3	
SMOTHERING	**.82**	.26	.21	.79
SUFFOCATING	**.79**	.22	.34	.79
HUNGER FOR AIR	**.61**	.48		.63
EFFORT	.24	**.90**	.20	.91
WORK	.38	**.71**		.68
TIGHT	.32		**.77**	.71
CONSTRICTED		.47	**.64**	.65
Initial Eigenvalues[c]	4.16	.90	.87	
Rotation sums of squares	2.00	1.89	1.27	
Percent of variance explained	28.5%	27.0%	18.1%	
Cronbach's α[d]	.87	.87	.74	

Bold type indicates primary factor loading for each item.
[a]Factor 1: Smothering/Suffocating/Hunger for air; Factor 2: Effort/Work; Factor 3: Tight/Constricted Loadings <.20 not shown.
[b]h^2 = extraction (final) communalities (row sums of squared loadings).
[c]Eigenvalues = prerotation column sums of squared loadings.
[d]Cronbach's α reported for primary loadings (bold type).
From Parshall, M. B. (2002). Psychometric characteristics of dyspnea descriptor ratings in Emergency Department patients with exacerbated Chronic Obstructive Pulmonary Disease. *Research in Nursing and Health, 25,* p. 339.

explained variance of factor *Tight/Constricted* was twice as high in the reduced analysis (from 9.3% to 18.1%). These results were consistent with qualitative data that were also collected. Ratings describing the 1 week earlier timepoint did not follow the same pattern. It is concluded that this shorter list of items can be used to reliably measure dyspneic sensations of COPD patients presenting in the ED.

In contrast to the tables presented here, sometimes reports of factor analysis present results not as a matrix, but simply as a list of factor names, with items and loadings listed under each name. The reader may consult Lake (2002), for an example of this type of presentation.

SUMMARY

The factor analysis techniques presented in this chapter are distinct from many other statistical techniques in the tremendous potential for researcher creativity to shape understanding of the results obtained. Through application of statistical techniques, you arrive at numbers that indicate groupings of variables in the data. These groups must then be named or described by the researcher, a creative process in which clinical wisdom, knowledge of the literature, and research sophistication must be integrated. This creative process is the key element on which the value of the factor analysis must rest. A factor analysis solution is well suited to inform the creative process. However, factor loadings and eigenvalues are only as valuable as the interpretation of the factors is insightful.

Application Exercises and Results

Exercise

There are many decisions to be made in any factor analysis, and it is common to run factor analysis more than one way in order to see how results compare. Do another factor analysis of the 30 items in the IPA scale. According to the developers of the scale, LIFE consists of the following 17 questions: items 1, 3, 4, 6, 8, 9, 11, 12, 13, 19, 20, 21, 23, 25, 27, 28, 30. CONFIDENCE consists of 13 questions: items 2, 5, 7, 10, 14, 15, 16, 17, 18, 22, 24, 26, 29. This suggests that you might restrict rotation to two factors in order to see how results compare.

Results

We reran the principal components factor analysis with Varimax rotation, again using SPSS, but this time we forced the number of factors to two. Results of our analysis are contained in Exercise Figure 14-1. You can compare your results with ours. You may have selected different rotation and extraction methods, or your printout may look different from ours if you selected different options for presentation or if you used different statistical software. To save space, we have printed only Communalities, Total Variance Explained, and Rotated Component Matrix. The KMO and Bartlett's Test and the Scree Plot would be the same as shown in Figure 14-1.

We see that first two factors together account for 49.1% of the variance between items. Variance explained by the two rotated factors are 8.2 and 6.5, respectively. The first factor contains 16 of the 17 questions associated with the life purpose and satisfaction scale. Only one item from the self-confidence scale (item 22—"*respond positively in most situations*") also loaded on this scale. This item also had a slightly smaller but still substantial loading (.48) on Factor 2. The second factor contains 12 of the 13 self-confidence items plus one item from the life purpose and satisfaction scale (item 19—"*sad things*"). This item also had a substantial loading (.42) on Factor 1. Thus, this analysis generally supported the structure proposed by the authors of the scale. The scree plot also suggests a potential for a two-factor solution, although some might argue that the high eigenvalue of the first factor, as well as multiple loadings of some items, indicates a unidimensional scale. Conceptually, does the two factor solution make good sense to you? Which provides a better conceptual fit—this two factor solution or the four-factor solution presented previously? Helping us to see how the items of an instrument fit together is among the most important purposes of this statistical technique.

Communalities

	Initial	Extraction
energy level	1.000	.353
reaction to pressure	1.000	.477
characterization of life as a whole .	1.000	.561
daily activities	1.000	.469
experience anxiety	1.000	.523
expectations of every day	1.000	.318
fearful	1.000	.487
think deeply about life	1.000	.500
productivity of life	1.000	.530
making mistakes	1.000	.415
value of work	1.000	.510
wishing I was different	1.000	.521
defined goals for life	1.000	.498
worrying that bad things will happen	1.000	.426
concentration during stress	1.000	.512
standing up for myself	1.000	.369
adequacy in most situations	1.000	.453
frustration to problems	1.000	.530
sad things	1.000	.510
worthwhile life	1.000	.606
satisfaction of present life ·	1.000	.618
respond positively in difficult situations	1.000	.543
joy in heart	1.000	.610
when relaxing	1.000	.444
trapped by life	1.000	.553
panic in frightening situations	1.000	.593
thinking about past	1.000	.376
feeling loved	1.000	.533
worry about future	1.000	.314
thinking about problems	1.000	.588

Extraction Method: Principal component analysis.

EXERCISE FIGURE 14-1. Factor analysis of IPA items.

Total Variance Explained

Component	Initial Eigenvalues			Extraction Sums of Squared Loadings			Rotation Sums of Squared Loadings		
	Total	% of Variance	Cumulative %	Total	% of Variance	Cumulative %	Total	% of Variance	Cumulative %
1	12.633	42.110	42.110	12.633	42.110	42.110	8.235	27.451	27.451
2	2.107	7.023	49.133	2.107	7.023	49.133	6.504	21.681	49.133
3	1.233	4.111	53.243						
4	1.176	3.921	57.164						
5	.947	3.158	60.322						
6	.843	2.811	63.134						
7	.777	2.592	65.725						
8	.714	2.379	68.104						
9	.674	2.246	70.350						
10	.648	2.159	72.509						
11	.630	2.101	74.610						
12	.573	1.909	76.519						
13	.536	1.788	78.307						
14	.534	1.780	80.086						
15	.513	1.710	81.796						
16	.475	1.582	83.378						
17	.450	1.500	84.878						
18	.446	1.486	86.364						
19	.425	1.417	87.781						
20	.406	1.354	89.134						
21	.396	1.321	90.456						
22	.376	1.254	91.709						
23	.373	1.242	92.952						
24	.342	1.142	94.093						
25	.335	1.116	95.210						
26	.323	1.077	96.287						
27	.295	.982	97.269						
28	.293	.977	98.246						
29	.273	.909	99.155						
30	.254	.845	100.000						

Extraction Method: Principal component analysis.

EXERCISE FIGURE 14-1. (*Continued*)

Rotated Component Matrix (a)

	Component	
	1	2
satisfaction of present life	.741	.261
worthwhile life	.730	.271
joy in heart	.710	.325
productivity of life	.701	.196
characterization of life as a whole	.696	.275
value of work	.689	.187
think deeply about life	.687	.170
defined goals for life	.682	.180
feeling loved	.680	.265
trapped by life	.666	.331
daily activities	.660	.183
thinking about problems	.622	.448
wishing I was different	.581	.428
respond positively in difficult situations	.562	.476
expectations of every day	.536	.174
energy level	.478	.353
thinking about past	.464	.400
panic in frightening situations	.161	.753
experience anxiety	.213	.691
reaction to pressure	.109	.682
concentration during stress	.218	.682
frustration to problems	.312	.658
fearful	.248	.652
worrying that bad things will happen	.128	.640
sad things	.418	.579
making mistakes	.312	.563
adequacy in most situations	.400	.541
standing up for myself	.305	.525
when relaxing	.442	.498
worry about future	.346	.441

Extraction Method: Principal component analysis. Rotation Method: Varimax with Kaiser Normalization.
a Rotation converged in 3 iterations.

EXERCISE FIGURE 14-1. (*Continued*)

Confirmatory Factor Analysis

Karen J. Aroian and Anne E. Norris

Objectives for Chapter 15

After reading this chapter, you should be able to do the following:

1. Describe the various uses for confirmatory factor analysis.
2. Discuss the advantages of using confirmatory over exploratory factor analysis.
3. Identify the five steps of conducting a confirmatory factor analysis.
4. Critique a confirmatory factor analysis of a factor model on the basis of the fit statistics and parameter estimates.
5. Discuss the advantages of using confirmatory factor analysis over more traditional approaches for estimating convergent and divergent validity, test–retest reliability, and other types of psychometric evaluation.

Confirmatory factor analysis (CFA) replaces the more traditional technique of exploratory factor analysis (EFA) because it allows more precise tests of an instrument's factor structure (Long, 1988). CFA can also be used to address other issues in instrument development.

CFA is a special application of structural equation modeling (SEM). Currently, there are three popular software programs that are available to conduct CFA (and SEM): LISREL, EQS, and AMOS. LISREL is the most complex to use and understand because it relies on matrix terminology and Greek notation. However, most texts on CFA use the Greek terminology notation in their discussion of this technique. Therefore, we introduce you to some of the terminology in this chapter. We will also use LISREL in the computer examples. Chapter 17, Structural Equation Modeling, will use EQS in its examples so that you can gain greater familiarity with more than one software program. For more in-depth knowledge of CFA and LISREL terminology, read one or more of the following: Hayduk (1996), Long (1988), and Mueller (1996).

RESEARCH QUESTION

CFA enables the researcher to investigate three key issues in instrument development. First, it provides a theory-driven method for addressing construct validity. For example, CFA enables the researcher to assign the items in an instrument to their respective factors according to theoretical expectations. (With CFA, it is even possible to assign an item to more than one factor.) Then the researcher can use model fit statistics to evaluate whether the collected data are consistent with the factor model they are specifying (Mueller, 1996). Similarly, convergent and divergent validity can be examined by assigning items in an instrument to their respective factors and then indicating, according to theoretical expectations, which factors should be correlated across instruments and which should not. Model fit statistics will tell you, in general, how consistent the item assignments and factor correlations that you have specified are with relationships inherent in the actual data (ie, item covariances). In addition, model fit and other CFA statistics will tell you whether the items belong on the factors as you have indicated, whether the factors are correlated (or not correlated) as you have indicated, and the magnitude of these correlations. Second, CFA enables the researcher to evaluate the reliability (internal consistency, test–retest) of research instruments. What makes the CFA approach different from traditional assessment of internal consistency (eg, Cronbach's alpha) is that measurement error is partialed out of the assessment in CFA. In contrast, in CFA test-retest reliability is examined in terms of the consistency in measurement error over time as well as the factor structure. However, the estimates of measurement error being made in these and other CFA can be biased if the assumptions for CFA are not met. These assumptions are discussed later in this chapter.

Third, CFA can be used to compare factor structures across groups to see whether an instrument works differently in different groups of subjects. Thus, for example, if one wonders about gender or ethnic differences in the factor structure, CFA can be used to determine whether the structure changes or is invariant across such groups. If group differences in measurement error are a concern (eg, one group may be more susceptible to concerns about social desirability than another), this can also be investigated because measurement error is always estimated in CFA.

TERMINOLOGY

Before talking about the type of data and assumptions required for CFA, it is necessary to discuss some of the terms used in CFA. These terms are also used in SEM because, as stated previously, CFA is a special case of SEM. The discussion here focuses on the meaning of these terms in the context of CFA. For a broader explanation of these and other SEM terms, see Chapter 17.

Latent Variables

In CFA, factors are often referred to as *unmeasured* or *latent variables* because they are not measured directly by the researcher. In fact, the latent variable is regarded

TABLE 15-1 *Greek Letters Used in LISREL to Refer to Confirmatory Factor Analysis Variables and Parameters*

Variables/Parameters	Symbol	Greek Letter
Latent variables or factors	ξ	xi
Observed variables or items	X	
Residual or measurement error	δ	delta
Correlation between factors	ϕ	phi
Factor loading	λ	lambda

as a cause of the item score: the quantity of the underlying construct is presumed to cause an item or a set of items to take on a certain value (De Vellis, 2003). In LISREL, latent variables are represented by the lowercase Greek letter ξ (xi) and are shown as circles (Table 15-1).

Observed Variables

The term *observed variables* is used in CFA to refer to the items in an instrument. This is because the effect of a latent variable (or factor) can be observed only indirectly through its influence on those things that can be measured (ie, responses to an instrument). These observed variables are also referred to as indicators because they indicate the presence of the latent variable.

A universal way of designating a variable as an observed variable is to represent it with an uppercase X and enclose it in a square. Hence, we would say that there are six observed variables in Figure 15-1. These six observed variables are considered indicators of the latent variable, competence, and are all theorized to load on this factor. Note in Figure 15-1 how the relationships between latent and observed variables are represented with arrows pointing to the observed variables to indicate that the latent variable is the cause of the observed variable.

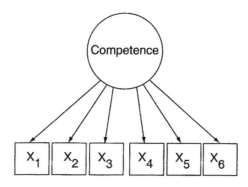

FIGURE 15-1. One latent variable, competence, with six observed variables.

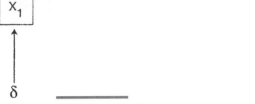

FIGURE 15-2. One observed variable and its residual.

Residuals

Classical measurement theory states that the observed score (the score obtained from the items) represents the true score or the quantity associated with the latent variable plus measurement error. This measurement error is referred to as the residual score. It represents the imprecision inherent to some extent in any research instrument.

Residual is the term used in CFA to refer to this residual score or measurement error. In CFA diagrams, residuals are represented by the lowercase Greek letter δ (delta). Residuals are also referred to as unique factors (Long, 1988) because they are unique to the measurement process and unrelated to the underlying latent constructs. Figure 15-2 illustrates how the residual for an observed variable is diagrammed in CFA. Note the arrow from the residual δ_1 to the observed variable X_1 indicates that the residual is influencing the observed score.

Residuals are estimated in CFA. They are interpreted as an indication of the reliability of the observed variables or items.

Parameters

The relationships between and among latent variables, observed variables, and residuals can all be estimated in CFA. For example, a researcher may theorize that certain latent variables (ie, factors) are correlated. Similarly, she may expect that some of the residuals (ie, measurement error) are correlated. In addition, there will be hypotheses about which observed variables are the indicators for which factors. These relationships are the structural links (or paths) in the factor model. LISREL software uses a system of Greek letters to categorize parameters according to the paths they define. For example, the parameter for a correlation between two latent variables (ie, factors) is ϕ (phi). The parameter for a correlation between the residuals (ie, measurement error) is θ (theta). The factor loadings are represented by the lowercase Greek letter λ (lambda). For example, Figure 15-3 displays a two-factor model (ie, two latent variables, ξ_1 and ξ_2) with seven observed variables (X_1 to X_7) and seven residuals (δ_1 to δ_7). The latent variables are correlated with each other, and two of the residuals are correlated (δ_6 and δ_7). Parameters are often referred to as fixed or free. A fixed parameter is not estimated in CFA. Instead, the researcher assigns it a particular value. Fixing a parameter to zero indicates the absence of a relationship. For example, the researcher fixes a λ parameter (ie, the factor loading)

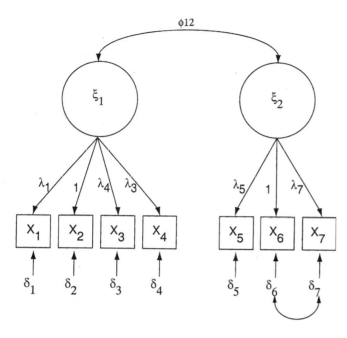

FIGURE 15-3. Diagram of a two-factor model where factors are intercorrelated and items #6 and #7 have correlated measurement errors. X_2 and X_6 are reference indicators.

to be equal to zero when the parameter represents the relationship between an item and a factor that the item is not expected to load on. Thus, in Figure 15-3, there is no $\lambda_{7,1}$ because X_7 is not hypothesized to serve as an indicator for ξ_1. By not including this relationship in the diagram, the researcher indicates that the parameter associated with it is set equal to zero.

It is fairly common practice to fix the λ parameter for one of the observed variables that serves as an indicator for a latent variable to be equal to one. This observed variable then becomes a reference variable because it and the latent variable have the same scale. Thus, if responses range from one to five for a particular item that has been made the reference variable, the latent variable will similarly range in magnitude from one to five. Note in Figure 15-3 that X_2 and X_6 are the reference variables for their respective latent variables.

Only free parameters are estimated in CFA. The computer calculates the value as part of the analysis using the covariances of the various indicators. LISREL, EQS, and AMOS all provide significance tests of these parameters as part of the analysis.

TYPE OF DATA REQUIRED

CFA requires the data to have two characteristics. First, the data should be continuous and normally distributed. However, special estimation methods and scaled statistics are available that are robust to violations of normality (Byrne, 1994; Hu & Bentler, 1995).

Second, the data should be numerous. Like traditional factor analysis, CFA requires a large sample size. The most common method for estimating the parameters in CFA is maximum likelihood (ML). For the ML method, a typical past recommendation has been a minimum of 100 to 200 subjects (or 100 to 200 subjects per group, if the researcher wants to compare the properties of the instrument in different groups). However, there are at least three reasons why this recommended sample size minimum should be revised to 500 or more. First, Fan and Wang's (1998) work with computer simulations suggests that sample sizes of 100 and 200 are more likely to generate models with statistically impossible values such as negative variances. These impossible values were not generated in their computer simulations when the sample size was greater than 500. Second, larger sample sizes decrease the effects of non-normality on model fit statistics and parameter estimates (West, Finch, & Curran, 1995), and non-normality frequently occurs in nursing and health-related research data sets. Third, a parameter's standard error (used for significance tests of parameters) can vary across equivalent models tested with the same data when sample sizes are less than 500 (Gonzalez & Griffin, 2001). This means that different conclusions could be reached about the significance of factor loadings (ie, lambda parameters) when testing competing factor models for a particular instrument.

ASSUMPTIONS

Two types of assumptions must be considered with CFA: general statistical and estimation method-specific assumptions. A discussion of each type follows.

General Statistical Assumptions

There are three types of general statistical assumptions in CFA. Violating these assumptions makes it difficult to identify a model that fits the data well and typically results in poorer fit indices. In other words, you run the risk of concluding that your factor structure is wrong when in fact it might be correct—you increase the risk of making a type II error.

The first type of assumptions should already be familiar to you. These are the assumptions of normal distributions, homoscedasticity, and linear relationships discussed in Chapters 11 and 12 for regression analysis. These assumptions arise because CFA involves solving a series of regression equations, much like what occurs in path analysis.

Second, there are assumptions regarding the error terms in CFA. These assumptions are similar to those made in regression regarding the residuals and are typically met in the course of meeting other SEM assumptions. Specifically, it is assumed that error terms in the model are (1) not correlated with any of the latent variables, (2) independent of one another, and (3) normally distributed (Fox, 1984). Although these assumptions are violated when the data are not multivariate normal, they are robust when the sample size is large (Chou & Bentler, 1995).

The third type of assumption pertains to sample size. It is assumed that the sample is asymptotic—so large as to approach infinity (Bollen, 1989). Smaller sample sizes (eg, less than 100 for a simple model when ML is used to estimate parameters) increase the probability of rejecting a true model (one that fits the data) (West et al., 1995). In other words, smaller sample sizes also increase the risk of making a type II error.

Estimation Method-Specific Assumptions

In addition to general statistical assumptions, there are distributional assumptions associated with the method used to estimate the parameters in CFA. This discussion will be limited to the ML method because it is the most commonly used estimation method (Chou & Bentler, 1995) and performs, on average, better than most other estimation methods even when its assumptions are violated. (See Bollen, 1989, and West et al., 1995, for a discussion of other estimation methods and their robustness.) ML assumes that (1) no single item or group of items perfectly explains another in the data set (Bollen, 1989) and (2) the items have a distribution that is multivariate normal (West et al., 1995). This first assumption is why instrument items cannot be redundant (ie, highly intercorrelated). ML is not very robust to violations of this first assumption: instruments with items that correlate at or above .90 cannot be evaluated with CFA.

Although the multivariate normal assumption is difficult to meet in practice, fortunately ML is fairly robust to violation of multivariate normality (Chou & Bentler, 1995). An important exception is when the sample size is small and the model is complex. Under these conditions, ML is not robust to violations of this multivariate normal assumption. Hence, researchers are encouraged to go beyond the 100 to 200 (or 500) minimum if they are evaluating instruments with more than three factors.

Exploratory Versus Confirmatory Factor Analysis

Both EFA and CFA are methods for organizing items into factors or, stated alternately, grouping observed variables that belong together under their respective latent variables. However, EFA has four statistical assumptions that are not necessary in CFA. The flexibility of CFA with respect to these assumptions is what makes it a preferred technique for analyzing the psychometric properties of an instrument. Note, however, that the assumptions of multivariate normality required in CFA (see earlier) are not necessary in EFA when it is performed using traditional factor analysis techniques, as discussed in Chapter 14.

The four assumptions that the researcher is forced to make in EFA have been referred to as *procrustean* because they force the data to fit circumstances that many view as unrealistic. First, the researcher is forced to assume that either all or none of the factors in an instrument are correlated with each other. For example, it is not possible to specify that only two out of three factors in an instrument are correlated with each other. Second, the researcher is forced to assume that all items are directly affected by all factors, even if the relationships between certain items and certain factors are trivial. In other words, all of the items must be forced to load on all of the factors even if some of these loadings are too small to be of statistical significance (ie, load less than ±.40). In other words, it is not possible in EFA to assign certain items to a particular factor and not to another. Third, the researcher must assume that none of the measurement error associated with the items is correlated. So, for example, if a researcher was assessing behaviors after myocardial infarction, she would have to assume that the measurement error associated with sensitive questions about the quality and quantity of sexual intercourse was not correlated. Even worse, there would be no way to test the validity of this assumption, whereas direct testing of this assumption is possible in CFA. Fourth, the researcher must assume that all items are equally affected by measurement error. Again, given the previous example, we can see how such an assumption can be at odds with the reality of the instrument being analyzed.

The researcher using EFA has only three choices to test hypotheses about the structure of the factor model: (1) to decide which items (observed variables) to include in the analysis, (2) to choose which type of EFA and rotational solution (eg, varimax, oblimen, or oblique) to use, and (3) to specify or constrain the number of factors to the desired or theoretically expected number. The lack of flexibility to relax the earlier-mentioned assumptions and the inability to specify correlational relationships in the factor model when using EFA has led to EFA being called a "data-driven" technique. In addition, the findings of EFA can be ambiguous or misinterpreted, particularly when the factors correlate at moderate to high levels. Erroneous conclusions can be drawn from EFA if an orthogonal rotation, such as varimax, is used when the factors are truly correlated. However, using an oblique rotation that assumes that the factors are correlated does not necessarily resolve the problem. There are an infinite number of oblique rotational solutions, and the estimated factor correlations can be dramatically different depending on the type of rotation (Hertzog, 1989).

CFA allows you to relax the assumptions imposed by EFA when it makes theoretical sense to do so. Rather than being limited by strict statistical assumptions, CFA gives you flexibility to specify a model according to your theoretical expectations. You can use CFA to specify the structure of the factor model and directly test whether the hypothesized structure fits the obtained data. For this reason, CFA is considered a "theory-driven" approach.

Figure 15-4 illustrates how a researcher could specify the factor structure for an instrument composed of three factors (latent variables) and seven items (observed variables). Note how the items are assigned to their respective factors: X_1 and X_2 are indicators of factor 1 (ξ_1), X_3 to X_5 are indicators of factor 2 (ξ_2), and X_6 and X_7 are indicators of factor 3 (ξ_3). Correlations among the factors are as follows: factor 2 is correlated with both factors 1 and 3; factors 1 and 3 are not correlated with each other. The measurement error terms associated with two items (δ_1 and δ_2) are also correlated. Correlated measurement error occurs when a variable that is not identified explicitly in the model or measured directly (eg, response bias such as social desirability) is theorized to influence item responses (Mueller, 1996).

Note how one of the items assigned to factor 3 (X_6) is theorized to have perfect reliability (ie, be perfectly measured). Thus, there is no error term for that particular observed variable. So, for example, if factor 3 was measuring age, X_6 could represent a person's chronologic age as determined from the medical record and

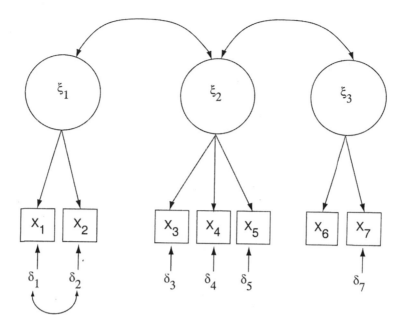

FIGURE 15-4. Diagram of a three-factor model where factors 1 and 3 are correlated with factor 2. Items #1 and #2 have correlated measurement error. Item #6 is assumed to have no measurement error.

X_7 might represent the physiologic age as determined by a score based on skin tenting, respiration rate, pulse, and so forth. Although measurement error could be present in the measure of chronologic age, it is generally assumed that such error is likely to be infinitesimally small (ie, approximately equal to zero).

Another advantage of CFA is that interpreting findings from CFA is much less ambiguous than interpreting findings from EFA. Various statistical tests or fit indices are available in CFA to determine whether the sample data are consistent with the specified structural relationships between the factors, items, and error terms. In other words, the fit indices provide information about whether the data confirm the hypothesized factor model. If the fit indices suggest that the model is misspecified (ie, it does not fit the sample data), the model can be respecified or modified and tested for a better fit.

The limitations of EFA are illustrated by Wagnild and Young's (1993) use of EFA to explore the factor structure of their Resilience Scale (RS). Findings from their original EFA of the RS were equivocal with regard to whether the measure was uni- or multidimensional. Specifically, the EFA and scree plot supported a unidimensional measure. However, the criterion of exploring all factors with eigenvalues greater than 1 led the authors to conclude that a two-factor solution was interpretable and also fit the data.

Because these findings were equivocal with regard to whether the RS was a uni- or multidimensional scale, Aroian and colleagues (1997) used CFA to test the hypothesis of uni- or multidimensionality of the Russian version of the RS. They were particularly concerned that the two-factor solution Wagnild and Young obtained with EFA yielded several items that loaded highly on both factors. Specifically, half of the items from one of the subscales (Acceptance of Self and Life) also loaded at more than .35 on the other subscale (Personal Competence). CFA provided the tools to test directly whether the Russian version of the RS was better conceptualized as a one- or two-factor measure. CFA allowed them to specify a one- and two-factor model and to use the nested chi-square to test which model provided a better fit for the data. Findings from the CFA suggested that the two-factor model provided a better fit than the one-factor model of the Russian version of the RS.

In sum, CFA offers several advantages over EFA: CFA can test the hypothesized configuration of the factor structure, assess measurement error in detail, and directly test hypotheses about factor structure. In contrast, EFA lets a particular dataset dictate underlying factors and can yield ambiguous findings (Hertzog, 1989; Mueller, 1996). (See Bollen, 1989, for a more in-depth discussion of the differences between CFA and EFA.)

Although CFA gives the researcher the statistical tools necessary for precise hypothesis testing, it is ultimately up to the researcher to decide which procedure to use and toward what end. Researchers with well-specified expectations can and do use EFA. Still others choose to use CFA in a highly exploratory manner. However, the latter approach can increase the risk for type II error (see the section on power in Chapter 17).

STEPS IN CONDUCTING A CFA

There are five steps to conducting a CFA: model specification, identification, estimating the parameters of the measurement model, evaluating the data-model fit, and model modification or respecification to improve the fit (Bollen, 1989).

Specification

Model specification involves specifying the structural relationships among the component parts of the model. Specification of the factor model is largely a theoretical issue and is best displayed by drawing a path diagram to illustrate the researcher's expectations. In practice, the researcher may not have a single factor model in mind; perhaps a handful of different factor models are theoretically plausible. Similar to the notion of testing competing hypotheses, Mueller (1996) suggests formulating some alternative models before performing data analysis rather than considering a single model.

For example, Aroian et al. (1997) specified a one-factor and a two-factor model of the Russian version of Wagnild and Young's (1993) RS. The specifications for these two models are illustrated in Figures 15-5 and 15-6.

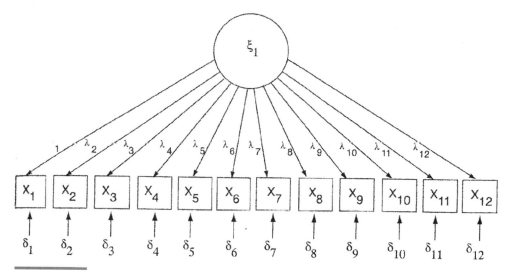

FIGURE 15-5. Single-factor structure model of Wagnild and Young's (1993) Resilience Scale.

The model that is being tested in Figure 15-5 has one latent variable or factor (ξ_1) with 12 observed variables (X_1 through X_{12}) and 12 residuals (δ_1 through δ_{12}). The model that is being tested in Figure 15-6 has two latent variables or factors (ξ_1 and ξ_2). Observed variables X_1 through X_9 and their respective residuals are assigned to the first latent variable (ξ_1). Observed variables X_{10} through X_{12} and their respective residuals are assigned to the second latent variable (ξ_2).

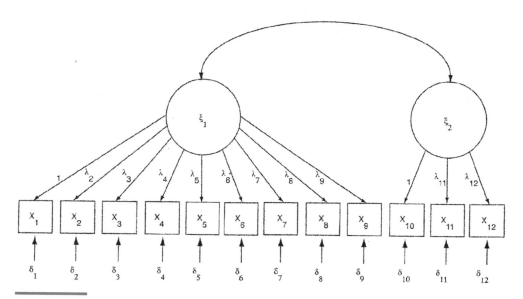

FIGURE 15-6. Two-factor structure model of Wagnild and Young's (1993) Resilience Scale.

CFA can also be used in an exploratory fashion. In this instance, a model is specified according to the results of a prior examination of the data (Long, 1988). Specifying a model based on prior examination of the data is an example of the "gray area" between EFA and CFA. The researcher is exploring or searching for viable hypotheses about the factor structure and is using the tools available from CFA to evaluate which hypotheses are plausible. When CFA is used in this exploratory fashion, the model should be developed with one sample (a *calibration* sample) and tested on another sample (a *validation* sample) for confirmation (Leamer, 1978).

The specification of the factor models displayed in Figures 15-5 and 15-6 was based on findings from Wagnild and Young's EFA of the original English version of the RS. In other words, prior research findings as well as Wagnild and Young's hypotheses about the factor structure of the RS dictated the specification of the two CFA models of the Russian version of the RS. From this perspective, CFA was used in a confirmatory rather than an exploratory manner.

Identification

Identification is a statistical rather than a theoretical issue. As in path analysis (see Chapter 16), the researcher wants the model being tested to be overidentified, that is, to have the information in the data (ie, the known values: variances and covariances of the instrument items) exceed the information being estimated in the CFA (ie, the unknown values: factor loadings, measurement error, and so forth). If the unknowns exceed the knowns, the model is said to be underidentified. If the knowns and unknowns are equal, the model is just identified. LISREL and other CFA computer programs cannot evaluate underidentified models and cannot provide the statistics needed to determine whether a just identified model fits the data well. Consequently, factor models tested with CFA need to be overidentified. As a first step toward specifying a model that is overidentified, researchers try to have at least three observed variables (or indicators) per latent variable. (This is sometimes referred to as the "three indicator rule.") They then pick a reference variable for each latent variable (see the earlier section on parameters) or standardize the scale of the latent variable by fixing its variance to be equal to one. The models depicted in Figures 15-5 and 15-6 have reference variables and more than three indicators per latent variable; thus, both models appear to be overidentified.

Unfortunately, the issue of identification is quite complex in CFA and involves several tests. Even then, overidentified factor models can become underidentified during the estimation process as a result of properties of the data. In such a case, researchers are often forced to make certain assumptions about the observed variables (eg, their measurement error is correlated) or to drop an observed variable from the analysis. A thorough discussion of identification is beyond the scope of this chapter. Readers interested in conducting CFA should consult one of the following texts for a more comprehensive treatment of identification: Bollen (1989), Hayduk (1996), and Long (1988).

Estimation

Estimation is the procedure for testing the model. It is performed by the computer. Estimation involves using a sample of observed data (ie, variances and covariances of observed variables or instrument items) to make estimates of population parameters (eg, factor loadings [λ], residuals or measurement error [δ], factor correlation [ϕ]).

Two questions are central to the estimation process. The first question pertains to bias, or whether in general the estimates are equal to the true parameters. The significance tests of the parameters estimated in the CFA (ie, the factor loadings) are used to address this question. These significance tests indicate how likely it is that the estimated parameter values could have been obtained by chance.

The second question concerns efficiency, or whether the sample data are being used in the most effective way (Long, 1988). In other words, does this factor model fit the data well, or might another model fit the data even better? The model fit statistics generated in CFA are used to answer this question. Evaluating these statistics occurs in the next step of conducting a CFA.

Evaluating Fit

The researcher evaluates the fit of the factor model by examining various statistics provided in the CFA computer output. The key question is whether the results provide empirical evidence that the specified model fit the data well, or suggest a data–model misfit. In the latter case, the hypothesis about the factor structure should be rejected, and the researcher may use the statistics provided in the CFA to guide decision making about modifying or respecifying the factor model.

As a first and rudimentary assessment of fit, the researcher inspects the parameter estimates on the computer output to determine whether they seem reasonable and consistent with theoretical expectations. There is a good chance that at least part of the factor model has been misspecified if these parameters have (1) a positive value when they should have a negative one (eg, a positive factor loading where a negative one is expected) or vice versa, (2) inappropriately large or small values (eg, a factor with a variance close to zero), (3) unusually large standard errors, or (4) reliability estimates of the observed variables that are negative, close to 0, or greater than unity.

However, the researcher must also examine various model fit statistics (also known as fit indices) because models with seemingly reasonable parameters may still not fit the data well (Mueller, 1996). A variety of fit indices are available to assess data–model fit. Unfortunately, there is no consensus on which indices are best, and major statistical packages such as LISREL, EQS, and AMOS automatically include in their default options indices that are known to have undesirable properties (Marsh, Bella, & Hau, 1996). We review here some of the fit indices seen in the literature. Interested readers should see Bollen and Long (1993), Hu and Bentler (1995), and Marsh et al. (1996) for extensive reviews of various model fit indices.

Traditionally, the most commonly reported fit statistic has been the chi-square goodness of fit statistic. The chi-square assesses the difference between the observed data and the hypothesized factor model (Byrne, 1994). A nonsignificant chi-square is an indication of fit because the researcher seeks to confirm the null hypothesis (ie, there is no difference between the data and the model). This use of the chi-square in CFA differs from the customary use of the chi-square statistic in bivariate statistics.

The chi-square goodness of fit has been falling out of favor because it is greatly influenced by sample size and violations of multivariate normality (Wang, Fan, & Willson, 1996). This statistic is more likely to suggest rejection of a plausible model when the sample size is large (ie, ≥ 500) because with larger sample sizes it is easier for trivial differences between the hypothesized factor structure and the actual data model to be rendered statistically significant (Wang et al., 1996). For this reason, the chi-square statistic should not be the sole method used for drawing conclusions about data–model fit (Bollen & Long, 1993). The relative chi-square is used as an informal measure of fit (Mueller, 1996). The relative chi-square is the ratio of chi-square to degrees of freedom (χ^2/df). There is no consensus on what value constitutes a good fit (Bollen, 1989). Generally, relative chi-squares less than 3.00 are preferred, but in practice some researchers interpret ratios as high as 3.00, 4.00, or even 5.00 as representing "good" data–model fit (Mueller, 1996).

A nested chi-square or the chi-square difference test is particularly useful when testing competing models. A nested chi-square is calculated by subtracting the chi-square and degrees of freedom for one model from the chi-square and degrees of freedom associated with another competitive model. The significance level associated with this nested chi-square is used to determine whether the fit of one model differs significantly from that of the other. When the chi-square difference is statistically significant, the model with the smaller chi-square is considered to fit the data better than the model with the higher chi-square. Table 15-2 shows how a chi-square difference test was used to test the two competing models of the Russian version of the RS displayed in Figures 15-5 and 15-6. As you can see, the chi-square difference was statistically significant, indicating that the two-factor model fit the data significantly better than the one-factor model (Aroian et al., 1997).

Other commonly used fit statistics, GFI (goodness of fit index), CFI (comparative fit index), and IFI (incremental fit index), usually range between 0 and 1, with values greater than .90 considered to indicate good fit. However, with certain

TABLE 15-2 *Calculation of Nested Chi-Square Used to Test Two Competing Models for the Russian Version of the Resilience Scale*

	Model Chi-Square	Degrees of Freedom
One-factor model	223.48	54
Two-factor model	167.50	53

Nested chi-square, $p < 0.0001$.

sample sizes, estimation methods, and distributions (eg, non-normal), this cutoff may not be high enough (Hu & Bentler, 1995). In addition, some researchers recommend the CFI over the GFI because Monte Carlo simulation studies suggest it is less influenced by sample size (eg, Wang et al., 1996). However, neither of these statistics takes into account how many parameters are included in the model, and model fit can be enhanced (ie, made closer to 1.0) by merely adding additional parameters (Bollen & Long, 1993). The IFI attempts to correct for this problem. Nonetheless, Marsh et al. (1996) indicate that the IFI is positively biased (ie, inflated) when the model is misspecified. This bias is exacerbated by small sizes (eg, <200).

The root mean square residual (RMR) and the Root Mean Square Error of Approximation (RMSEA) are two other measures of fit which range from 0 to 1, but in contrast to the GFI, CFI, and IFI, the closer these indices are to zero, the better. Values greater than .10 justify rejecting the model (Bachand & Beard, 1995) with values less than .05 indicating a good fit (Hu & Bentler, 1995). The RMSEA differs from the RMR in that it attempts to correct for the number of parameters in the model being tested. However, the RMR has certain advantages because, unlike the RMSEA and the other fit indices discussed here, it is based on the residual matrix, not the chi-square statistic. Unfortunately, neither the RMR or the RMSEA has not been extensively studied through Monte Carlo simulation, so little is known about the effects of sample size, non-normality, and so forth on these two indices.

Experts generally recommend that a variety of fit indices be used so that the weakness of a particular index is offset by the strength of another (Gonzalez & Griffin, 2001). For example, Aroian and colleagues (1997) reported several fit indices when they evaluated the data–model fit of the two-factor model of the Russian version of the RS. The chi-square obtained for the two-factor model was statistically significant, suggesting that the data did not fit the hypothesized factor model. However, the sample was relatively large (N = 450), which could mean that the chi-square test was overpowered and not the best index to use. Therefore, more credence was given to the relative chi-square, GFI, and IFI. These indices suggested that the two-factor model provided a reasonable fit for the data. Specifically, the relative chi-square = 3.15, GFI = .94, and IFI = .91.

Even when fit indices are acceptable, a researcher may not be able to confirm that the hypothesized factor model is correct if the dataset fits other alternative models equally well. In other words, a hypothesized model can be rejected when there is no data–model misfit, but the specified model cannot be confirmed as being the single "right" model (Mueller, 1996). Rather, the researcher has identified a *possible* factor structure that could have given rise to the dataset under investigation.

Model Modification

If the fit indices indicate a possible data–model misfit, the researcher can choose to modify the initially hypothesized model and test the resulting newly proposed model for an improved data–model fit. Misfit can arise because relationships have been omitted from the model. For example, the researcher may have hypothesized that an item only loaded on one of the factors, when in fact it loads on more than one. Alternatively, factors that were hypothesized to correlate with one another may not in fact be correlated. The researcher can use certain statistical information produced in the CFA to determine what relationships to add or drop from the factor model. LISREL and AMOS provide tests called modification indices that indicate which parameters should be dropped or added to improve the fit of the model. EQS provides the Lagrange multiplier test, which indicates which parameters should be added, and the Wald test to indicate which parameters should be dropped. In addition to these tests, researchers examine the residuals (ie, the measurement error being estimated in CFA) for each observed variable. Large residuals can be readily identified by using the standardized estimates so that all measurement error is on the same scale. Large residuals may indicate problems with how the relationship between the observed variable and the latent variable have been specified.

Any posthoc modifications to a model must make substantive sense and must be congruent with theoretical expectations. Otherwise, the CFA is reduced to a data-driven process. Moreover, as the initial factor model is modified and reanalyzed with the same dataset, the data–model fit will usually improve simply because the model has been fitted to the same dataset. In other words, the improved fit is not necessarily because the model is truly better, but because the researcher is capitalizing on chance. One solution to the problem of posthoc model modification is to test the factor model on a new and independent sample. Alternatively, if the initial sample is large enough, it can be split into calibration and validation subsamples. For example, Aroian and colleagues (1998) conducted a specification search to identify the "best-fitting" factor model for the Demands of Immigration Scale. The specification search was conducted on a calibration sample of 792 Russian immigrants. Once they achieved an adequate fit with their sample data, the modified or respecified model was confirmed on a validation sample of 857 Russian immigrants.

COMPUTER EXAMPLE: MEASURE OF ENGLISH ABILITY

The computer example is a CFA of a measure of English ability that was developed by Tran and Aroian (1999). They conceptualized English ability as multidimensional. The instrument was hypothesized to have three factors: Basic Language Ability, Ability to Use Language for Fun, and Ability to Use Language for Survival. They administered this measure to 300 elderly Russian immigrants. LISREL 8.12 was used to test the hypothesized factor model.

The hypothesized factor structure being tested is displayed in Figure 15-7. The three latent variables (or factors) are labeled Basic (ξ_1), Fun (ξ_2), and Survival (ξ_3). There are 13 observed variables because the instrument contains 13 items. The first five observed variables are the indicators for Basic: "Notice," or ability to read notices in English (X_1); "Read," or ability to read in English (X_2); "Understand," or ability to understand spoken English (X_3); "Write," or ability to write in English (X_4); and "Speak," or ability to speak in English (X_5). Observed variables six through nine are the indicators for Fun: "Travel," or English ability for travel or sightseeing (X_6);

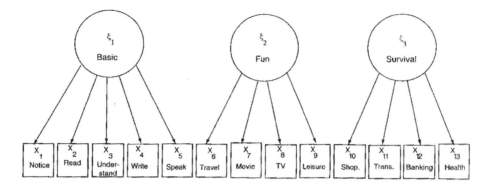

FIGURE 15-7. Factor model being tested in the computer example.

"Movie," or ability to understand movies or plays in English (X_7); "TV," or the ability to understand TV in English (X_8); and "Leisure," or ability to participate in other leisure activities in English (X_9). Observed variables 10 through 13 are the indicators for Survival: "Shopping," or adequacy of English for shopping (X_{10}); "Transportation," or English ability for taking public transportation (X_{11}); "Banking," or English ability for conducting banking business (X_{12}); and "Health," or ability to use English for obtaining health care services (X_{13}). Selected parts of the LISREL output are displayed in Figures 15-8 to 15-11. Figure 15-8 displays the nonstandardized factor loadings that LISREL estimated. (Standardized factor loadings are provided in Fig. 15-11.) This part of the output is entitled "LAMBDA-X" because l is the parameter that links the observed variables (X) to the latent variables. Each row in Figure 15-8 corresponds to an observed variable. For example, the first row provides the estimates for the first item, Notice (X_1). The first line in this row displays the number 0.760. This number is the factor loading for Notice. Below it is the standard error in the estimate (0.050). Below the standard error in the estimate is the *t* value used to determine whether the estimate is statistically significant (15.223). Generally, *t* values greater than 2 imply statistical significance, so this factor loading or l is statistically significant (as are all the l estimates in this CFA). No values are listed for Notice under Fun and Survival because these parameters were not estimated; they were fixed at zero.

Figure 15-9 displays the portion of the LISREL output that contains estimates of the correlations between the factors. The correlations are in a matrix labeled PHI because Phi (ϕ) is the parameter representing correlation between latent variables. As would be expected, the correlation between Basic and itself = 1. Consistent with the hypothesized factor model in Figure 15-7, LISREL estimated f for every pair of latent variables. The correlation (ϕ) appears first. The standard error in the estimate is listed next, under ϕ. The *t* value is listed under the standard error in the estimate. The correlation between Survival and Fun appears to be small (0.146) and not significant (*t* value = 2.178, $p > 0.05$). This suggests that, as might be expected, the relationship between basic English ability and ability to use the language for survival

(text continues on page 370)

LISREL ESTIMATES (MAXIMUM LIKELIHOOD)

LAMBDA-X

	Basic	Fun	Survival
notice	0.760 (0.050) 15.223	- -	- -
read	0.919 (0.045) 20.512	- -	- -
understd	0.812 (0.048) 16.783	- -	- -
write	0.876 (0.046) 18.917	- -	- -
speak	0.842 (0.047) 17.765	- -	- -
travel	- -	0.725 (0.055) 13.184	- -
movie	- -	0.839 (0.053) 15.806	- -
tv	- -	0.656 (0.056) 11.653	- -
leisure	- -	0.634 (0.057) 11.168	- -
shopping	- -	- -	0.828 (0.050) 16.516
transpor	- -	- -	0.820 (0.050) 16.309
banking	- -	- -	0.798 (0.051) 15.703
health	- -	- -	0.432 (0.059)

FIGURE 15-8. LISREL estimates (maximum likelihood).

```
PHI

                   Basic        Fun    Survival
                 --------   --------   --------
        Basic      1.000

          Fun      0.230      1.000
                  (0.063)
                   3.675

     Survival      0.639      0.146      1.000
                  (0.041)    (0.067)
                  15.532      2.178
```

FIGURE 15-9. Phi.

STANDARDIZED RESIDUALS

	notice	read	understd	write	speak	travel
notice	0.000					
read	-0.405	0.000				
understd	1.971	-4.143	0.000			
write	-3.637	10.476	-4.487	0.000		
speak	1.664	-4.682	7.492	-3.788	0.000	
travel	1.368	1.413	2.304	2.387	2.897	0.000
movie	-4.511	-3.973	-0.327	-2.844	-1.714	1.623
tv	0.802	0.205	4.836	0.185	3.324	-4.937
leisure	0.998	0.145	2.371	1.107	2.213	2.484
shopping	3.575	0.130	0.253	-0.583	1.782	-0.019
transpor	0.651	-2.446	-0.833	-1.586	-0.190	0.221
banking	0.882	-1.408	0.245	0.255	0.208	3.195
health	1.104	-0.092	3.934	1.753	3.620	5.460

MODIFICATION INDICES FOR THE THETA-DELTA

	notice	read	understd	write	speak	travel
notice	- -					
read	0.164	- -				
understd	3.884	17.167	- -			
write	13.225	109.750	20.135	- -		
speak	2.768	21.917	56.125	14.350	- -	
travel	2.078	0.060	2.697	2.115	0.261	- -
movie	14.214	2.452	0.001	0.186	1.675	2.634
tv	0.468	6.952	22.789	8.000	7.063	24.375
leisure	1.831	3.758	0.175	0.007	0.793	6.169
shopping	10.353	0.644	1.023	3.812	0.687	0.566
transpor	0.000	0.174	0.105	0.072	0.001	0.402
banking	0.444	0.936	0.079	2.327	0.611	1.132
health	1.139	15.019	14.178	0.196	9.342	6.568

FIGURE 15-10. Standardized residuals/modification indices for the theta-delta.

Measure of English Ability- a Factor Analysis
COMPLETELY STANDARDIZED SOLUTION

LAMBDA-X

	Basic	Fun	Survival
notice	0.760	- -	- -
read	0.919	- -	- -
understd	0.812	- -	- -
write	0.876	- -	- -
speak	0.842	- -	- -
travel	- -	0.725	- -
movie	- -	0.839	- -
tv	- -	0.656	- -
leisure	- -	0.634	- -
shopping	- -	- -	0.828
transpor	- -	- -	0.820
banking	- -	- -	0.798
health	- -	- -	0.432

FIGURE 15-11. Factor loadings for items from the measure of English ability.

needs is stronger than the relationship between the ability to use the language for survival and fun.

The fit of this model could be improved. Although the statistical significance of the chi-square (χ^2, 62 *df* = 313.31, *p* = .00) could be due to sample size, other fit statistics suggest that the model does not provide the best fit for the data. Specifically, the relative chi-square (313.31/62 = 5.05) is high and the GFI is low (.85). In addition, the RMR (.09) exceeds the preferred value, although it is less than .1. The standardized residuals and modification indices displayed in Figure 15-10 help identify problems with how the model was originally specified. (We have included only some of the standardized residuals and modification indices for the sake of clarity.) Notice the large positive standardized residual for Read and Write (10.476). This residual is higher than the standardized residuals for all other pairs of observed variables. When a standardized residual is large and positive such as this, it indicates that there is a relationship between the two variables that has not been accounted for in the model as it is currently specified (Bachand & Beard, 1995). In other words, this type of residual suggests that these two variables have correlated measurement error. This suggestion needs to be confirmed by looking at the modification indices for theta delta. (Remember that LISREL terminology uses delta [δ] to refer to measurement error.) As you can see in the lower part of Figure 15-10, the modification index associated with Write and Read is very large (109.750). This large value indicates that if the measurement error associated with these two variables was assumed to be correlated, the improvement in model fit would be substantial. (The model as it is currently specified assumes that there is no correlation between these variables.) The researcher must now decide whether assuming that the measurement error for items measuring the ability to read and write in English is theoretically justified. If so, the model would be respecified and the analysis redone.

In addition to providing statistics about the fit of the model and ways to improve this fit, statistics are provided that are estimates of the factor loadings. These statistics, the standardized Lambda-X parameters, indicate the relative importance of the observed variables to the measurement of their latent constructs. The LISREL output in Figure 15-11 shows the factor loadings for the three factors Basic, Fun, and Survival. Note how this part of the output is labeled Lambda-X because lambda (l) is the parameter that links the observed variables (X) to the latent variables.

The output in Figure 15-11 indicates that all of the items load highly on their respective factors with the exception of Health (0.432). Modification indices for Lambda-X (not shown) suggest that model fit could be improved if Health were treated as an indicator for Fun instead of Survival. However, this change in the model does not seem to be theoretically justified, so it is doubtful that the researcher would respecify the model in this matter.

USING CFA TO ADDRESS OTHER ISSUES IN PSYCHOMETRIC EVALUATION

Internal Consistency

The LISREL output for the Measure of English Ability discussed previously also provides information about this measure's internal consistency. In CFA, it is common practice to interpret the squared multiple correlations, or R^2, for each observed variable as descriptive reliability estimates (Mueller, 1996). The R^2 is the proportion of variance in the observed variable that is accounted for by the latent variable(s) for which it is an indicator (Bollen, 1989). Figure 15-12 contains the portion of the LISREL output that provides the R^2 for each observed (or X) variable. With one exception, the reliability estimates for most of the observed variables range from acceptable to good ($R^2 = .40$ to $.84$). However, the R^2 for Health is low ($R^2 = .19$). This is consistent with the low factor loading noted for this variable at the end of the previous section.

```
SQUARED MULTIPLE CORRELATIONS FOR X - VARIABLES

    notice        read    understd       write       speak      travel
  --------    --------    --------    --------    --------    --------
     0.577       0.844       0.659       0.767       0.709       0.526

SQUARED MULTIPLE CORRELATIONS FOR X - VARIABLES

     movie          tv     leisure    shopping    transpör     banking
  --------    --------    --------    --------    --------    --------
     0.704       0.430       0.401       0.685       0.673       0.637

SQUARED MULTIPLE CORRELATIONS FOR X - VARIABLES

    health
  --------
     0.187
```

FIGURE 15-12. Squared multiple correlations for X-variables.

Test–Retest Reliability

If test–retest data are collected for a sufficiently large sample (ie, 200, or 500 or more, per time point), CFA can be used to provide a more sophisticated approach to the issue of test–retest reliability. The focus of this more sophisticated approach is measurement invariance over time.

The traditional approach to test–retest reliability requires administering the measure to the same respondents on more than one occasion and computing a reliability coefficient (Pearson's *r*) of the relationship between the scores obtained at the different administrations. However, this traditional approach assumes that measurement error associated with the repeated measurements is truly random. The more likely possibility is that a component of the error term is unique to the respondent, and this unique component is likely to be stable during each administration of the instrument because the same observed variables are measured over time with the same respondents (Strommel et al., 1992). This component of the error term that is unique to the respondent produces autocorrelations among the residuals associated with the observed variables at the different time points. In other words, the error terms associated with the observed variables are autocorrelated.

CFA takes advantage of the likelihood that measurement error over time is not random. With CFA, the researcher specifies and evaluates autocorrelated measurement error. This allows the researcher to look at both the stability of measurement error over time as well as stability in the factor structure (ie, factor loadings, factor intercorrelations). This more sophisticated approach to test–retest reliability is particularly useful in nursing, where drawing valid conclusions about intervention effects requires distinguishing real change in the construct of interest from the effects of unreliability of measurement. Establishing that an instrument is invariant across time is a critical first step to measuring real change.

Stability of the Factor Structure in Different Population Subgroups

In addition to establishing that an instrument is invariant across time, it is also critical to establish that it is invariant across groups, particularly if a researcher is interested in using an instrument to assess the effects of a nursing intervention in different populations. Moreover, drawing valid conclusions about group differences requires that research instruments are measuring the same constructs in the same ways in the groups that are being compared. Before the development of CFA, it was not really possible to address the issue of measurement invariance in any substantive fashion. Traditional factor analysis did not allow the determination of whether the factor loadings in two different groups were statistically different from one another, let alone making comparisons of measurement error.

The notion of nested models is a central part of using CFA to test hypotheses about measurement invariance. A specific model is said to be nested within a less restricted model if it is a special case of the second model. For example, there are three conditions that are essential for measurement invariance across groups, and each of the three conditions are increasingly more stringent: (1) each subscale (or latent variable) must be based on the same observed variables across comparison populations, (2) the unstandardized factor loadings must be the same, and (3) the covariances among the factor subscales or latent variables must be the same (Schaie & Hertzog, 1985). Each of these conditions can be specified as a set of nested CFA models: model 3 is nested within model 2, and model 2 is nested within model 1. The nested chi-square (see Chapter 17 for a discussion of this fit index) is used to evaluate which of the three competing models provides the best fit to the data.

Convergent and Divergent Validity

CFA is also well suited for the multimethod–multitrait approach to construct valida-tion. The multimethod–multitrait approach addresses issues of both convergent and divergent validity. Convergent and divergent validity involves developing valid-ity hypotheses about how the measure of interest *converges* and *diverges* with other measures of constructs that are theoretically related and theoretically unre-lated, respectively.

The multimethod–multitrait approach is an extension of convergent and diver-gent validity. Multiple traits or constructs are measured more than once on the same occasion using multiple methods (eg, interviews, summated rating scales, and visual analog scales) so that method variance can be separated from trait variance. Hypotheses about how scores on measures of the same trait are related, and how scores on measures of different traits are not, can then be tested.

Like the advantages of CFA over traditional EFA, CFA offers more information about convergent and discriminant validity. These advantages include detailed assessment of measurement error and the availability of fit indices to test the corre-spondence between theoretically derived hypotheses and empirical results. For example, the traditional approach of using the validity coefficient (Pearson's *r*) to estimate convergent validity is based on the assumption that the criterion measure (a comparison measure of the same or a similar construct as the instrument in question) has no measurement error. However, there are few established research instruments that meet this gold standard. Thus, in practice, the validity coefficient is usually a function of error in the measure of interest as well as error in the criterion measure or the measure being used for comparison. CFA, however, estimates the error vari-ance in both the measure of interest and the criterion measure. Interested readers are encouraged to read Pedhazur and Schmelkin (1991) or Wothke (1996) for further dis-cussion of using CFA for multitrait–multimethod approaches to construct validation.

SUMMARY

This chapter has given an overview of CFA and introduced the reader to its various uses and advantages. CFA is a powerful and complicated procedure. Readers who are interested in learning more about this technique are encouraged to consult more advanced texts on the topic and to follow the computer manual for the specific software package they are using.

Application Exercises and Results

Exercises

1. Draw the measurement model for the Inventory of Positive Psychological Attitudes (IPPA). Is the model that you have specified over- or underidentified according to the three indicator rule?

2. We attempted to analyze this two-factor model using LISREL. The analysis could not be run (the determinate of the matrix was not positive definite). We deleted items that were identified in Kass and colleagues (1991) as loading on more than one factor (ie, respecified the model). However, we were again unable to test this model (the determinate of the matrix was not positive definite). What alternative measurement model(s) should we test with these data?

Results

1. Your measurement model should have two factors (latent variables) that are correlated with each other, Life Purpose and Self-Confidence. Seventeen items load on Life Purpose (ie, Life Purpose latent variable has 17 indicators) and thirteen items load on Self-Confidence (ie, Self Confidence latent variable has 13 indicators). Because there are well more than three indicators per latent variable, the measurement model is overidentified, according to the three indicator rule. See also Exercise Figure 15-1. Note: Kass and colleagues'

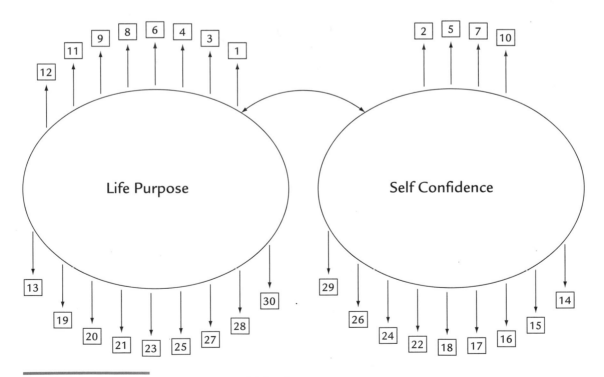

EXERCISE FIGURE 15-1. Measurement model for the IPPA.

(1991) EFA identified two factors with some items loading on more than one factor. However, they encouraged researchers to use the IPPA as either a single or two factor measure.

2. Both the original two-factor model and the respecified one are not statistically identifiable due to how we have specified relationships among the measured variables (IPPA items). One alternative model to test would be a single factor model to see if this fit the data any better than the two-factor model. Additionally, we might want to review the results obtained using traditional SPSS factor analysis (Chapter 14) to explore the factor structure of the IPPA in the current data set. Based on these results we might want to further respecify the two-factor model by deleting any additional items that loaded on more than one factor in the SPSS output generated for a PC extraction with a varimax rotation.

Path Analysis

Anne E. Norris

Objectives for Chapter 16

After reading this chapter, you should be able to do the following:

1. State the three conditions necessary for causality.
2. Draw a recursive path model.
3. Identify which independent variables are theorized to have indirect effects in addition to direct effects on the dependent variable.
4. Identify the appropriate regression analyses needed to calculate the path coefficients in a model.
5. Calculate the direct and indirect effects of an independent variable in a model.

RESEARCH QUESTION

Path analysis is used to answer questions regarding the relationships between a set of independent variables and a dependent variable. Path analysis is based on simple regression techniques, but by looking at these relationships it takes the researcher a step beyond the traditional regression analysis discussed in Chapters 11 and 12. Path analysis moves beyond testing whether a set of independent variables predicts a phenomenon to examining the relationships among those variables. Asher (1983) argues that by taking this step beyond regression analysis, we achieve a richer understanding of our phenomena. For example, Robinson (1995) used path analysis to examine how social support, income and education, spiritual beliefs, and coping influenced the grief response of widows (Fig. 16-1). Path models are considered a type of causal model, and path analysis is referred to as a causal modeling technique. Path models depict theorized, directional relationships among a set of variables. For example, in Robinson's model in Figure 16-1, social support, income

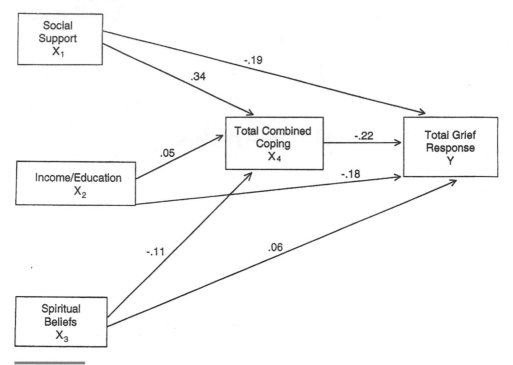

FIGURE 16-1. Robinson's (1995) path model.

and education, and spiritual beliefs are depicted as influencing or "causing" the widow's total combined coping.

Path analysis is literally an analysis of the paths or lines in a model that represent the influence of one variable on another. It is used to answer research questions about the effect of a given independent (X_1) variable on the dependent variable (Y) in the model. As you learn in this chapter, independent variables may have both direct $(X_1 \rightarrow Y)$ and indirect effects. Indirect effects arise when the independent variable is theorized to influence other independent variables in the model. In Robinson's path model, social support, income and education, and spiritual beliefs influence coping, which in turn influences the widow's grief response. Thus, the diagram indicates that these variables have indirect effects on the dependent variable (grief response) through their influence on coping. The direct lines between these three variables and the dependent variable, grief response, indicate that these variables have direct effects on the dependent variable as well.

By analyzing the paths, path analysis provides information about the consistency between data and a theorized path model. If the data do not fit the theorized relationships in the model, this suggests that the model (and the theory that generated it) may warrant revision. However, data that are consistent with the model are supportive but not definitive; such data merely indicate that the model (and the theory) was not disconfirmed.

Ideally, the path model should be drawn before the data are collected. However, in secondary data analysis, the model is drawn after the data are collected but before the analysis is conducted. In both primary and secondary data analysis, the model may also be drawn after completing a regression analysis because the researcher wishes to examine the relationships between the independent variables. In either case, Asher (1983) recommends working with a model based on an a priori theoretical or substantive understanding of the relationships between variables in the model. Although it is important to modify a model in response to statistical results, the path analysis should not become a mindless attempt to find a model that best fits the data. Such attempts result in models that may not replicate and may have questionable theoretical value.

TYPE OF DATA REQUIRED

Path analysis requires the same type of data as for linear multiple regression. In other words, you need a dependent variable that is continuous and normally distributed. Ideally, the independent variables are also continuous. Some researchers use the coding techniques (dummy, effect, orthogonal) discussed in Chapter 11 to include categorical variables, but by doing so they violate a statistical assumption underlying path analysis (see the discussion of assumptions later) and jeopardize the validity of their findings. In addition, the researcher should strive to have a large enough dataset to follow Nunnally and Bernstein's (1994) recommendation of 30 subjects per independent variable in the model to increase the likelihood that findings can be replicated and are not mere artifact.

Although path analysis is considered a causal modeling technique, it can be performed with either cross-sectional or longitudinal data. For example, Robinson's data were cross-sectional. Hence, it is important to understand some of the theoretical assumptions underlying path analysis, namely those pertaining to causation.

ASSUMPTIONS

There are two types of assumptions that must be considered with path analysis: theoretical and statistical.

Theoretical Assumptions

In the strictest sense, causation is investigated with experimental designs in which the independent variable is manipulated, the subsequent effects of this are measured, and variables that could confound or influence the effect of the independent variable are controlled for (eg, subjects are randomized to condition). However, path analysis typically involves testing a causal or path model with data that do not result from an experimental design. For example, path analysis can be done with survey data, data produced by a review of medical records, and so forth. Given this, many researchers have reservations about using such models to imply causation (Pedhazur, 1997). Hence, although the notion of causation is implicit, careful terminology is used. For example, independent variables may be referred to as predictor variables but are described as influencing rather than causing the dependent variable.

Nevertheless, theoretical assumptions of causation are implicit in path analysis, and such assumptions are strengthened when three conditions of causation are met (Kenny, 1979). First, there must be an observed and measurable relationship between X_1 and Y. In other words, X_1 and Y must be correlated. Second, X_1 should precede Y in time; that is, it must be possible to temporally order X_1 and Y such that X_1 occurred first in time. This condition may seem easy to meet, but it can be quite complicated. Consider a cross-sectional dataset concerning a health behavior such as engaging in regular exercise, and predictors of this behavior, such as education and beliefs about exercise. For education, the matter is straightforward. It is safe to assume that education temporally precedes current exercise. For beliefs, it is less clear. Do we assume that beliefs about exercise were present first? This would be consistent with hypothesizing that these beliefs lead to engaging in regular exercise. However, could the exercise have occurred before the beliefs developed or were fully formed? This would be consistent with hypothesizing that engaging in regular exercise changes or alters beliefs about exercise. Unfortunately, the researcher must take a stand on the hypothesized causal direction; otherwise, the model would be nonrecursive, and nonrecursive path models cannot be tested with cross-sectional data.

This example illustrates the problem with using causal modeling techniques to imply causation. It also underscores the importance of theory: We can use theory to resolve the dilemma of whether the belief or the behavior came first. For example, Pender's (1987) Health Promotion Theory and Fishbein and Ajzen's (1975) Theory of Reasoned Action both specify that beliefs guide behavior. Therefore, we can use these theories to guide us in assigning a direction between beliefs and behaviors such that beliefs are theorized to influence engaging in exercise (Fig. 16-2).

Third, X_1 and Y should have a nonspurious relationship. This means that the observed, measurable, and temporally ordered relationship between X_1 and Y will not disappear when the effects of other variables on this relationship are controlled. For example, suppose in our predictors of exercise analysis, we found that the

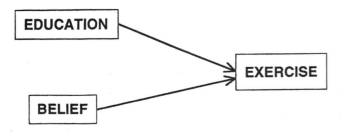

FIGURE 16-2. Education influences exercise. Belief influences exercise.

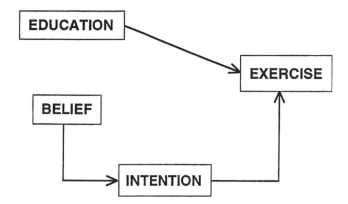

FIGURE 16-3. Intention confounds the relationship between belief and exercise because belief influences intention, which in turn influences exercise.

relationship between beliefs and engaging in exercise disappeared when the effects of intention to exercise were controlled for statistically (ie, we entered intention into a regression analysis predicting exercise behavior first, with belief entered on the second step, and found that the beta for belief was no longer significant). This would mean that the earlier relationship between belief and exercise was spurious—it only appeared to exist because both belief and exercise were correlated with intention. Another way to say this is that the relationship was confounded by intention. If we found this, we would modify the diagram of our causal model from the one in Figure 16-2 to the one in Figure 16-3.

This third condition of causation seems straightforward. We can use regression to test whether the data meet this assumption, but the problem is that we can do this only if we have measured the right confounding variable. It is difficult (perhaps impossible) to identify and rule out all the variables that could confound the observed relationship between X_1 and Y. The solution is to use theory, existing literature, and discussions with colleagues to identify the variables that seem clearly likely to confound the relationships in the model, and then include measures of such variables in the analysis (Asher, 1983). Unfortunately, in secondary data analysis, the researcher works with an existing dataset and can include only the variables that are contained in the dataset. Thus, such researchers may need to recognize this as a limitation of their results.

Statistical Assumptions

RELATED TO MULTIPLE REGRESSION

The statistical assumptions in path analysis are of two types. The first you are already familiar with: the assumptions of normal distributions, homoscedasticity, and linear relationships discussed in Chapters 11 and 12 for multiple regression analysis. These assumptions arise because path analysis consists of a series of regression equations.

UNIQUE TO PATH ANALYSIS

The second type of assumption is unique to path analysis. This type is necessary if we want to use path analysis to calculate the direct and indirect effects of variables in the path model. There are four such assumptions:

1. When two independent variables are correlated with one another and diagrammed as having no other variables influencing them, their relationship cannot be analyzed, and it is assumed that the magnitude of this relationship is represented by the correlation coefficient (Pedhazur, 1997).
2. It is assumed that the flow of causation in the model is unidirectional (Pedhazur, 1997). The model is recursive: If we start with any independent variable in a model and move our fingers along the straight lines in the direction of the arrows from one variable to the next, we will not come back to the independent variable we started with; we will not find ourselves moving in a circle.
3. It is assumed that the variables in the model are measured on an interval scale (Pedhazur, 1997). However, Asher (1983) argues that this assumption can be somewhat relaxed with ordinal variables, particularly as the number of categories in the ordinal variable increases.
4. All variables in the model are measured without error; measurement error is assumed to be zero (Pedhazur, 1997). This last assumption underscores the importance of having reliable measures of variables in the path model.

POWER

Power analyses in path analysis are the same as those discussed in Chapter 11 for multiple regression and so are not discussed in detail here. As you see later in the examples in this chapter, path analysis involves more than one regression analysis. Hence, the power analysis should be calculated for the regression equation that involves the smallest effect size (or requires the largest number of subjects because it contains the most variables). This will ensure that you have enough power to detect the significance of important paths in the model.

KEY TERMS

Path analysis brings with it a set of terms that are common to causal models in general. We have already discussed recursive and nonrecursive models and direct and indirect effects. In this next section, we will discuss these terms in more detail and then introduce some additional ones.

Recursive and Nonrecursive Models

As discussed earlier in this chapter, an assumption in path analysis is that the model is recursive; that is, there is a one-way flow of causation in the model. Another way of thinking about this is that in a recursive model, all the paths between variables are one-way roads. The only exception is when theory and previous research is insufficient to support a direction being assigned to the "road." In this case, a correlational rather than a directional relationship is assumed, indicated by a curved line with an arrow at each end. In a nonrecursive model, at least one of the paths between two variables is a two-way road, or there is a set of paths in the model that are circular. These models do not meet the assumptions necessary for standard path analysis. There is a way to use longitudinal data to translate some theoretical models that are inherently nonrecursive into a recursive form that can then be tested with path analysis (see Asher, 1983, and Pedhazur, 1997, for examples of this and other ways to approach recursive models).

Indirect and Direct Effects

A given independent variable in a model can be diagrammed as having one of three kinds of effects on the dependent variable, depending on its relationships with other variables in the model: only direct, only indirect, or both direct and indirect. Let us return to a path model of factors influencing engaging in regular exercise. In Figure 16-4, intention has only a direct effect on the dependent variable. This effect is reflected in the direct line between intention and exercise that points toward exercise. In this same figure, age and education also have direct effects on exercise, and age and education are correlated.

In Figure 16-5, education has only an indirect effect on exercise through its relationship with intention. There is no direct line between education and exercise, as there was in Figure 16-4. However, there is a direct line between education and intention that points toward intention, and between intention and the dependent variable.

In Figure 16-6, education has both direct and indirect effects on the dependent variable. As in Figures 16-4 and 16-5, intention has only a direct effect.

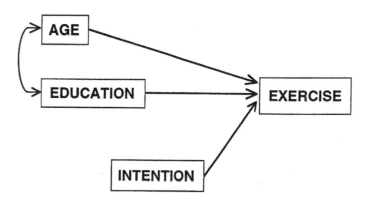

FIGURE 16-4. Age, education, and intention have direct effects.

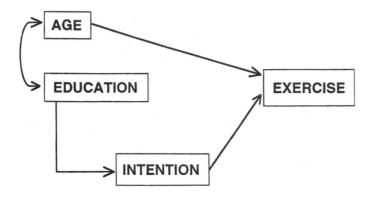

FIGURE 16-5. Education has an indirect effect. Age and intentions have direct effects.

Endogenous and Exogenous Variables

All variables in a path model can be described as either endogenous or exogenous. This is an important distinction, because to do path analysis you need to perform a regression analysis for every endogenous variable in the model. Endogenous variables are variables that are diagrammed as being influenced by other variables in the model. The variables diagrammed as independent of any influence are the exogenous variables (Bollen, 1989).

Dependent variables are always endogenous, but some independent (or predictor) variables can be endogenous if they are themselves being influenced by other independent variables in the model. Thus, in Figure 16-6, intention is both an independent variable and an endogenous variable. This means that to analyze the path model depicted in Figure 16-6, we need two regression analyses—one with exercise regressed onto age, education, and intention and one with intention regressed onto education. This second regression only involves one independent variable. Hence the path coefficient is simply the correlation between intention and

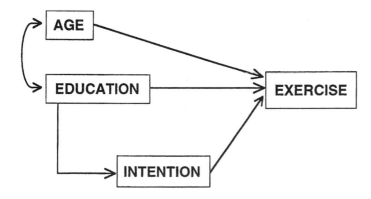

FIGURE 16-6. Education has direct and indirect effects.

education. Age is not included in this second regression because it has no direct or indirect effect on this intention. Note that for any given endogenous variable, all variables that are exogenous to it (i.e., any that have direct or indirect effects) need to be entered into the regression equation for that specific endogenous variable.

In the diagrams you have seen in this chapter, both endogenous and exogenous variables are indicated with a square drawn around them. This square is used to indicate that these variables correspond to a subject's response or score in a particular dataset. Variables demarcated with a square are referred to as measured variables or indicators of specific theoretical constructs. As you will learn in Chapter 17, circles are used to indicate that a variable is an unmeasured, theoretical construct.

Path Coefficients

Path coefficients are produced by the various regression analyses used in the path analysis. They represent the magnitude of the influence of one variable on another in the path model. The subscripts used in the notation for path coefficients are ordered such that the letter or abbreviation representing the variable being influenced is always listed first and the one for the variable doing the influencing is listed second. Thus, in Figure 16-6, the path coefficient for the path between intention and exercise is $p_{e,i}$.

Either the standardized (beta) or the nonstandardized (b) regression coefficient can be used as the value for the path coefficient, but use of the former is more common. Use of the standardized coefficient allows comparison of the magnitude of one path in the model with that of other paths in the model. Thus, use of the standardized coefficient makes it possible for the reader to determine which independent variable has the greatest direct effect on the dependent variable. In contrast, use of the nonstandardized coefficient makes it possible to evaluate how the magnitude of a particular path varies in different sample subgroups or study populations. Pedhazur (1997) recommends that both coefficients should be reported; if only standardized coefficients are reported, then the standard deviations of all the variables should be reported as well, so that interested readers can calculate the nonstandardized value. Use of standardized path coefficients may be more common because these coefficients are needed to determine the direct, indirect, and total effect of an independent variable. The determination of these effects is discussed later (see the sections on determining direct and indirect effects, and conducting a path analysis).

Identification

Causal models can be overidentified, just identified, or underidentified. Visually, just identified models are easy to recognize because all the variables in the model are interconnected with each other by a path (Pedhazur, 1997). Such models can become overidentified through the process of "theory trimming" or the deletion of nonsignificant paths in the model (Heise, 1969). Note how the overidentified model in Figure 16-7 becomes the just identified model in Figure 16-8 with the addition of

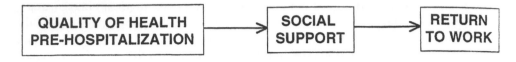

FIGURE 16-7. Overidentified model.

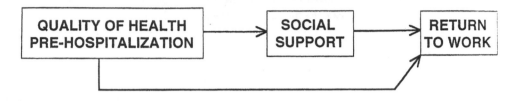

FIGURE 16-8. Just identified model.

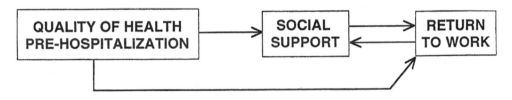

FIGURE 16-9. Underidentified model.

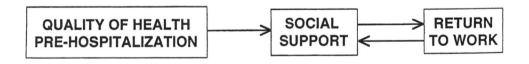

FIGURE 16-10. Partially underidentified model.

the direct path between quality of health pre-hospitalization and return to work ($p_{r,q}$). The just identified model becomes underidentified in Figure 16-9 when the path $p_{s,r}$ is added and the model becomes nonrecursive. In Figure 16-10, the addition of this same path to the overidentified model in Figure 16-7 results in a nonrecursive model that is partially underidentified.

An advantage of overidentified models is that unlike just identified or underidentified models, the model as a whole can be statistically evaluated for its fit to the data. The results of this statistical test can be used to support the validity of the path model, although this is not commonly done in the published literature. A discussion of this statistic is beyond the scope of this chapter, but if readers are interested in learning more about it, Pedhazur (1997) is an excellent resource.

DETERMINING DIRECT AND INDIRECT EFFECTS

Being able to determine the direct and indirect effects of an independent variable is an important advantage of path analysis (Asher, 1983). It allows you to know the total effect of an independent variable, which could be important in deciding which independent variables you might want to target in an intervention. Being able to determine these effects also allows you to compare them. For example, an independent variable can have an indirect effect that is greater than its direct effect, or vice versa. It is also possible that the two effects may cancel each other out, in the sense that they could be similar in magnitude but opposite in direction (one positive, the other negative).

Pedhazur (1997) presents a method for using matrix algebra to ease the calculation of direct and indirect effects for more complex models (ie, models with many variables and many paths). However, for simplicity an alternative method developed by Wright (1934) is presented in this chapter that does not require a knowledge of matrix algebra. Using Wright's method, you can work directly from the diagram of the path model and identify the simple (direct effect) and compound (more than one path is involved) paths relevant to a particular variable. These compound effects can either be meaningful (indirect) or nonmeaningful (noncausal).

According to Wright, the value of any one compound path is equal to the product of the simple paths that make it up. Thus, in the hypothetical model in Figure 16-11, the compound path from quality of health prehospitalization to return to work through social support is equal to $p_{s,q}$ multiplied by $p_{r,s}$. In the hypothetical model in Figure 16-12, there are two possible meaningful compound paths between quality of health prehospitalization and return to work: $(p_{s,q})(p_{r,s})$, and a new one that takes us from quality of health prehospitalization to return to work through social support and adherence. The value of this new compound path is $(p_{s,q})(p_{ad,s})(p_{r,ad})$. There is also a nonmeaningful compound (or noncausal) path between quality of health prehospitalization and return to work through age: This

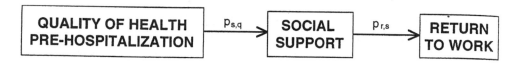

FIGURE 16-11. Model with one compound path from quality of health prehospitalization to return to work through social support.

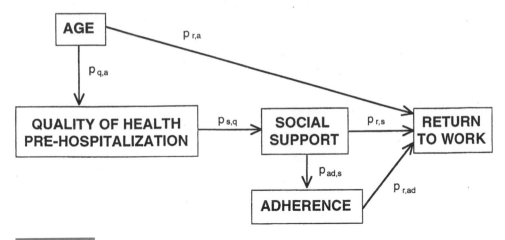

FIGURE 16-12. Model with two meaningful and one nonmeaningful compound paths from quality of health prehospitalization to return to work.

compound path is equal to $(p_{r,a})(p_{q,a})$. This compound path ignores the direction of the relationships specified by the path model. This is why it is noncausal and is considered nonmeaningful. However, it is an important component of the correlation between quality of health prehospitalization and return to work.

Wright found that when a path model is correctly specified, the correlation between two variables is equal to the sum of the simple (direct effect) and all possible compound paths (indirect effect and noncausal) between these two variables. Measurement error may enter in and cause the correlation to be approximately, rather than exactly, equal to the sum of the direct effect, indirect effect, and noncausal component. However, incorrect specification of the model could cause the sum of the direct and indirect effects and noncausal component to be noticeably less than the correlation. This noticeable difference between the sum and the correlation is an indication that the model may need revision (Asher, 1983).

Thus, in Figure 16-12 we could describe the correlation between quality of health prehospitalization and return to work with the following equation:

$$r = (p_{s,q})(p_{r,s}) + (p_{s,q})(p_{ad,s})(p_{r,ad}) + (p_{r,a})(p_{q,a})$$

In this equation, there is no direct effect, $(p_{s,q})(p_{r,s}) + (p_{s,q})(p_{ad,s})(p_{r,ad})$ is the sum of the total indirect effect of the variable, and $(p_{r,a})(p_{q,a})$ is the noncausal component of the correlation.

It is important to identify all the compound paths in a model that are relevant to the correlation between two variables. Otherwise, one might, through error, conclude incorrectly that a path model needs respecification. Fortunately, Wright has provided three rules that, if followed, result in the identification of all possible compound paths between two particular variables. These rules guide the researcher in looking at a diagram of a path model and tracing the possible compound paths. The goal is for the researcher to identify compound paths that are meaningful (indirect effects) and not meaningful (noncausal), because both are part of the correlation.

Wright's three rules for identifying all compound paths are as follows:

1. No compound path involves going through the same variable more than once.
2. No compound path involves going forward with the direction of an arrow through a variable and then backward against the direction of a second arrow through a second variable (although it is perfectly acceptable to go backward first and then forward).
3. No compound path involves going through a curved, double-headed arrow line (ie, a diagrammed relationship between two variables that has been left as a correlation) more than once.

The second rule sounds complicated, but we have already been applying it to identify the nonmeaningful compound path in Figure 16-12 for the variables quality of health prehospitalization and return to work. Look back over the diagram in Figure 16-12 and trace this path once more. The third rule hints at the problem with including a correlation in a path model; namely, that the correlation may get in the way of determining the indirect effect of an independent variable. For this reason, researchers should assign a direction to hypothesized relationships between variables whenever possible, but not at the expense of theory or logic and reason.

CONDUCTING A PATH ANALYSIS

Conducting a path analysis involves preparation, analysis, and a consideration of the analysis' limitations. In this section we go through the steps needed to conduct a path analysis, using two examples: a computer example of a study of factors influencing individuals' perceptions of their overall state of health, and an example from the published literature, Kurlowicz's (1998) test of conceptual framework for family well-being.

Computer Example: A Study of Factors Influencing Individuals' Perceptions of Their Overall State of Health

This example illustrates how researchers can use path analysis to move a step beyond traditional regression analysis. Here, the researchers start the path analysis after completing a regression analysis in which the factors that influence an individual's perception of health have been identified. These data are taken from the dataset included with this book.

The independent variables in this example are satisfaction with current weight, frequency of exercise, and scores on an inventory of personal attitudes about self, life, and work. Age and education were tested for inclusion as independent variables but were not significant in this final regression model and were dropped. The sample size is 659, and the independent variables are continuous and fairly normally distributed. We are comfortable in continuing with the analysis because we know that multiple regression is somewhat robust to (ie, able to tolerate) mild to moderate violations of normality, particularly as the sample size increases. The only information we have about measurement error is that the Cronbach's alpha for the inventory of personal attitudes is 0.95.

PREPARATION

The first step is to draw the model to be tested with path analysis. This path model is drawn after having used regression analysis to identify which variables from a theoretical framework are significantly related to the dependent variable of interest. The results of this regression analysis are depicted in Table 16-1. To draw the model we will also need a table of correlations among the variables in the regression

TABLE 16-1 *Regression Results Used to Create Path Model in Computer Example*

Model Summary

Model	R	R Square	Adjusted R Square	Std. Error of the Estimate
1	.580[a]	.336	.333	1.143

a. Predictors: (Constant), satisfaction with current weight, personal attitudes, exercise.

ANOVA[b]

Model		Sum of Squares	df	Mean Square	F	Sig.
1	Regression	663.461	3	221.154	110.725	.000[a]
	Residual	1308.247	655	1.997		
	Total	1971.709	658			

a. Predictors: (Constant), satisfaction with current weight, personal attitudes, exercise.
b. Dependent Variable: overall state of health.

Coefficients[a]

Model		Unstandardized Coefficients		Standardized Coefficients		
		B	Std. Error	Beta	t	Sig.
1	(Constant)	2.690	.312		8.634	.000
	exercise	.375	.059	.220	6.314	.000
	personal attitudes	.023	.002	.370	10.990	.000
	satisfaction with current weight	.124	.022	.193	5.546	.000

a. Dependent Variable: overall state of health.

TABLE 16-2 *Correlations Among Variables in Computer Example*

		Overall state of health	Exercise	Satisfaction with current weight	Total
Pearson Correlation	Overall state of health	1.000	.394	.369	.482
	Exercise	.394	1.000	.363	.281
	Satisfaction with current weight	.369	.363	1.000	.260
	Personal attitudes	.482	.281	.260	1.000

(Table 16-2); familiarity with the research findings and theory pertinent to this topic; logic and reason to assign, where possible, a temporal order to the independent variables that are correlated with one another and for which research findings and theory are not available; and awareness of the need to maintain a one-way flow of causation to meet the assumptions necessary for path analysis.

An examination of the correlations listed in Table 16-2 reveals that all the independent variables are correlated with one another. This means that we must now attempt to assign a direction to these relationships. Theories about health behavior hold that attitudes guide behavior (Norris & Ford, 1995). Therefore, we can assign a direction to the relationship between personal attitudes and frequency of exercise and draw a path ($p_{f,p}$) to represent this (Fig. 16-13). Research on exercise suggests

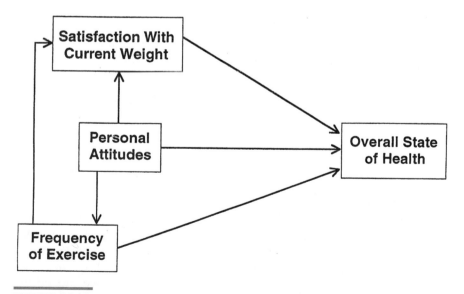

FIGURE 16-13. Diagram of initial path model.

that people who exercise moderately and regularly may be more satisfied with their weight (Tucker & Maxwell, 1992), and there is no evidence that those in our sample exercise excessively. Consequently, we draw a path ($p_{s,f}$) in Figure 16-13 to represent the influence of frequency of exercise on satisfaction with current weight. Research and theory are not available for assigning a direction to the relationship between personal attitudes and satisfaction with current weight, so here we use logic and reason and awareness of the need to maintain a one-way flow of causation. It seems reasonable to hypothesize that a general set of attitudes should influence satisfaction with something specific such as current weight. So we assign a direction to the path between these two variables ($p_{s,p}$) to represent this. There is in fact only one direction that can be assigned to this relationship that will ensure that the model meets the necessary assumption of a one-way flow of causation. If we instead hypothesized that satisfaction with current weight influenced personal attitudes, the model would have a component that is circular or nonrecursive. You can see this if you redraw the model in Figure 16-13 such that it contains the path $p_{p,s}$ in place of $p_{s,p}$.

The second step is to identify the regression analyses needed to calculate the path coefficients and test the paths in the model. Look at the model in Figure 16-13 and count the number of endogenous variables to determine the number of regression analyses needed. You should come up with three endogenous variables: the dependent variable, overall state of health; frequency of exercise, which is endogenous to personal attitudes; and satisfaction with current weight, which is endogenous to frequency of exercise and personal attitudes. Checking to be sure that we have identified all the variables that have direct or indirect effects on a specific endogenous variable, we identify the three regression analyses needed for this model as follows:

1. Overall state of health (o) regressed on satisfaction with current weight (s), frequency of exercise (f), and personal attitudes (p);
2. Frequency of exercise regressed on personal attitudes; and
3. Satisfaction with current weight regressed on frequency of exercise and personal attitudes.

The second regression analysis is nothing more than the correlation between frequency of exercise and personal attitudes. It is always the case that the path between an endogenous and an exogenous variable is equal to the correlation between these two variables whenever (1) there is an endogenous variable with only one variable exogenous to it, and (2) the exogenous variable is fully exogenous and has no other variables influencing it.

ANALYSIS

The first step is to calculate the path coefficients. This is easy! We actually know what many of these coefficients are from our prior work. Figure 16-14 shows what we know using information from Tables 16-1 and 16-2. We are using the betas or the standardized coefficients for our diagram because we are not looking at group differences.

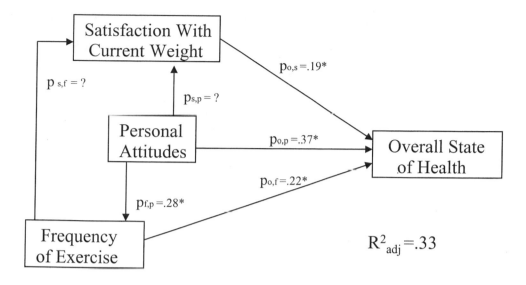

FIGURE 16-14. Diagram of model prior to running third regression analysis to test paths to endogenous variables. (*Path coefficient is significant at $p < .001$.)

To calculate the remaining coefficients, we run the third regression analysis we identified in our preparation earlier—the one with satisfaction with current weight as the dependent variable. The results of this third regression analysis are shown in Table 16-3.

From the results in Table 16-3, we see that the remaining paths ($p_{s,p}$, $p_{s,f}$) are statistically significant ($p < 0.001$). Hence, there is no need to modify our model, and we can proceed to calculating the direct and indirect effects of the independent variables. Figure 16-15 depicts our final path model. We will need to refer to this model to complete this second step of the analysis.

The second step is to determine the direct, indirect, and total effects of the independent variables. Now we construct Table 16-4 to help us use Wright's work about the components of a correlation. We fill in Table 16-4 using the correlation values from Table 16-2 for the left column and the beta weights from Table 16-1 for the simple paths column. These beta weights are the direct effects of the independent variable on overall state of health.

Figure 16-15 is used to identify the paths that need to be multiplied to determine the values for the compound paths. Wright's rules are used to trace the paths needed to calculate these compound paths. For example, the second rule tells us that the coefficients for $p_{f,p}$ and $p_{o,p}$ should be multiplied to determine the noncausal component of $r_{f,o}$. Note that the compound paths are sorted into (1) indirect effects, which are the sums of products for meaningful compound paths, and (2) noncausal components, which are the sums of products for compound paths that are meaningless.

TABLE 16-3 *Regression Results for Paths to Endogenous Independent Variables in Computer Example*

Model Summary

Model	R	R Square	Adjusted R Square	Std. Error of the Estimate
1	.399[a]	.159	.157	2.459

a. Predictors: (Constant), personal attitudes, exercise.

ANOVA[b]

Model		Sum of Squares	df	Mean Square	F	Sig.
1	Regression	751.371	2	375.686	62.116	.000[a]
	Residual	3967.591	656	6.048		
	Total	4718.962	658			

a. Predictors: (Constant), personal attitudes, exercise.
b. Dependent Variable: Satisfaction with current weight.

Coefficients[a]

Model		Unstandardized Coefficients		Standardized Coefficients	t	Sig.
		B	Std. Error	Beta		
1	(Constant),	1.423	.539		2.638	.009
	exercise,	.830	.098	.315	8.455	.000
	personal attitudes	.016	.004	.172	4.598	.000

a. Dependent Variable: satisfaction with current weight.

Table 16-5 contains the value of the direct and indirect effects as determined by using Wright's formula for the components of a correlation coefficient and his rules for calculating compound paths. Personal Attitudes appears to have the greatest effect (0.48) on the overall state of health. Also, all but one of the sums of the total effect and noncausal components match the magnitude of the respective correlation coefficient. The one sum that does not (satisfaction with current weight) is very close (within .01).

Consideration of the Analysis' Limitations

Now that we have a final path model, it is important to review the assumptions underlying path analysis to be aware of the limitations of the analysis we have just conducted.

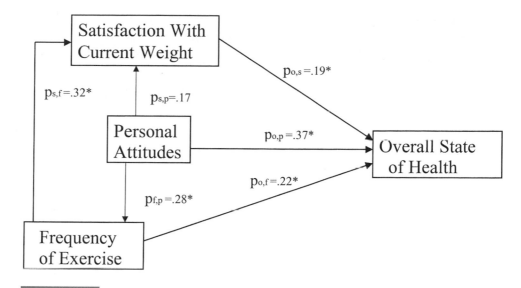

FIGURE 16-15. Final path analysis results for computer example. (*Path coefficient is significant at $p \leq .001$.)

First, we need to consider whether any of the relationships in the model may be spurious (ie, violate the third condition of causation). Are there potentially confounding variables that we should have included? Second, can we assume that there is no measurement error in our measures? What evidence do we have to support the reliability of our measures? Finally, we should also remind ourselves of the need to

TABLE 16-4 *Table Used to Determine Direct and Indirect Effects of Independent Variables in Figure 16.15*

r = **DIRECT** +		(INDIRECT) compound + $\cdots$ + compound	+ +	(NON-CAUSAL) compound + $\cdots$ + compound
$r =$ **simple** +				
$r_{f,o} = p_{o,f}$	+	$(p_{s,f})\,(p_{o,s})$	+	$(p_{f,p})(p_{o,p}) + (p_{f,p})\,(p_{s,p})\,(p_{o,s})$
$.39 = .22$	+	$(.32)(.19)$	+	$(.28)(.37) + (.28)(.17)(.19)$
$r_{p,o} = p_{o,p}$	+	$(p_{f,p})\,(p_{o,f}) + (p_{f,p})(p_{s,f})(p_{o,s}) + (p_{s,p})(p_{o,s})$	+	none
$.48 = .37$	+	$(.28)(.22) + (.28)(.32)(.19) + (.17)(.19)$	+	0
$r_{s,o} = p_{o,s}$	+	none	+	$(p_{s,f})\,(p_{o,f}) + (p_{s,p})(p_{o,p}) +$
				$(p_{s,p})(p_{f,\,p})(p_{o,f}) + (p_{s,f})(p_{f,p})(p_{o,p})$
$.37 = .19$	+	0	+	$(.32)(.22) + (.17)(.37) +$
				$(.17)(.28)(.22) + (.32)(.28)(.37)$

TABLE 16-5 *Table of Direct Effects, Indirect Effects, and Noncausal Components Associated with Each Independent Variable in Figure 16.15*

	DIRECT	+	INDIRECT	TOTAL EFFECT	TOTAL EFFECT + NONCAUSAL
Frequency of exercise (r = .39)	.22	+	.06	.28	.39
Personal attitudes (r = .48)	.37	+	.11	.48	.48
Satisfaction with current weight (r = .37)	.19	+	0	.19	.36

replicate this model with longitudinal data. In this example, we were forced to make assumptions regarding the directions between the variables in our model because we were working with cross-sectional data. For example, it may be the case that having a positive perception of their overall state of health causes individuals to exercise more, but we have no way of knowing this. Path analysis does not allow us to evaluate the correctness of the directions we have assigned. Rather, we have assumed that these are the correct directions. Path analysis can only tell us that given our assumptions, this particular path is or is not statistically significant.

Example of Published Path Analysis

This example illustrates Grimes-Holsinger's (2002) use of path analysis to demonstrate the effect of an infusion skills checklist with a standardized teaching tool on time required for instruction and the number of teaching visits engaged in by infusion nurses working with patients in their home. Study participants were 105 patients receiving antibiotic therapy in their home with 52 patients receiving instruction with a standardized skills checklist and 53 receiving a nonstandardized intervention. The investigator analyzed the nursing activity record and off-hour call log to determine the number of teaching visits and length of time spent teaching. No reliability information was given with respect to this coding. Standard deviations and ranges for teaching visits and length of time spent teaching were not given, so it is not possible to determine if these continuous variables were normally distributed or if they were skewed.

PREPARATION

1. Draw the model to be tested with path analysis.

   Grimes-Holsinger was interested in testing the just identified model depicted in Figure 16-16. Note that the intervention or treatment variable (standardized skills checklist, nonstandardized), which is categorical (ie, dichotomous), is

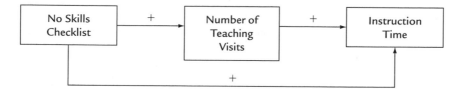

FIGURE 16-16. Theoretical model tested by Grimes-Holsinger (2002). Adapted from Figure 1 in Grimes-Holsinger, V. (2002). Comparing the effect of a skills checklist on teaching time required to achieve independence in administration of infusion medication. *Journal of Infusion Nursing, 25*(2), 109–120.

included in the model to be tested, but is coded as 1 for "nonstandardized" and 0 for "standardized." As can be seen from the figure, Grimes-Holsinger is hypothesizing that not using the standardized skills checklist will result in an increased number of teaching visits and an increased amount of instruction time. The number of teaching visits is also expected to increase the amount of instruction time. According to the model, not using the standardized checklist is hypothesized as having both direct and indirect effects on amount of instruction time.

2. Identify the regression analyses needed to calculate the path coefficients and test the paths in the model.

The model in Figure 16-16 specifies two endogenous variables, number of teaching visits and instruction time. Only one variable is involved in predicting teaching visits, the variable representing the effect of not using the skilled checklist ("no skills checklist"). Hence, the regression analysis for teaching visits can be reduced to the correlation between teaching visits and no skills checklist. Thus, only one regression analysis needs to be conducted to identify the path coefficients in the model: instruction time is regressed on number of teaching visits and no skills checklist.

ANALYSIS

1. Calculate the path coefficients.

The path coefficients reported by Grimes-Holsinger are shown in Figure 16-17. However, as can be seen from the data in Table 16.6, the values reported in her article as path coefficients (or betas from the regression) are all correlation coefficients. Grimes-Holsinger did not use the values produced in the regression analysis predicting instruction time for the paths involving direct effects on this variable. Given this is not possible to determine whether the paths involving instruction time are significant. It is likely that these coefficients would remain positive in the regression analysis, assuming there is no suppression (see Cohen & Cohen, 1983).

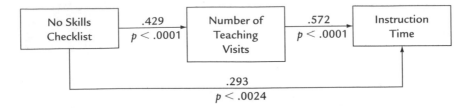

FIGURE 16-17. Results of path analysis for theoretical model tested by Grimes-Holsinger (2002). Adapted from Figure 4 in Grimes-Holsinger, V. (2002). Comparing the effect of a skills checklist on teaching time required to achieve independence in administration of infusion medication. *Journal of Infusion Nursing, 25*(2), 109–120.

2. Determine the direct, indirect, and total effects of the independent variables.

    Unfortunately, we cannot do this given the data reported by Grimes-Holsinger in her article. Grimes-Holsinger does report some R^2 values in her article, but it is not clear how these were produced. A table of regression results is also provided but the coefficients are the same as the correlation coefficients because only one variable appears to have been entered into each regression analysis that was reported.

Consideration of the Analysis' Limitations

On the surface, Grimes-Holsingers' (2002) analysis would initially appear to meet many of the theoretical and statistical assumptions for path analysis. Her sample size is appropriate. Her model is just identified, but it has a one-way flow of causation. However, she includes a dichotomous variable in the model and the reliability of her measures is not clear which by itself would argue for the need to replicate these results before using them to guide practice.

Unfortunately, Grimes-Holzemer made a mistake that many beginning researchers make in testing the path model by using correlation coefficients instead of regression

Table 16-6 Regression Analysis

Variables	Predictors	b	B	t	p
Teach Time	Number of teaching visits	75.90	0.572	7.07	<.0001
Teach time	No Skills Checklist	76.12	0.293	3.11	.0024*
Number of teaching visits	No Skills Checklists	0.84	0.429	4.82	<.0001

Table 7 in Grimes-Holsinger, V. (2002). Comparing the effect of a skills checklist on teaching time required to achieve independence in administration of infusion medication. *Journal of Infusion Nursing, 25*(2),119

coefficients where an endogenous variable has more than one variable influencing it. This is why it is so important to identify the regression equations needed to conduct the path analysis and to keep in mind that all variables having a direct or indirect effect on a particular endogenous variable need to be included as predictors in the regression equation. Moreover, this is a good example of how important it is to review correlation tables, regression results, and the final path model in an article to be sure that the results reported in the final model were created with the appropriate statistical methods.

Grimes-Holzemer's analysis highlights a challenge many researchers face: What to do with a categorical variable in a path analysis? Such variables may be included, but then the rules regarding the calculation of indirect and direct effects may not hold because the relationship between such variables and other continuous variables is not linear. Thus, a full path analysis cannot be done.

In data analysis situations such as the one presented here by Grimes-Holsinger, where the researcher is interested in the relationship between two variables in two or more groups of individuals, and whether this relationship differs in the groups, ANOVA may be more appropriate. Correlations are calculated for each group as part of the descriptive data needed to interpret the results. Then an ANOVA is conducted in which the two correlated variables are entered as a pair of repeated measures, representing one within subjects factor, "measure," and the group variable is the between subjects factor. A significant interaction term between Group and Measure indicates that the magnitude of the correlation is different in the groups being analyzed.

SUMMARY

Path analysis is a data analysis technique that can be used to inform our understanding of phenomena. It is useful because, at the very least, it challenges us to think of the effects of independent variables in more complex ways (Asher, 1983). Although on the surface it may appear complex, path analysis is a relatively simple data analysis technique. It is nothing more than a series of regression analyses and some hand calculations. The difficulty is in thinking through the relationships among a set of variables, and correctly specifying the regression equations to be tested.

Path analysis, like any statistic, is just a tool in the hands of the researcher. The validity of the model testing and theory building it produces depends on the quality of the data and the thinking that accompanies the use of the statistic.

Application Exercises and Results

Exercises

1. Identify the regression analyses needed to conduct a path analysis of the model depicted in Exercise Figure 16-1. Run the regression analyses. Delete any paths that are not significant at the .01 level and rerun regressions if necessary, adding the new betas to the model.

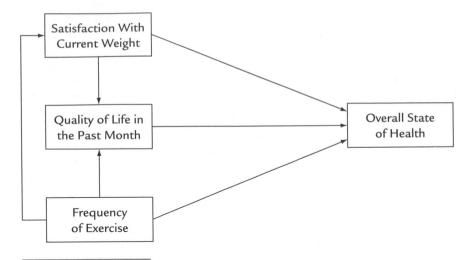

EXERCISE FIGURE 16-1. Path model for testing in Application Exercises.

2. Calculate the direct, indirect, and noncausal components of the correlations between each Overall State of Health and the predictor variables in the model.
3. What is the rationale for using a .01 alpha level as compared to a .05 level for determining significance? Would you feel more comfortable with a .005 level? Why or why not?
4. Discuss the limitations of this analysis.

Results

1. There are three endogenous variables in the model depicted in Exercise Figure 16-1. This means three regression equations are needed:
   a. Overall State of Health regressed on Frequency of Exercise, Current Satisfaction with Weight, and Quality of Life in Past Month.
   b. Quality of Life in Past Month regressed on Frequency of Exercise and Current Satisfaction with Weight.
   c. Current Satisfaction with Weight regressed on Frequency of Exercise.

   Notice that equation c. above only involves one independent variable. This means we can take a shortcut because in this case the correlation between Current Satisfaction with Weight and Frequency of Exercise is the same value as the beta that would be produced if we regressed Current Satisfaction with Weight on Frequency of Exercise. Hence, in Exercise Figure 16-2, you see a correlation matrix produced when regression equation a. was analyzed, and regression results for equations a. and b.

   When you write all the values for the standardized path coefficients in the model, your model should be like the one depicted in Exercise Figure 16-3. Note that the coefficients have all been rounded to two digits. All are significant at the .01 level so there is no need to delete paths from the model and run any additional regressions.

2. Exercise Figure 16-2 provides the numbers used to calculate the direct and indirect effects for the predictors in the path model. The specific calculations specified by Wright's rules are depicted in Exercise Table 16-1. Working these calculations through, we find that the total effect for frequency of exercise is .40, the total effect for quality of life in the past

Correlations

		overall state of health	exercise	satisfaction with current weight	quality of life in past month
Pearson Correlation	overall state of health	1.000	.391	.372	.401
	exercise	.391	1.000	.365	.260
	satisfaction with current weight	.372	.365	1.000	.251
	quality of life in past month	.401	.260	.251	1.000
Sig. (1-tailed)	overall state of health	.	.000	.000	.000
	exercise	.000	.	.000	.000
	satisfaction with current weight	.000	.000	.	.000
	quality of life in past month	.000	.000	.000	.
N	overall state of health	698	698	698	698
	exercise	698	698	698	698
	satisfaction with current weight	698	698	698	698
	quality of life in past month	698	698	698	698

Coefficients[a]

Model		Unstandardized Coefficients		Standardized Coefficients	t	Sig.
		B	Std. Error	Beta		
1	(Constant)	3.978	.253		15.734	.000
	exercise	.407	.060	.239	6.810	.000
	satisfaction with current weight	.138	.023	.214	6.109	.000
	quality of life in past month	.477	.056	.285	8.470	.000

[a.] Dependent Variable: overall state of health.

Coefficients[a]

Model		Unstandardized Coefficients		Standardized Coefficients	t	Sig.
		B	Std. Error	Beta		
1	(Constant)	3.368	.112		29.968	.000
	exercise	.199	.040	.195	5.029	.000
	satisfaction with current weight	.069	.015	.180	4.635	.000

[a.] Dependent Variable: quality of life in past month.

EXERCISE FIGURE 16-2. SPSS output for correlation and regression analyses used in application exercise 1.

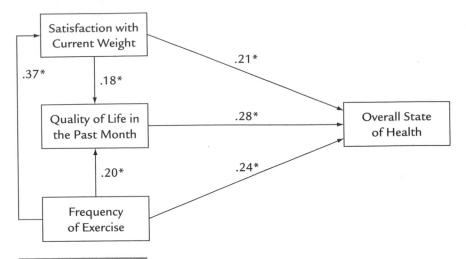

EXERCISE FIGURE 16-3. Results for final path model tested in Application Exercises. * Path coefficient in statistically significant at $p < .01$.

month is .29, and the total effect for satisfaction with current weight is .26. If we add in the noncausal components, we see that the total effect and the noncausal sum to a value that is within .01 to .02 of the correlation for a given predictor and the dependent variable, overall state of health.

3. The rationale for using an alpha of .01 for the significance level relates to power. Our sample size is 698 so we have more than adequate power to detect moderate to moderately small effect sizes. To determine if you would prefer an even stricter significance level, you need to decide what size effect you would consider clinically meaningful in this data set, given the phenomenon being studied and the measurement issues present.

EXERCISE TABLE 16-1 *Table Used to Determine Direct and Indirect Effects of Independent Variables in Exercise Figure 16-1*

r = DIRECT r = simple	+ +	(INDIRECT) compound + ··· + compound	+ +	(NON-CAUSAL) compound + ··· + compound
Frequency of Exercise				
.39 = .24	+	(.20)(.28) + (.37)(.21) + (.37)(.18)(.28)	+	0
Quality of Life in Past Month				
.40 = .28	+	0	+	(.24)(.20) + (.21)(.18)
			+	(.21)(.37)(.20)
Satisfaction with Current Weight				
.37 = .21	+	(.18)(.28)	+	(.24)(.37) + (.37)(.20)(.28)

4. There are at least three limitations in this analysis. First the model is underidentified, but this is a minor problem as we are not attempting to test model fit here.

Second, the variables are all measured with single indicators so it is unclear how reliably they are measured. However, random measurement error should obscure relationships so this limitation does not threaten the theoretical conclusions we might wish to make. It only suggests that it is possible that our path coefficients represent an underestimate of the magnitude of the relationships in the model. A more serious concern is whether there is any systematic measurement error present which would affect the validity of these single item measures. Is it possible that frequency of exercise might have been over reported? Is it possible that the relationships between quality of life in the past month, current satisfaction with weight, and overall state of health are in part due to the participant's mood and sense of well-being when completing the questionnaire used to collect these data? The answers to these questions are not known. We need to consider the likelihood that these types of systematic measurement errors may be present, and then weigh their importance based on how we think they might be influencing the results if in fact they are present.

Third, and perhaps most important is that these data are cross-sectional. Given this, we do not know if it is quality of life in the past month that influences current satisfaction with weight or vice versa. We need to use theory and prior research to try to justify the direction used for this path.

CHAPTER

17

Structural Equation Modeling

Anne E. Norris

Objectives for Chapter 17

After reading this chapter, you should be able to do the following:

1. Describe at least three types of research questions that can be addressed with structural equation modeling (SEM).
2. Identify three dataset requirements for conducting SEM.
3. Describe the relationship between the measurement model and the theoretical model in SEM.
4. Describe the role of theory in the SEM process.
5. Critique an SEM analysis on the basis of the model fit statistics and description of the modeling process.

A GENERAL INTRODUCTION

This chapter is intended as an introduction to structural equation modeling (SEM) and assumes an understanding of the concepts and issues discussed in Chapter 16 with respect to path analysis. The purpose of this chapter is to acquaint readers with the possibilities SEM offers and aid them in interpreting SEM results published in the literature. Readers who are interested in gaining a more in-depth knowledge of SEM are encouraged to read one or more of the following sources: Bollen (1989), Byrne (1994), Hayduk (1996), or Hoyl (1995).

SEM is a relatively new statistical technique: The first computer program that could perform SEM was not developed until the late 1970s. Like path analysis, SEM is used to test theoretical models. Over the years, SEM has been referred to as covariance structure modeling, because covariances are analyzed in SEM; latent variable analysis, because SEM analyzes relationships between latent (ie, unmeasured)

405

variables; and a LISREL analysis, because LISREL was the name of the first software available for conducting SEM.

SEM challenges us to think about how we measure theoretical constructs. In fact, it allows us to use multiple measures of theoretical constructs. For example, researchers do not have to settle for one measure of health. They can use psychological, performance, and physiological measures, and the response options for these measures can vary with the measure. Alternatively, they can use a health attitudes questionnaire, but instead of totaling item responses into one lump sum, each item is treated as a different measure of health.

The measurement of theoretical constructs is critical in SEM. SEM tests two models simultaneously: a measurement model and a theoretical model. Together these two models are referred to as the full model. The measurement model is a model of how theoretical constructs are measured. The theoretical model is a model of the hypothesized relationships between the theoretical constructs. Valid tests of the theoretical model are dependent on a good fit of the measurement model to the data. The statistics produced in SEM help the researcher determine how good this fit is.

RESEARCH QUESTION

SEM allows us to ask old questions in new and more powerful ways, and new questions that could not have been addressed without the technology and thinking that underlie SEM. The latter sort of questions are only just beginning to be identified and pursued.

There are at least three types of "old" questions that can be addressed with SEM. First, like path analysis, SEM can be used to test a causal model. However, unlike path analysis, measurement error is estimated and removed from the relationships between theoretical constructs. Thus, it is possible to get a more precise test of theories. In addition, SEM can be used to analyze nonrecursive models (ie, models with two-way paths).

Second, as discussed in Chapter 15, SEM provides a new way to examine the factor structure of an instrument and to address other psychometric issues. For example, test–retest reliability takes on a whole new level of sophistication when the consistency in both factor loadings and measurement error is examined over time.

Third, SEM provides a new way to look at group differences. With SEM it is possible to determine whether the same theoretical model works equally well for explaining the data in different sample subgroups. For example, Norris and Ford (1995) predicted that different theoretical models for explaining condom use were needed for young African American and Hispanic men and women. They used SEM to compare the models depicted in Figures 17-1 through 17-4 (measurement model and error terms are not included for the sake of simplicity). They found that the four models were significantly different: The same model could not be used to explain

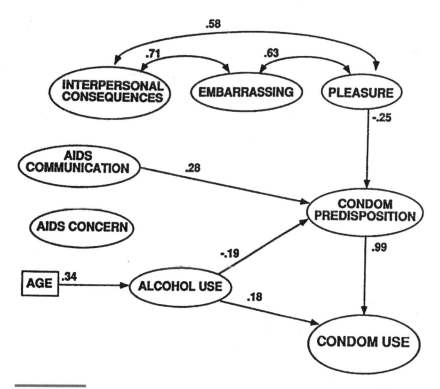

FIGURE 17-1. Model of African American males. (From Norris, A. E., & Ford, K. [1995]. Condom use by low-income African-American and Hispanic youth with a well-known partner: Integrating the Health Belief Model, Theory of Reasoned Action, and Construct Accessibility Model. Reprinted with permission from *Journal of Applied Social Psychology, 25*(20), 1801–1830. © V.H. Winston & Son, Inc., 360 South Ocean Blvd., Palm Beach, FL 33480. All rights reserved.)

condom use in all four groups. Moreover, four of the paths that were common to two or more models (eg, the paths age and alcohol use in Figs. 17-1 and 17-2) differed significantly in magnitude as well.

In addition, SEM opens the door to new questions. For example, with SEM it is possible first to assume that different levels of measurement error are present in data and then to test the effect of these different levels on the theoretical relationships specified in the model. Thus, conclusions could be made about the robustness of these relationships to problems such as subjects' poor memories, tendency to alter responses to make a better impression, misreading the question, and so forth. For example, Rigdon (1994) found that the nonrecursive relationship between stressful life events and depression specified in Ferguson and Horwood's (1984) model became recursive when different assumptions about measurement error were made (Ferguson and Horwood assumed no measurement error). Thus, the notion that

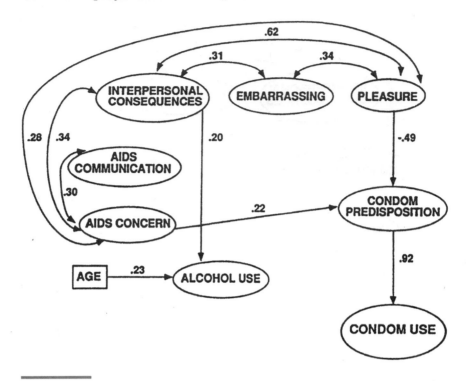

FIGURE 17-2. Model for African American females. (From Norris, A. E., & Ford, K. [1995]. Condom use by low-income African-American and Hispanic youth with a well-known partner: Integrating the Health Belief Model, Theory of Reasoned Action, and Construct Accessibility Model. Reprinted with permission from *Journal of Applied Social Psychology, 25*(20), 1801–1830. © V.H. Winston & Son, Inc., 360 South Ocean Blvd., Palm Beach, FL 33480. All rights reserved.)

stressful life events contribute to depression, which in turn contributes to stressful life events (ie, nonrecursive relationship), is not robust to measurement error: Perhaps the effect of depression on stressful life events found by Ferguson and Horwood is nothing more than depressed people perceiving their life more negatively. Regardless, Rigdon found that the only relationship that appeared robust was the effect of stressful life events on depression.

KEY TERMS

Before talking about the type of data and assumptions required for SEM, we must discuss some of the terms used in SEM. Frequently, different names have evolved to refer to the same term. These different names result from differences in the software used for SEM and in the orientation to SEM. Currently, the most commonly used

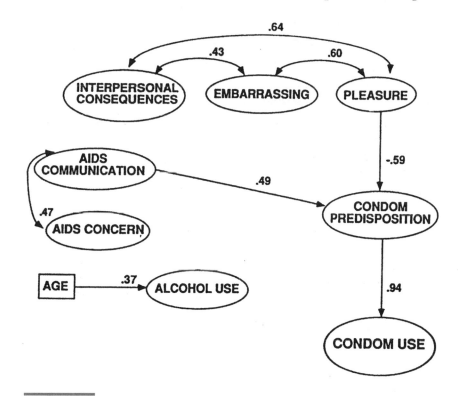

FIGURE 17-3. Model for Hispanic males. (From Norris, A. E., & Ford, K. [1995]. Condom use by low-income African-American and Hispanic youth with a well-known partner: Integrating the Health Belief Model, Theory of Reasoned Action, and Construct Accessibility Model. Reprinted with permission from *Journal of Applied Social Psychology, 25*(20), 1801–1830. © V.H. Winston & Son, Inc., 360 South Ocean Blvd., Palm Beach, FL 33480. All rights reserved.)

software programs are LISREL, AMOS, and EQS. In this section, names for terms that are unique to these programs will be noted. (See also Chapter 15 for an introduction to the Greek letters used as part of LISREL terminology.)

Indicators, Measured Variables, Proxies, and Manifest Variables

Indicators, measured variables, proxies, and manifest variables are different terms used in SEM to refer to the same thing: measures of a theoretical construct. For simplicity, *indicator* will be used in the remainder of this chapter to refer to these measures. Indicators are directly measured by the researcher: They correspond to a specific response on a questionnaire or piece of data in a dataset. In LISREL the letters X and Y are used to refer to indicators for theoretical constructs that are exogenous

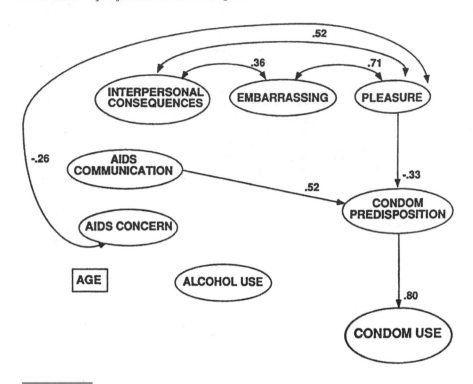

FIGURE 17-4. Model for Hispanic females. (From Norris, A. E., & Ford, K. [1995]. Condom use by low-income African-American and Hispanic youth with a well-known partner: Integrating the Health Belief Model, Theory of Reasoned Action, and Construct Accessibility Model. Reprinted with permission from *Journal of Applied Social Psychology, 25*(20), 1801–1830. © V.H. Winston & Son, Inc., 360 South Ocean Blvd., Palm Beach, FL 33480. All rights reserved.)

and endogenous, respectively. (As you may recall from Chapter 16, endogenous variables are influenced by other variables in the model, whereas exogenous variables are independent of such influences.) In EQS, the letter V is used for all indicators. A universal way of designating a variable as an indicator is to enclose it in a square in the SEM diagram. Hence, we could say that the construct health in Figure 17-5 has six indicators: well-being, happiness, Karnofsky's Performance Status, percentage of activities of daily living (ADLs), treadmill performance, and resting heart rate.

Residuals and Measurement Error

Residuals and measurement error represent the imprecision inherent to some extent in any research measure, whether it is an item on a questionnaire or the results of an HIV viral load test. For simplicity, *measurement error* is used in the remainder of this chapter to refer to this inherent imprecision. Measurement error

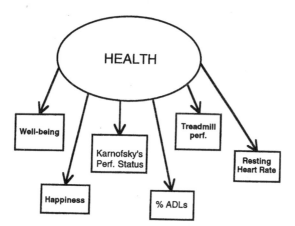

FIGURE 17-5. Measurement model for the construct, health.

may be theorized to be correlated if some systematic (ie, nonrandom) error is expected in the data. This might occur if certain items in a questionnaire elicit social desirability concerns, or when the same measure is used at different points in time.

In LISREL, measurement error is represented by the lowercase Greek letter δ (delta) if the theoretical construct is exogenous and ϵ (epsilon) if the construct is endogenous. In EQS the letter E is used for the measurement error associated with both types of theoretical constructs. Although measurement error is sometimes left out of SEM diagrams, it is always estimated in SEM analyses unless an indicator is assumed to have no measurement error. An indicator is assumed to have no measurement error if it is the only indicator used to measure a theoretical construct. This often occurs when a theoretical construct is low in abstraction (eg, age or height) or when multiple measures of the construct are not available.

Measurement Model

The measurement model is a model of how theoretical constructs are measured. For example, Figure 17-5 is a measurement model for the construct health. The model, as diagrammed, indicates that we are hypothesizing that well-being, happiness, Karnofsky's Performance Status, percentage of ADLs self-completed, treadmill performance, and resting heart rate are all indicators for the construct health. Some measurement error is expected for each of these six indicators, but this has not been included in the diagram.

Sometimes the focus of the SEM is on the measurement model, as when SEM is used for confirmatory factor analysis (see Chapter 15) to examine an instrument's construct validity. Other times the measurement model receives little attention because the researcher is focused on examining relationships between theoretical constructs. However, the validity of any theory testing that SEM provides is dependent on the fit of the measurement model to the data. If the measurement model does

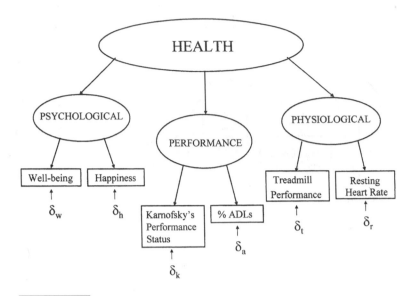

FIGURE 17-6. Measurement model for the health construct as a second-order factor with error terms included.

not fit the data well, we cannot determine whether a failure to find a hypothesized relationship is due to a problem with the theory or a problem with measurement.

Theoretical Constructs, Unmeasured Variables, and Latent Variables

In SEM, theoretical constructs are often called unmeasured or latent variables because they are not measured directly by the researcher. To minimize confusion, theoretical constructs will be referred to as latent variables for the remainder of the chapter. Latent variables are free of the random or systematic measurement error inherent in indicator variables (Bollen, 1989). A universal way of identifying a theoretical construct as a latent variable is to demarcate it with a circle in a diagram of an SEM model. Thus, it can be said that the model in Figure 17-5 has one latent variable—health.

In LISREL, latent variables are designated as ξ (xi) or η (eta), depending on whether the latent variable is exogenous or endogenous. In EQS, all latent variables are designated with an F for factor. Let us revisit our measurement model for health. Figure 17-5 represents health as a single latent variable with psychological, performance, and physiological indicators. Alternatively, we could hypothesize that health is a multidimensional construct with psychological, performance, and physiological indicators measuring its different dimensions. This hypothesis would be consistent with a model for health such as that shown in Figure 17-6. The advantage of SEM is that we can test both models (or hypotheses) and see which one fits the data better before going on to test a larger theoretical model about factors that influence health. (Measurement error would be estimated for both models, although it is only included in the diagram for Fig. 17-6.)

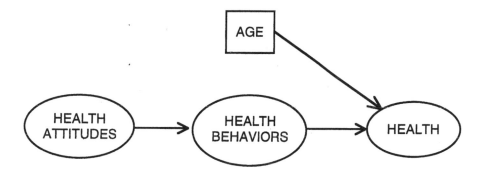

FIGURE 17-7. Hypothetical model predicting health as a function of age, health attitudes, and health behaviors.

Disturbance

The disturbance is the error in the prediction of an endogenous latent variable by other latent variables in the model. It is analogous to the error variance (ie, residual) in linear regression analysis. The disturbance is often left out of SEM diagrams. If present, it is designated by a short arrow pointing at the endogenous latent variable. In LISREL, ζ (zeta) is used to refer to the disturbance; EQS uses the letter D.

Theoretical Model

The theoretical model is a model of the hypothesized relationships between latent variables. For example, in Figure 17-7, we are hypothesizing that health is influenced by age, health attitudes, and health behaviors. Health attitudes are diagrammed as having only an indirect effect on health. Within the theoretical model, variables are designated as endogenous or exogenous, just as they are in path analysis. Thus, in Figure 17-7, health behaviors and health are endogenous variables. In EQS, endogenous and exogenous latent variables are referred to as factors (eg, F1, F2, F3). In LISREL, Greek letters are used: ξ (xi) for endogenous and η (eta) for exogenous latent variables.

Coefficients, Parameters, and Parameter Estimates

Researchers refer to path coefficients in the measurement and theoretical model as coefficients, parameters, or parameter estimates. These words are often used interchangeably because they mean the same thing, but for the sake of clarity, the word *parameter* will be used for the rest of the chapter. Unlike EQS, which uses no special notation to denote parameters, the LISREL software uses a system of Greek letters to categorize parameters according to the paths they define. Consequently, researchers (regardless of the software they use) may talk about lambda parameters (λ) when referring to paths in the measurement model, beta parameters (β) when referring to paths between endogenous variables, or gamma (γ) when referring to paths between two exogenous variables or one exogenous and one endogenous variable. Researchers further define these parameters by using the same subscript notation discussed in Chapter 16 (eg, $\gamma_{1,2}$).

Parameters are often referred to as fixed or free. A fixed parameter is not estimated in the SEM analysis; instead, the researcher assigns it a particular value. For example, researchers typically fix a parameter in the measurement model to 1.0. This allows a measurement scale (eg, 0 to 10 or 1 to 4) to be determined for the latent variable. Other parameters are fixed to zero to represent the absence of a path between two latent variables or between an indicator and a latent variable.

A free parameter has no value assigned to it. Free parameters are estimated in the SEM analysis: The computer calculates the value as part of the analysis using the covariances of the various indicators. Both standardized and nonstandardized parameters (ie, path coefficients) are estimated in SEM. SEM computer programs provide significance tests of these parameters as part of the analysis. It is possible to use the standardized parameter estimated and Wright's (1934) method to compute the indirect and total effects of latent variables, just as you would in path analysis (see Chapter 16).

Model Fit Statistics

SEM software programs produce a variety of statistics pertaining to the fit of the model. Unfortunately, the major statistical packages, including LISREL, EQS, and AMOS, automatically include in their default options indices that are known to have undesirable properties (Marsh et al., 1996). We try to restrict our discussion here to those indices that are most commonly used in the literature and review any undesirable properties that have been identified. There is currently no consensus on which indices are best, and research on the properties of these indices is ongoing.

Two indexes commonly reported in the literature are the GFI (goodness of fit index) and the CFI (comparative fit index). Both the GFI and CFI can range from 0 to 1.0. Historically, a good-fitting model is one that has a GFI or CFI greater than 0.90 (Bentler & Bonnett, 1980). However, recent work suggests that even this cutoff may not be high enough in all cases given certain sample sizes, estimation methods, and distributions (Hu & Bentler, 1995). Values equal to or greater than .95 may be more desirable because they decrease the chance of making a type II error. Some researchers recommend the CFI over the GFI because Monte Carlo simulation studies suggest it is less influenced by sample size (Tanguma, 2001; Wang et al., 1996). However, neither of these indices takes into account how many parameters are included in the model, and model fit can be enhanced (ie, made closer to 1.0) by merely adding additional parameters (Bollen & Long, 1993). Unfortunately, many indices developed to reward parsimony (eg, IFI, PGFI, AIC) have not proved satisfactory for a variety of reasons and are not recommended for general use (Marsh et al., 1996). Two indices that reward parsimony and appear to have some promise, based on recent work with Monte Carlo simulations, are the nonnormed fit index (NNFI) and the normed Tucker Lewis index (NTLI) (Marsh et al., 1996).

Consequently, these indices may begin appearing more frequently in the literature. These indices range, like the CFI and the GFI, between 0 and 1.0, with values greater than 0.90 indicating a good fit.

The root mean squared residual (RMR) is an absolute misfit index that differs from many other fit indices (eg, GFI, NFI) in that it is not based on the chi-square. The RMR is solely based on the residual matrix and unlike the GFI and NFI, the RMR decreases as the fit improves with zero indicating a perfect fit. In contrast, an RMR greater than .10 argues for the model being rejected due to a poor fit to the data (Bachand & Beard, 1995). Generally a good RMR value is found when chi-square based fit indices such as the CFI or GFI are greater than .95. However, on occasion, the RMR may suggest that the model fits very well, but the CFI or GFI may indicate poor model fit (Browne et al., 2002). This occurs when measurement is very precise, making error variance low—a rare phenomenon in health behavior research, but more common in physiological research. In such cases, one should include that the model being tested does provide a good fit to the data despite the discrepancy between the RMR and the chi-square based fit indices (Browne et al., 2002).

The root mean square error of approximation (RMSEA) is also a misfit index. Like the RMR, values close to zero indicate a good fit with values less than .05 indicating a very good fit (Hu & Bentler, 1995). The RMSEA is a little different from the RMR in that it attempts to correct for the number of parameters in the model being tested, and is based on the chi-square. Unfortunately, little is known about the effects of sample size, non-normality, and so forth on either the RMSEA or the RMR.

All SEM programs produce a model chi-square. This chi-square assesses the difference between observed data and a restricted structure resulting from the full (ie, measurement and theoretical) model (Byrne, 1994). This means that in SEM, the researcher wants the chi-square test to be nonsignificant: the researcher seeks to confirm the null hypothesis (ie, there is no difference between the data and the model).

A limitation of the model chi-square is that it is greatly influenced by sample size and violations of multivariate normality (Jöreskog & Sörbom, 1988). In fact, Bollen and Long (1993) say that any work that uses only the model chi-square to draw conclusions about model fit should be greeted with skepticism.

Two hand-calculated statistics are also used to assess model fit. One of these, Carmines and McIver's (1983) relative chi-square (ratio of chi-square to degrees of freedom) is calculated by dividing the model chi-square by its degrees of freedom. There is no consensus on what value constitutes a good fit (Bollen, 1989), but Carmines and McIver recommend that relative chi-squares be less than 3. A second type of hand-calculated statistics, the nested chi-square, is used to determine which of two competing models fits the data significantly better. This is the test we would use to determine which measurement model of health, Figure 17-5 or Figure 17-6, is better. A nested chi-square is calculated by subtracting the chi-square and degrees of freedom for one model from those associated with another competitive model. The significance level associated with this nested chi-square is used to determine whether the fit of one model differs significantly from that of the other. Table 17-1 contains an example of how to calculate the nested chi-square to determine if one

TABLE 17-1 *Example of How to Calculate a Nested Chi-Square*	
Chi-square statistic for model of health depicted in Figure 17-6:	2,006.37, df = 1,202
Chi-square statistic for model of health depicted in Figure 17-5:	2,021.58, df = 1,200
nested chi-square:*	−15.21, df = 2

*Sign (negative or positive) of the nested chi-square does not matter.

measurement model for health fits the data significantly better than the other. Note that the chi-square for Figure 17-6 (second-order factor model) is smaller than the one for Figure 17-5. This suggests that the second-order factor model fits the data better (remember, in SEM we want the chi-square to be nonsignificant). The significance level associated with the nested chi-square confirms this: $\chi^2 = |15.21|$, $df = 2$, $p < 0.001$.

In general, a variety of fit statistics should be used to evaluate model fit (Gonzalez & Griffin, 2001). For example, a researcher may choose to report the CFI, chi-square test, and relative chi-square ratio. A model may be interpreted as fitting the data even when the chi-square is statistically significant if the CFI or GFI is greater than 0.90 and the relative chi-square is less than 3.

Identification

Identification of both the measurement model and the theoretical model is critical to the estimation of parameters and testing of model fit that occurs in SEM. Just as in path analysis, these models can be overidentified (eg, when the number of covariances or known information exceeds the number of parameters being estimated), just identified (eg, when the number of covariances or known information is equal to the number of parameters being estimated), or underidentified (eg, when the number of parameters being estimated exceeds the number of covariances or known information). In SEM, the measurement and theoretical models being tested must be overidentified. The computer program cannot generate model fit statistics if the model is just identified; if the model is underidentified, the program either will not run or will run only after the software chooses specific parameters in the model to constrain to be equal to zero.

Unfortunately, identification (ie, delineating a model that is overidentified) is not an easy or straightforward task. For example, it is possible for a model to be overidentified on paper but empirically underidentified on the computer due to the statistical properties of the indicators (eg, problems with normality, high intercorrelations). Templin and Peters (2002) provide a simple method to make sure a model is at least overidentified on paper based on calculation of the model's degrees of freedom. According to this method, it is only when the model's degrees of freedom are positive that the model is overidentified. The model's degrees of freedom is equal to the unadjusted degrees of freedom minus the number of parameters in the model (ie, all variances, disturbances, free paths in both measurement and theoretical model, free covariances (specified correlations)). The unadjusted degrees of freedom is equal to the number of distinct variances and covariances in the model to be tested or:

$$P * [(p+1)/2]$$

where p is equal to the number of manifest variables.

Thus, the formula for calculating a model's degrees of freedom can be written as:

$$Model\ df = (P * [(p + 1)/2]) - k$$

where k is the number of parameters that will be estimated when the model is analyzed in SEM.

Modification Indices

In addition to model fit statistics and parameter estimates, SEM programs provide statistics predicting the potential change in model fit (change in chi-square) associated with adding or deleting parameters. Researchers may use these statistics to guide them in making changes in their model. Two specific types of modification indices produced by EQS are the Lagrange multiplier test (for adding parameters) and Wald test (for deleting nonsignificant parameters). The modification indices produced by LISREL are simply referred to as modification indices or MI and indicate only whether specific parameters should be added.

Multiple Group Analysis

Multiple group analysis is a type of analysis in which group differences in measurement and theoretical models are tested. A researcher could use this type of analysis to determine whether the factor structure of an instrument is the same in different sample subgroups (eg, different age, gender, or ethnic groups). Group differences in theoretical models are explored when the measurement model is equivalent or at least partially invariant across groups (Byrne, 1994). An equivalent measurement model means that the free parameters are not significantly different across groups. A partially invariant measurement model has at least one free parameter that is equivalent across groups (ie, the difference is not statistically significant). It is important to establish that the measurement model is equivalent or partially invariant to avoid having group differences in the theoretical model confounded by measurement differences.

TYPE OF DATA REQUIRED

SEM requires data to have three characteristics. First, the data should be continuous and normally distributed. However, new techniques are being developed for categorical data (Muthén, 1993; Von Eye & Clogg, 1994; West et al., 1995). In addition, special estimation methods and scaled statistics are available that are robust to violations of normality (Byrne, 1994; Hu & Bentler, 1995).

Second, the data should contain multiple indicators of latent variables. At least three indicators of a latent variable are needed for its measurement model to be just identified. Fixing the parameter for one of the three indicators to be equal to 1.0 makes the model overidentified. As noted earlier, this is a common practice because it also allows a measurement scale to be determined for the latent variable. Measurement models with less than three indicators can become overidentified if the researcher makes certain assumptions (ie, fixes certain parameters), such as assuming a measure has no measurement error. It is important that these multiple indicators capture different aspects or characteristics of a latent variable. Indicators cannot be so redundant (ie, highly correlated) that one can be used to predict another perfectly or nearly perfectly. This type of redundancy is called linear dependency. It prevents the model from being empirically identified (Chou & Bentler, 1995). This means that although the model as diagrammed looks identified, high intercorrelations in the data render it empirically underidentified. Third, the data should be numerous: SEM requires a large sample size. Assuming the most common method for estimating the parameters in SEM (maximum likelihood [ML]), a past recommendation has been a minimum of 100 to 200 subjects (100 to 200 per group in a multiple group analysis). However, there are at least four reasons why this recommended sample size minimum should be revised to 500 or more. First, Fan and Wang's (1998) work with computer simulations of a simple, three-factor model suggests that sample sizes of 100 and 200 are more likely to lead to improper solutions (ie, those with statistically impossible values such as negative variances). Sample sizes of 500 did not produce improper solutions. Second, Curran and colleagues (2002) found that even models with only small to moderate misspecification had biased mean and variance estimates when the sample size was 200 or less. Third, larger sample sizes decrease the effects of non-normality on model fit statistics and parameter estimates (West et al., 1995), and non-normality frequently occurs in nursing and health-related research datasets. Fourth, a parameter's standard error (used to compute parameter significance tests) varies across equivalent models when sample sizes are less than 500 (Gonzalez & Griffin, 2001). This means that different conclusions about a parameter's significance may be arbitrarily reached when testing equivalent or competing models. It is disturbing to realize that much of the research demonstrating problems when sample sizes dip below 500 was conducted using simple models. It is unclear whether similar problems would arise for sample sizes of 500 or more when models are more complex (ie, have more theoretical variables and hence more parameters to be estimated)! We do know that as theoretical models become more complex, a larger sample size is needed. And as discussed later in this chapter, one approach to power analysis suggests that power is likely to be inadequate when models are tested in sample sizes of 200 or less. Therefore, until additional research is conducted, a minimum sample size of 500, even for fairly simple models seems advisable, particularly when data are not normally distributed.

Although SEM is considered a causal modeling technique, it can be performed with either cross-sectional or longitudinal data and is not typically used to analyze data produced from an experimental design. For example, the data used by Norris and Ford (1995) in their multiple group analysis (results depicted in Figs. 17-1 through 17-4) are from a survey and are cross-sectional. Thus, it is important to be aware of theoretical assumptions pertaining to causation in SEM.

ASSUMPTIONS

There are three types of assumptions that must be considered with SEM: theoretical, general statistical, and estimation method-specific.

Theoretical Assumptions

In SEM the importance of using theory to guide your work cannot be emphasized enough. As in path analysis, theoretical (or causal) assumptions are made in the process of identifying a model to be tested. However, with SEM, assumptions of causation are made regarding both measurement of latent variables (eg, this indicator measures this construct) and relationships between latent variables (eg, attitudes influence behavior). Assumptions are made when paths are drawn (ie, parameter does not equal zero) and not drawn (ie, parameter equals zero). For example, in Figure 17-6 there are no paths connecting well-being, happiness, treadmill performance, and resting heart rate with the performance construct; thus, it is assumed that the parameters between these indicators and the performance construct are equal to zero.

As in path analysis, it is important to consider the three conditions of causation: the presence of an observed and measurable relationship between variables, temporal ordering, and nonspuriousness (see Chapter 16 for a discussion of these three conditions). Bollen (1989), and others writing specifically about SEM, use the terms *association, direction of influence*, and *isolation* to refer to these three conditions of causation. Bollen talks about meeting a condition of pseudoisolation to emphasize the researcher's inability to be certain that a relationship between two latent variables is nonspurious. Further, he emphasizes the need to recognize the tentativeness of any claims made through SEM about causality, and argues for replication as an important check on whether the conditions of association and isolation have been met.

General Statistical Assumptions

There are three types of general statistical assumptions in SEM. Violating these assumptions makes it difficult to identify a model that fits the data well and typically results in poorer fit indices.

The first type of assumptions should already be familiar to you. These are the assumptions of normal distributions, homoscedasticity, and linear relationships discussed in Chapters 11 and 12 for regression analysis. These assumptions arise because, like path analysis, SEM also involves solving a series of regression equations. Although SEM is somewhat robust to violations of normality, including categorical variables can bias significance tests of parameters and the model chi-square test by increasing the likelihood that they will be significant (West et al., 1995). The effect of categorical variables is contingent on their correlation with other variables in the measurement model and must be examined on a case-by-case basis (Bollen, 1989). Variables should be transformed so that their relationships are linear, and a multiple group analysis should be conducted when interactions are predicted. For example, Norris and Ford (1995) used a multiple group analysis to show that different models of condom use were needed for each gender or ethnic subgroup in their sample. Their findings confirmed the effect of a gender-by-ethnicity interaction on condom use.

Second, there are assumptions regarding the error terms in SEM. These assumptions are similar to those made in regression regarding the residuals, and are typically met in the course of meeting other SEM assumptions.[1] Although these assumptions are violated when the data are not multivariate normal, they are robust when the sample size is large (Chou & Bentler, 1995).

The third type of assumption pertains to sample size. It is assumed that the sample is asymptotic—so large as to approach infinity (Bollen, 1989). Smaller sample sizes (eg, less than 100 for a simple model when ML is used to estimate parameters) increase the probability of rejecting a true model (one that fits the data) (West et al., 1995).

Estimation Method-Specific Statistical Assumptions

In addition to general statistical assumptions, there are distributional assumptions associated with the method used to estimate the parameters in SEM. This discussion is limited to ML because it is the most commonly used estimation method (Chou & Bentler, 1995) and performs, on average, better than most other estimation methods, even when its assumptions are violated. See Bollen (1989) and West and colleagues (1995), for a discussion of other estimation methods and their robustness. ML assumes that no single variable or group of variables perfectly explains another in the dataset (Bollen, 1989) and that indicators have a distribution that is multivariate normal (West et al., 1995). This first assumption is why indicators cannot be redundant (ie, highly intercorrelated). ML is not very robust to violations of this first assumption: models with variables that correlate at or above 0.90 cannot be estimated.

Although the multivariate normal assumption is difficult to meet, ML is fortunately fairly robust to violation of this assumption (Chou & Bentler, 1995). However, there are two exceptions: when the sample size is small and the model is complex, and when categorical or dichotomous variables are used. Special techniques and estimation methods for models with categorical variables are available, although the sample size requirement can become so large as to be impractical (Hoyle & Panter,

---

[1] Specifically, it is assumed that error terms in the model are not correlated with any latent variables, are independent of one another, and are normally distributed (Fox, 1984).

1995; see Muthén, 1993, Von Eye & Clogg, 1994, and West et al., 1995, for a discussion of these techniques and estimation methods). In addition, it often makes more theoretical (as well as statistical) sense to perform a multiple group analysis when dichotomous variables represent group differences such as gender or employment status.

Power

Power is an important issue in SEM in two respects. First, given the same model, a larger sample is more likely to generate a significant model chi-square and hence rejection of the model regardless of its truth (Bollen, 1989; Kaplan, 1995) unless multiple measures of fit are used (Gonzalez & Griffin, 2001). Even models that fit the data well have small specification errors because it is difficult, if not impossible, to specify a model perfectly. Large sample sizes magnify the effects of these small specification errors, leading to a significant chi-square (ie, chi-square test is overpowered). Conversely, a small sample size will mask the effect of large specification errors, generating a nonsignificant chi-square and acceptance of a model when it should be rejected.

Second, the probability of committing a type II error (ie, accepting a model that should be rejected—accepting the null hypothesis) increases as models are respecified and tested (Kaplan, 1995). However, as is demonstrated later in this chapter in the computer examples, respecifying and retesting models is an inherent part of conducting an SEM analysis. Undue inflation of type II error can be avoided when the SEM analysis is guided by theory and modifications are selected in model specification that result in the greatest change in model fit (ie, have the most power). In addition, Chou and Bentler (1995) recommend splitting a dataset in half (when the sample size allows this) and developing a model with one half. The final model can then be retested with the remaining half of the data.

Although power is an important consideration in SEM, evaluating how much power is available in a given SEM analysis is not a simple or straightforward matter. Power is influenced by both sample size and misspecification errors (Kaplan, 1995), but misspecification errors are not typically known to the researcher. Different methods of power analysis have been proposed, but a discussion of these and their various shortcomings is beyond the scope of this chapter. Interested readers are encouraged to consult Kaplan (1995) and Saris and Satorra (1993) for a discussion of specific methods of power analysis, or MacCallum et al. (1996) and Hancock and Freeman (2001) for a new approach that allows calculation of minimum sample sizes. Note, Hancock and Freeman (2001) provide select sample size and power tables for models with varying degrees of freedom (calculation described previously in identification section) based on the MacCallum and colleagues (1996) method. A review of these tables indicates that even using least-conservative assumptions, power is less than .80 for models with less than 70 degrees of freedom and a sample size of 200 or less. Moreover, a sample size of 100 only yields a power of .80 when the model has 225 or more degrees of freedom. These tables provide further support for raising the SEM minimum sample size well beyond 200.

CONDUCTING SEM

Like path analysis, SEM involves preparation (model specification), analysis (model estimation and testing), and a consideration of the analysis' limitations. Preparation involves drawing a full model (ie, delineating the measurement model for each latent variable as well as the hypothesized relationships between these constructs) and fixing parameters to either zero or a nonzero value (eg, 0.5, 1.0) for identification purposes. Once the full model has been specified (and the data have been collected), a computer program estimates the parameters and tests the fit of the model to the data. The measurement model is evaluated first, and once the researcher determines that the measurement model fits the data, the theoretical model can be tested.

Fitting the model to the data is rarely accomplished in a single analysis. More often, the computer output suggests that certain parameters are not statistically significant and could be dropped, or additional respecification of the model is needed (ie, GFI or CFI is less than 0.90). For example, modification indices (in EQS the Lagrange multiplier test) may suggest adding parameters to the model. If this makes good theoretical sense, the researcher makes the change, and then the fit of this respecified model is tested. Although it may make for more model testing, the addition of parameters (ie, paths) should be made incrementally to observe whether the parameter contributes substantively to the fit of the model (Kaplan & Wenger, 1993).

In the end, the limitations of the SEM analysis are considered to help put the results in the proper context. For example, the researcher might consider whether certain assumptions about measurement may have influenced the results in some way. Concern about the validity of the final model can also arise if many models were tested in the process of finding one that fit the data well.

In the remainder of this section, a computer example of SEM is discussed and a published example of SEM is summarized and critiqued. The computer example provides a flavor of the SEM analysis process, and the critique underscores the need to give SEM articles a careful review.

Computer Example: Testing a Theoretical Model of Condom Use

This example uses SEM to test a theoretical model of condom use for African American men with a partner they know well. Specifically, we use SEM to determine which parameters are significant and whether the model as a whole provides a good fit to the data. If additional parameters are added to the model, we need to be able to justify this on theoretical grounds.

The data and model testing results reported here are part of a larger multiple group analysis published by Norris and Ford (1995) in the *Journal of Applied Social Psychology*. The sample size is 203, and the data are cross-sectional. The SEM software is EQS (Bentler, 1992), and the method of estimation is ML. Variables are excluded from the analysis if they have skew or kurtosis of $|1.5|$ or more.

The theoretical model being tested is depicted in Figure 17-8. This model is an integration of three different health behavior models: Health Belief Model (Janz &

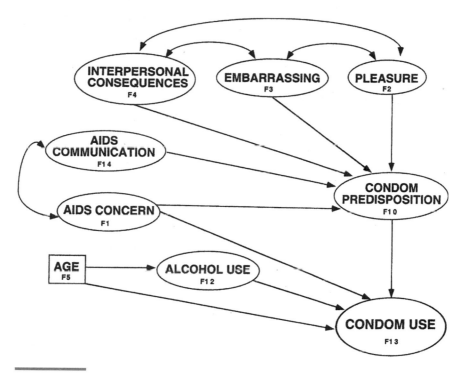

FIGURE 17-8. Initial theoretical model for computer example.

Becker, 1984), Theory of Reasoned Action (Fishbein & Ajzen, 1975), and Construct Accessibility Model (Norris & Devine, 1992). The effects of talking about AIDS, age, and alcohol use are also included in response to findings in the literature.

As can be seen in Figure 17-8, the theoretical model contains eight latent variables. Interpersonal consequences, embarrassing, and pleasure are three different types of condom beliefs (ie, three condom-belief factors). Condom predisposition is a new latent variable that combines concepts from the Theory of Reasoned Action (condom attitude, partner norm) and Construct Accessibility Model (state of information in memory). Other latent variables include AIDS communication, AIDS concern (AIDS susceptibility), alcohol use, and condom use. Age is also included: It is demarcated with a square because it has only one indicator and is assumed to be measured without error. This theoretical model is overidentified using criteria described elsewhere (Bollen, 1989, Wiley Interscience; Hayduk, 1987 Johns Hopkins).

The measurement model for the latent variables fit the data well. Separate measurement models were tested for each latent variable: The CFIs for these were 0.91 or more, and the relative chi-squares ranged from 0.20 to 1.80.

Although the model in Figure 17-8 is overidentified on paper, the computer found that the model was empirically underidentified when it estimated and tested the model. The computer made the model overidentified by constraining the error associated with condom predisposition to be equal to zero. This is indicated by the

| **TABLE 17-2** *Model Fit Statistics for Initial Theoretical Model in Computer Example* |

*** WARNING *** TEST RESULTS MAY NOT BE APPROPRIATE DUE TO CONDITION CODE

PARAMETER   CONDITION CODE

  D10,D10   CONSTRAINED AT LOWER BOUND

GOODNESS OF FIT SUMMARY

CHI-SQUARE =   371.158 BASED ON   242 DEGREES OF FREEDOM

PROBABILITY VALUE FOR THE CHI-SQUARE STATISTIC IS LESS THAN 0.001

THE NORMAL THEORY RLS CHI-SQUARE FOR THIS ML SOLUTION IS   338.987.

BENTLER-BONNETT NORMED   FIT INDEX =   0.7.55

BENTLER-BONNETT NONNORMED FIT INDEX =   0.881

COMPARATIVE FIT INDEX   =   0.896

Note: Bentler (1992) recommends the CFI over the other fit indices provided above.

warning in Table 17-2 that test results may not be appropriate due to condition code, and that the parameter D10,D10 (the error term for condom predisposition) is constrained at lower bound.

The computer's constraining of the error term associated with condom predisposition (D10,D10) gives us some direction as to how to respecify the model to improve the likelihood that it can be empirically overidentified. The computer's choice of this particular constraint suggests there are too many latent variables diagrammed as influencing condom predisposition. But how do we know which parameters to drop? The answer is in the Wald test results presented in the top half of Table 17-3. The Wald test predicts whether dropping a particular parameter would significantly worsen the fit of the model. The Wald predicts that three parameters in the model that involve condom predisposition (F10) could be dropped without worsening the fit of the model: F10,F4; F10,F3; and F10,F1. None of these parameters are associated with a significant change in the chi-square (ie, probability associated with the change is ≥.46). Dropping the paths represented by these three parameters results in the respecified model in Figure 17-9, and should have no effect on the overall fit of the model. Note, we ignore results for the Lagrange multiplier test in the bottom half of Table 17-3 because the constraint imposed by the computer on D10,D10 may affect their validity. We also do not make any further changes in the model because our goal is to create a model that is statistically overidentified without needing to constrain any variance terms to zero before we make any additional changes. At this point in the analysis, we only know that there are identification problems with respect to the regression equation predicting the condom predisposition variable in the theoretical model.

We proceed directly to testing the respecified model in Figure 17-9. The Lagrange multiplier test for this next analysis will tell us whether any of the parameters we have dropped should be added back to the model. Although the Wald test in Table 17-3 argues against these parameters being in the model, it is good to

TABLE 17-3 *Results of Wald and Lagrange Multiplier Tests for Initial Theoretical Model in Computer Example*

WALD TEST (FOR DROPPING PARAMETERS)

*** WARNING *** TEST RESULTS MAY NOT BE APPROPRIATE DUE TO CONDITION CODE

MULTIVARIATE WALD TEST BY SIMULTANEOUS PROCESS

		CUMULATIVE MULTIVARIATE STATISTICS		
STEP	PARAMETER	CHI-SQUARE	D. F.	PROBABILITY
1	F13,F5	0.036	1	0.850
2	F10,F4	0.382	2	0.944
3	F10,F3	0.658	3	0.956
4	D13,D13	1.449	4	0.919
5	F13,F12	2.871	5	0.825
6	F13,F1	4.861	6	0.677
7	F10,F1	7.712	7	0.462

MULTIVARIATE LAGRANGE MULTIPLIER TEST BY SIMULTANEOUS PROCESS IN STAGE 1

		CUMULATIVE MULTIVARIATE STATISTICS		
STEP	PARAMETER	CHI-SQUARE	D. F.	PROBABILITY
1	V11,F13	14.847	1	0.000
2	V22,F1	28.271	2	0.000
3	V23,F13	36.500	3	0.000
4	V34,F5	43.684	4	0.000
5	V7,F4	50.027	5	0.000
6	V30,F12	55.977	6	0.000
7	V26,F13	60.882	7	0.000
8	V13,F5	65.656	8	0.000
9	V9,F13	70.214	9	0.000
10	V8,F12	74.643	10	0.000
11	F14,F4	79.050	11	0.000
12	V9,F5	83.102	12	0.000
13	V1,F3	86.974	13	0.000

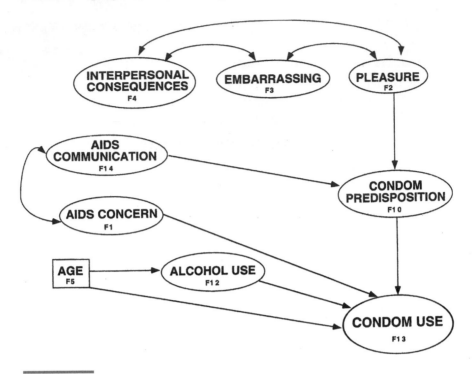

FIGURE 17-9. First respecified model for computer example.

review the Lagrange multiplier test for the respecified model to confirm the decisions we made earlier. It is important to confirm these decisions because the statistics that guided them (ie, those in Table 17-3) were created only after constraining the disturbance term or error in the regression equation predicting condom predisposition. This term needs to be estimated if we want to remove error variance from our estimates of the path coefficients for the latent variables we hypothesize to influence condom predisposition. Once we have estimated and have a good sense of the value of the disturbance term, we could choose to constrain it. However, constraining this term when we do not know its value is questionable and hence the statistics produced in the previous SEM may not be reliable.

Model fit statistics for the respecified model (Fig. 17-9) are provided in Table 17-4. Note there is no warning about a condition code: fortunately, we solved the identification problem. Also, the fit of this new model is acceptable. The model chi-square is significant, but the CFI equals 0.90. The relative chi-square (375.296/246) is 1.53. This also argues for the fit of the model because it is less than 3.0. Given acceptable model fit statistics, we want to know whether all the paths in this re-specified theoretical model are necessary. Would dropping any of the parameters representing these paths significantly affect the fit of the model? We want to minimize the probability of our making a type II error here so it is important to review the rest of the output.

The Wald test results in Table 17-5 indicate that there are three parameters that could be dropped: F13,F5; F13,F12; and F13,F1. These represent the paths from age

TABLE 17-4 *Model Fit Statistics for First Respecified Theoretical Model in Computer Example*

GOODNESS OF FIT SUMMARY

INDEPENDENCE MODEL CHI-SQUARE = 1517.312 ON 276 DEGREES OF FREEDOM

INDEPENDENCE AIC = 965.31161 INDEPENDENCE CAIC = −200.99448
MODEL AIC = −116.70398 MODEL CAIC = −1156.23766

CHI-SQUARE = 375.296 BASED ON 246 DEGREES OF FREEDOM
PROBABILITY VALUE FOR THE CHI-SQUARE STATISTIC IS LESS THAN 0.001
THE NORMAL THEORY RLS CHI-SQUARE FOR THIS ML SOLUTION IS 342.759.

BENTLER-BONETT NORMED FIT INDEX = 0.753
BENTLER-BONETT NONNORMED FIT INDEX = 0.883
COMPARATIVE FIT INDEX = 0.896

Note: Bentler (1992) recommends the CFI over the other fit indices provided above.

(F5), alcohol use (F12), and AIDS concern (F1) to condom use (F13). Dropping them results in a second respecified model, depicted in Figure 17-10.

Now we turn to the Lagrange multiplier test results in Table 17-5 and ask ourselves, should any parameters be added to the model? The answer to this question is "no." None of the parameters listed involve two latent variables (ie, there are no pairs of Fs). Instead they refer to potential changes in our measurement model that cannot be justified on theoretical grounds and therefore should not be made. Moreover, the measurement model has already been determined to fit the data well and is not the focus of analysis at this point.

The results of the Lagrange multiplier test in Table 17-5 support our earlier decision to drop the three parameters representing the influence of interpersonal consequences, embarrassing, and AIDS concern on condom use. The pattern of findings from this model testing and estimation argue for assuming these latent variables have no influence on condom predisposition (ie, the parameters are equal to zero). As can be seen in Table 17-6, the fit statistics for the second respecified model (see Fig. 17-10) differ little from those for the first respecified model in Table 17-4. This is good: We have simplified our model without sacrificing model fit. In Table 17-7, the Wald test does not suggest dropping any additional paths between the latent variables, and the Lagrange multiplier test does not suggest adding any such paths. Together with the model fit statistics, these two tests argue against any further respecification of the model. Also, the Lagrange multiplier test results in the context of these model fit statistics support assuming that the paths from age, alcohol use, and AIDS concern to condom use are equal to zero.

The SEM test of the theoretical model is concluded at this point. We now consider two limitations of the analysis. First, due to sample size constraints we did not randomly split the dataset in half, develop our model with one half, and then retest it with the remaining half of the data. Thus, it is possible that our findings could result from a type II error. However, only three models were specified and tested. This limited number of models argues against our findings being the result of a type II error. Second and more serious, the data are cross-sectional, but our model implies causal

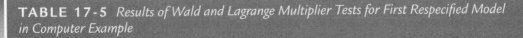

TABLE 17-5 *Results of Wald and Lagrange Multiplier Tests for First Respecified Model in Computer Example*

WALD TEST (FOR DROPPING PARAMETERS)
MULTIVARIATE WALD TEST BY SIMULTANEOUS PROCESS

| | | CUMULATIVE MULTIVARIATE STATISTICS | | |
STEP	PARAMETER	CHI-SQUARE	D. F.	PROBABILITY
1	F13,F5	0.040	1	0.841
2	D13,D13	0.790	2	0.674
3	F13,F12	2.141	3	0.544
4	F13,F1	4.599	4	0.331

MULTIVARIATE LAGRANGE MULTIPLIER TEST BY SIMULTANEOUS PROCESS IN STAGE 1

| | | CUMULATIVE MULTIVARIATE STATISTICS | | |
STEP	PARAMETER	CHI-SQUARE	D. F.	PROBABILITY
1	V11,F13	12.514	1	0.000
2	V23,F13	23.205	2	0.000
3	V22,F14	32.068	3	0.000
4	V7,F4	39.285	4	0.000
5	V34,F5	46.470	5	0.000
6	V29,F12	52.430	6	0.000
7	V26,F13	58.037	7	0.000
8	V9,F13	62.870	8	0.000
9	V1,F10	67.682	9	0.000
10	V13,F5	72.444	10	0.000
11	V9,F5	76.782	11	0.000
12	V8,F12	80.774	12	0.000

relationships (eg, talking about AIDS makes people more predisposed to use condoms). These theoretical relationships need to be validated with longitudinal data.

CRITIQUE OF PUBLISHED SEM ANALYSIS

Williams and colleagues (2002) used SEM to evaluate the effects of a smoking cessation intervention using self determination theory (SDT) as their conceptual framework. Their sample size for the analysis was 239 patients. These patients had been

TABLE 17-6 *Model Fit Statistics for Second Respecified Theoretical Model in Computer Example*

GOODNESS OF FIT SUMMARY

INDEPENDENCE MODEL CHI-SQUARE =   1517.312 ON   276 DEGREES OF FREEDOM

INDEPENDENCE AIC =   965.31161   INDEPENDENCE CAIC =   −200.99448
         MODEL AIC =   −118.75645   MODEL CAIC =   −1170.96737

CHI-SQUARE =   379.244 BASED ON   249 DEGREES OF FREEDOM
PROBABILITY VALUE FOR THE CHI-SQUARE STATISTIC IS LESS THAN 0.001
THE NORMAL THEORY RLS CHI-SQUARE FOR THIS ML SOLUTION IS   349.732.

BENTLER-BONETT NORMED   FIT INDEX =   0.750
BENTLER-BONETT NONNORMED FIT INDEX =   0.884
COMPARATIVE FIT INDEX   =   0.895

Note: Bentler (1992) recommends the CFI over the other fit indices provided above.

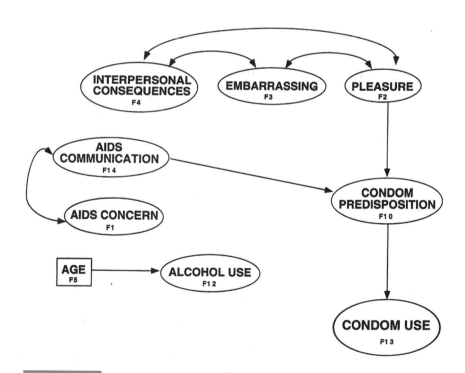

FIGURE 17-10. Second respecified model for computer example.

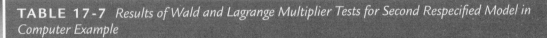

TABLE 17-7 *Results of Wald and Lagrange Multiplier Tests for Second Respecified Model in Computer Example*

WALD TEST (FOR DROPPING PARAMETERS)
MULTIVARIATE WALD TEST BY SIMULTANEOUS PROCESS

STEP	PARAMETER	CUMULATIVE MULTIVARIATE STATISTICS		
		CHI-SQUARE	D. F.	PROBABILITY
1	D13,D13	1.365	1	0.243

MULTIVARIATE LAGRANGE MULTIPLIER TEST BY SIMULTANEOUS PROCESS IN STAGE 1

STEP	PARAMETER	CUMULATIVE MULTIVARIATE STATISTICS		
		CHI-SQUARE	D. F.	PROBABILITY
1	V11,F13	12.213	1	0.000
2	V22,F14	23.845	2	0.000
3	V23,F13	32.416	3	0.000
4	V7,F4	39.514	4	0.000
5	V34,F5	46.056	5	0.000
6	V30,F12	52.014	6	0.000
7	V1,F13	57.443	7	0.000
8	V13,F5	62.278	8	0.000
9	V9,F12	66.804	9	0.000
10	V9,F13	71.246	10	0.000
11	V3,F12	75.267	11	0.000

randomized to one of two intervention conditions, automony supportive or controlling interpersonal style. The model that they tested is depicted in Figure 17-11. This model is overidentified as per the Templin and Peters (2002) method and the information in the article regarding measurement of the latent variables.

The latent variables in their analysis were each measured with three or more indicators. All indicators were continuous variables. The distributions of these variables is not described, but the estimation method was corrected for nonnormality. This suggests that the indicators may not have all been normally distributed.

Rated autonomy support and autonomous motivations were each measured with five separate indicators. Continuous abstinence was measured with three indicators. The intervention variable was a manifest variable (single indicator) and this indicator was categorical (autonomy supportive, controlling interpersonal).

Perceived competence was measured at two different time points, prior to and after exposure to the intervention. Four indicators were used to measure the variable

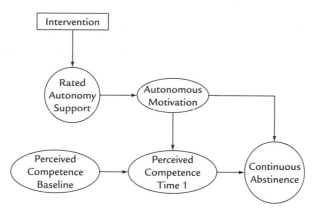

FIGURE 17-11. Hypothesized self-determination model of smoking cessation. (From Williams, G. C., Gagne, M., Ryan, R. M., & Deci, E. L. [2002]. Facilitating autonomous motivation for smoking cessation. *Health Psychology, 21*(1), 40–50.)

at each of these time points. The authors included correlations between the measurement error associated with the indicators for the two competence latent variables in their model. This makes good sense. One would expect the same items completed at two different time points to have correlated measurement error. However, it is unclear how the errors were correlated. Most likely measurement error was correlated for the individual items that parallel each other at the two time points. It is possible to correlate every potential pair of measurement error across the two time points. However, this is generally not done because it cannot be justified from a measurement standpoint and unduly inflates the number of parameters being estimated in the analysis. The data were analyzed with EQS, and the method of estimation was ML with robust correction for nonnormality. The chi-square for the measurement model was significant ($p < 0.05$). However, other model fit indices argued that the measurement model fit the data well (CFI = 0.95, RMSEA = .07). The model chi-square test was significant in the analysis for the full model, but other fit statistics argued that the full model fit fairly well: CFI = .95, RMSEA .06. These fit statistics might have been higher if the authors had deleted two nonsignificant paths in the theoretical model and rerun the analysis (see Fig. 17-12). Without rerunning the analysis, it is difficult to evaluate the final model reported in this article. The coefficients reported are for a misspecified model (a model with nonsignificant paths). The model needs to be respecified and then reanalyzed so that the path coefficients and their significance tests can be reestimated.

In sum, when we consider the limitations of this SEM analysis, we must begin by questioning certain aspects of how the data were analyzed. In addition to needing to respecify and re-analyze the model, there is concern about the inclusion of a dichotomous variable to represent the intervention effect. A better way to have analyzed these data would have been to do a multiple group analysis and then evaluate whether the magnitude of the theoretical relationships varied in the two intervention groups. However, the sample size would have been less than desirable (approximately ½ of 239). Given the sample size, the authors might have been wise to consider dropping the intervention variable from the analysis and relying on the autonomy support variable to capture the effect of the intervention. Although the data are interesting, it is difficult to make firm conclusions about the findings. It

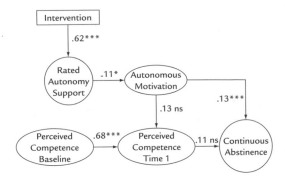

FIGURE 17-12. Standardized parameter estimates for the self-determination theory-based structural model (using the structural equation modeling software EQS Version 5.7a). *$p < .05$. ***$p < .001$. (From Williams, G. C., Gagne, M., Ryan, R. M., & Deci, E. L. [2002]. Facilitating autonomous motivation for smoking cessation. *Health Psychology, 21*(1), 40–50.)

might be unwise to use these data to guide practice unless the authors were contacted and able to make results available for analyses of a respecified model with and without the intervention variable. Even then, it could be argued that this model should not be used to guide practice without being replicated in a larger sample.

SUMMARY

SEM is a valuable data analysis tool in many respects. For example, SEM affords us greater precision in testing theories and in evaluating construct validity. However, SEM is still just a tool: SEM in and of itself cannot be used to imply causation or ensure construct validity. The use of theory to guide the analysis is essential, but the validity of the result is also influenced by the data and how SEM is used. A beautiful theory can be contradicted by the data, such as when the CFI or GFI is less than 0.90. Alternatively, the theory can be unnecessarily distorted as a result of type II error when too many models are run, and problematic data can also make the use of SEM unfeasible.

Application Exercises and Results

Exercises

1. Review the fit information listed in Exercise Figures 17-1 and 17-2. Which model provides a better fit to these data? Do any additional models need to be run? Does the model with the best fit still need to be respecified and reanalyzed?

Results

1. The model fit statistics for the model in Exercise Figure 17-1 are not acceptable. The GFI is equal to .89 and the CFI is equal to .76. Note also that the RMSEA is greater than .10. These results argue for this model being respecified. The authors did this and after testing three more models, they arrived at the model in Exercise Figure 17-2. The fit statistics for this model argue that it is a very good fit to the data. Thus, these statistics argue against the

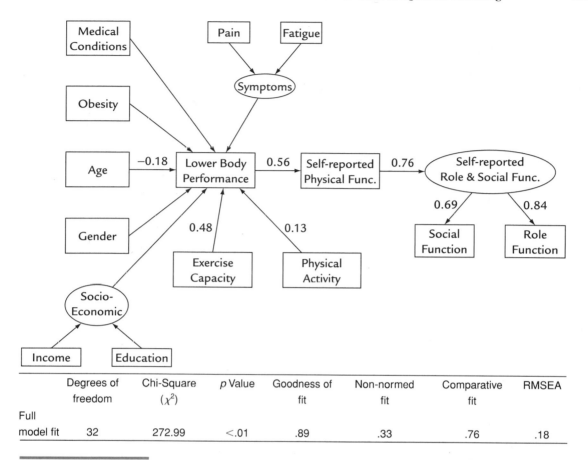

	Degrees of freedom	Chi-Square (χ^2)	p Value	Goodness of fit	Non-normed fit	Comparative fit	RMSEA
Full model fit	32	272.99	<.01	.89	.33	.76	.18

EXERCISE FIGURE 17-1. (Figure 1 from Bennett, J. A., Stewart, A. L., Kayser-Jones, J., & Glaser, D. (2002). The mediating effect of pain and fatigue on level of functioning in older adults. *Nursing Research, 51*(4), 259.)

model needing to be respecified and reanalyzed. However, look at the variables in the model. Do you see any variables that are categorical? There is one variable that is. Given this and the lack of effect this variable has on other variables in the model, it makes sense to rerun the analyses without this variable. The fit statistics should not change, but by meeting the statistical assumptions, you will get better estimates of the parameters in the model.

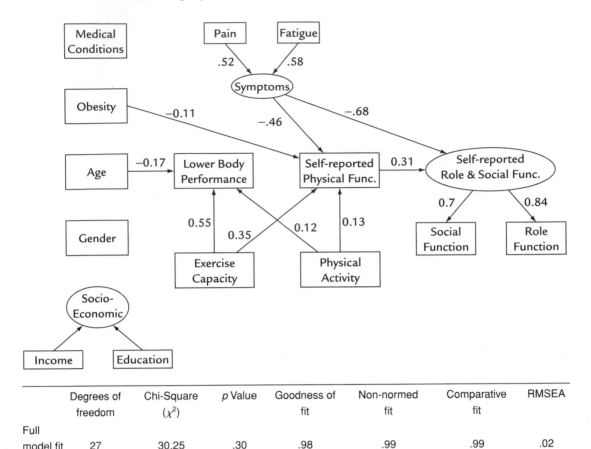

	Degrees of freedom	Chi-Square (χ^2)	*p* Value	Goodness of fit	Non-normed fit	Comparative fit	RMSEA
Full model fit	27	30.25	.30	.98	.99	.99	.02

EXERCISE FIGURE 17-2. (Figure 4 from Bennett, J. A., Stewart, A. L., Kayser-Jones, J., & Glaser, D. (2002). The mediating effect of pain and fatigue on level of functioning in older adults. *Nursing Research*, *51*(4), 262.)

Glossary

a: Intercept constant. The point at which the regression line intercepts the Y axis.

Adjusted group means: Group mean scores that have been adjusted for the effect of the covariate on the dependent variable.

Adjusted R^2: R squared adjusted for the number of subjects and variables.

Alpha: The probability of making a type I error.

Alternative hypothesis: Proposes there is a directional or nondirectional difference between groups or a relationship between variables.

Analysis of covariance (ANCOVA): A combination of regression and analysis of variance techniques that allows comparison of group means after adjustment for the effect of the covariate.

Analysis of variance (ANOVA): A parametric statistical test that compares between- and within-group variance to measure differences between two or more groups.

A priori contrasts: Planned comparisons based on orthogonal hypotheses.

b: Regression coefficient. In linear regression, it is the rate of change in Y with a one-unit change in X, and it is used to calculate predicted scores. In logistic regression, it is used to calculate probabilities.

Bar graph: A graph used for nominal or ordinal data. A space separates the bars.

Bartlett's test: A chi-square statistic used to test the significance of lambda.

Beta coefficients: In a regression equation, the weight associated with standardized scores on the variables; a partial correlation coefficient.

Between-group variance: A measure of the deviation of group means from the grand mean.

Biserial correlation: A technique used when one variable is dichotomized and the other is continuous to estimate what the correlation between the two variables would be if the dichotomized variable were continuous.

Blinding: Keeping subjects and observers unaware of treatment assignments.

Box plots: A graphic display that uses descriptive statistics based on percentiles.

Box's M: A measure of the multivariate test for homogeneity of variance. It is very sensitive to departures from normality.

Box's test of equality of covariance matrices: A test of the assumption that the variance–covariance matrices are equal across all levels of the between-subjects factor in a repeated measures analysis of variance.

Canonical coefficient: Equivalent to a *b*-weight in regression; can be used to calculate predicted scores based on actual scores.

Canonical correlation: A measure of the relationship between a set of independent variables and a set of dependent variables.

Canonical variate: A weighted composite of the variables in a set.

Canonical weights: Standard score weights generated in a canonical correlation; like betas in regression; used more for explanation than prediction.

Central limit theorem: When many samples are drawn from a population, the means of these samples tend to be normally distributed.

Centroid: The mean of the discriminant scores for a given group.

Chi-square: A statistical test used with categorical (nominal) data. It compares the actual number in each group with the expected number.

Coefficient of determination: The correlation coefficient squared (r^2); a measure of the variance shared by the two variables; a measure of the "meaningfulness" of the relationship.

Coefficient of variation: Measures the spread of a set of data as a proportion of its mean; usually expressed as a percentage.

Common factor analysis: Based on the assumption that there is systematic and random error in measurement. Analysis is based on common variance only.

Communality: The portion of item variance accounted for by the factors.

Compound symmetry: An assumption underlying the repeated measures analysis of variance. The correlations and variances across the measurements are equivalent.

Conditional probability: The likelihood that an event will occur given the knowledge that another event has already occurred.

Confidence interval: A range within which the population parameter is estimated to fall based on the statistic and the standard error.

Confirmatory factor analysis (CFA): A special application of structural equation modeling and a theory-driven method for testing an instrument's factor structure.

Contingency coefficient: A nonparametric technique to measure the relationship between two nominal-level variables.

Continuity correction (Yates correction): Used in chi-square analysis when the expected frequency in cells in 2×2 tables is less than 5.

Continuous variable: Any measure that can assume 11 or more dichotomous levels. With multicategory items, somewhat fewer categories are needed to qualify (Nunnally & Bernstein, 1994, p. 570).

Correlated *t* test (paired *t* test): A parametric test to compare two pairs of scores.

Correlation coefficient: The mathematical relationship between two variables. Values range from -1 to $+1$.

Correlation matrix: A square symmetric matrix containing correlations between pairs of variables.

Covariate: A continuous variable used to adjust the mean scores of groups; a method for control of extraneous variation.

Cramer's V: Modified phi, used to assess relationship between categorical variables; used with tables larger than 2×2.

Cronbach's alpha: A measure of internal consistency reliability.

Cross-validation: Checking the validity of R^2 by calculating it in a second sample.

Degrees of freedom: The freedom of a score's value to vary given what is known about the other scores and the sum of the scores.

Dependent variable: The response or outcome measure.

Deviance: In logistic regression, the comparison between the predicted probability of being in the correct group based on the model to the perfect prediction. Large values indicate poor model fit.

Deviation coding (effect coding): A method of coding nominal-level variables using 1s, -1s, and 0s; reflects the comparison of each group mean with the grand mean.

Directional hypothesis: States a relationship between the variables being studied or a difference between experimental treatments that the researcher expects to emerge.

Discriminant function: The mathematical function that combines information from predictor variables to obtain the maximum discrimination among groups.

Discriminant function analysis: A statistical technique that provides a prediction of group membership based on predictor variables.

Dummy coding (indicator coding): A method of coding nominal-level variables using 1s and 0s; reflects a comparison of the control group mean with other group means.

Effect coding (deviation coding): A method of coding nominal-level variables using 1's, −1s, and 0s; reflects the comparison of each group mean with the grand mean.

Effect size: The impact made by the independent variable on the dependent variable.

Efficiency: The degree to which the test result and the diagnosis agree, that is, the overall accuracy of a test in measuring true findings; expressed as a percentage.

Eigenvalue: The amount of variance explained by a factor or discriminant function.

Endogenous variables: Variables influenced by other variables in a model.

Epsilon: A correction used in repeated measures analysis of variance when the assumption of compound symmetry has not been met. Epsilon is multiplied by the degrees of freedom for the within-subjects factor(s), making them smaller, and thus making the test more conservative.

Equamax rotation: Combines the characteristics of Quartimax and Varimax rotation.

Estimation: The procedure for testing a model whereby a sample of observed data is used to make estimations of population parameters.

Eta: Sometimes called the correlation ratio. It can be used to measure a nonlinear relationship. The range of values is from 0 to 1.

Exogenous variables: Variables that are not influenced by other variables in a model.

Exp(B): The exponent of b or the odds ratio.

F: A measure of the ratio of between to within variance produced by analysis of variance.

Factor: A group of items that "belong" together.

Factor analysis: A statistical tool for analyzing scores on large numbers of variables to determine whether any identifiable dimensions can be used to describe many of the variables under study. Intercorrelations are treated mathematically in such a way that underlying traits are identified.

Factor loadings: Correlations of variables with a factor.

Factor matrix: Each row represents one variable; each column represents a factor.

Factor pattern matrix: A matrix produced by oblique rotation in factor analysis. It contains regression weights. It is generally preferable to the structure matrix for interpretation.

Factor scores: Actual scores weighted by factor loadings.

Factor structure matrix: A matrix produced by oblique rotation in factor analysis. It contains correlation coefficients.

Fisher's exact test: An alternative to chi-square for 2×2 tables when sample size and expected frequencies are small.

Fisher's Z_r: Transformation of correlation coefficients into Fisher's Z to create a normal distribution.

Friedman matched samples: A nonparametric analogue of repeated measures analysis of variance.

Goodness of fit statistic: A measure of how well the data fit the model; compares the observed probabilities to those predicted by the model.

Graphs: The visual representations of frequency distributions.

Greenhouse-Geisser: A conservative epsilon value used to alter the degrees of freedom for the within-subjects factor(s) in repeated measures analysis of variance when the assumption of compound symmetry has not been met.

Heteroscedasticity: Refers to situations in which the variability of the dependent variable is not equivalent across the values of the independent variable.

Hierarchical regression: The researcher determines the order of entry of the variables into the equation. Variables may be entered one at a time or in subsets.

Histogram: The appropriate graph for interval and ratio data. There is no space between the bars.

Homogeneity of regression: The direction and strength of the relationship between the covariate and the dependent variable must be similar in each group.

Homogeneity of variance: The variances of the dependent variable do not differ significantly between the groups.

Homoscedasticity: An assumption underlying correlation and regression. For every value of X, the distribution of Y scores must have approximately equal variability.

Hotelling-Lawley trace: The sum of the ratio of the between and within sum of squares for each of the discriminant variables.

Huynh-Feldt: A value for the epsilon correction factor in repeated measures analysis of variance that is less conservative than Greenhouse-Geisser.

Hypothesis: Formal statement of the expected relationships between variables or differences between groups.

Identification: A necessary condition for conducting confirmatory factor analysis and structural equation modeling, where the amount of information or known values in the data exceeds the information being estimated or unknown values.

Improvement: In logistic regression, the change in $-2LL$ between successive steps of building a model.

Imputation: Estimation of missing values in a dataset based on prior knowledge, mean or median substitution, or regression techniques.

Independent variable: The variable that is seen as having an effect on the dependent variable. In experimental designs, the treatment is manipulated.

Indicator: A measured variable in structural equation models; may also be called a manifest variable.

Indicator coding (dummy coding): A method of coding nominal-level variables using 1s and 0s. Reflects a comparison of the control group mean with other group means.

Intercept constant (a): The point at which the regression line intercepts the Y axis.

Interquartile range: The range of values extending from the 25th to the 50th percentile.

Interval-level measurement: A rank order scale in which the distances between the values are equivalent.

Just identified model: All variables in the model are interconnected with each other by a path.

Kendall's tau: A nonparametric measure of relationship between two ordinal variables.

Kruskal-Wallis H: Nonparametric analogue of analysis of variance; used to compare groups on an outcome measure.

Kurtosis: A measure of whether the curve is normal, flat, or peaked.

Lambda: Wilks' lambda varies from 0 to 1 and represents the error variance. $1 - \text{lambda} = R^2$.

Latency effect: Interaction between treatments in repeated measures designs.

Latent variable: A theoretical construct in structural equation models that is not directly measured but represented by measured variables.

Least significant difference test: A posthoc test that is a modified version of multiple t tests.

Levene's test of equality of error variances: A test of the assumption that the group means have equal variances.

Likelihood: The probability of the observed results given the parameter estimates.

Line chart: The preferred type of chart to show many changes over time for many periods of time, or to place emphasis on a particular factor.

Listwise deletion: Cases (subjects) are dropped from analysis if they have any missing data.

Logistic regression: A technique designed to determine which variables affect the probability of an event.

Lower-bound epsilon: The most conservative approach to "correcting" the degrees of freedom in repeated measures analysis of variance when the assumption of compound symmetry has not been met.

Maximum likelihood (ML) method: A method of estimation used in confirmatory factor analysis and structural equation modeling.

Mann-Whitney U: A nonparametric statistical test to compare two groups. It is analogous to the *t* test.

Mauchly's test of sphericity: A test of the assumption of compound symmetry in repeated measures analysis of variance.

McNemar: A nonparametric measure of difference between two paired dichotomous measures; used to measure change.

Mean: Arithmetic average.

Meaningfulness: The clinical or substantive meaning of the results of statistical analysis.

Mean replacement: Substitution of the mean of the distribution for missing values on a specific variable.

Measurement: The assignment of numerals to objects or events, according to a set of rules (Stevens, 1946).

Median: The middle value or subject in a set of ordered numbers.

Median replacement: Substitution of the median of the distribution for missing values on a specific variable. Often used if the variable distribution is skewed.

Mixed design: A study that includes between- and within-group factors.

Mode: The most frequently occurring number or category.

Model chi-square: In logistic regression, the difference between minus 2 log likelihood ($-2LL$) for the model with only a constant and $-2LL$ for the complete model; tests the null hypothesis that the coefficients for all the independent variables equal zero.

Model modification: Respecifying an initially hypothesized model in confirmatory factor analysis and structural equation modeling to test the newly proposed model for improved data–model fit.

Multicollinearity: Interrelatedness of independent variables.

Multiple correlation: The relationship between one dependent variable and a weighted composite of independent variables.

Multiple group comparisons: The two most common are a priori (before the fact) and posthoc (after the fact) comparisons of group means.

Multivariate analysis of variance: An analysis of variance with more than one dependent variable.

Mutually exclusive: An object or subject is in one, and only one, group in the design.

Negative predictive value: The proportion of people who do not have the disease who tested negative for the disease, that is, "true negatives"; expressed as a percentage.

Nominal: The lowest level of measurement; consists of organizing data into discrete units.

Nondirectional hypothesis: A specific statement that a difference exists between groups or a relationship exists between variables, with no specification of the direction of the difference or relationship.

Nonparametric statistics: "Distribution-free" techniques that are not based on assumptions about normality of data.

Nonrecursive model: A model in which causal flow is not unidirectional.

Normal curve: A theoretically perfect frequency polygon in which the mean, median, and mode all coincide in the center, and which takes the form of a symmetrical bell-shaped curve.

Null hypothesis: Proposes that there is no difference between groups or no relationship between variables.

Oblique rotation: The resulting factors are correlated with each other.

Observed variables: The indicators for the latent variable or the items on a research instrument.

Odds ratio: The probability of occurrence over the probability of nonoccurrence.

One-tailed test of significance: A test used with a directional hypothesis that proposes extreme values are in one tail of the distribution.

One-way analysis of variance: Analysis of variance with one factor (independent variable).

Ordinal-level measurement: The rank ordering of data points.

Orthogonal: Independent of each other.

Orthogonal coding: A method of coding orthogonal contrasts between groups. A priori contrasts can be tested through this method of coding.

Orthogonal rotation (Varimax): The resulting factors are not correlated with each other.

Outliers: Values that are extreme relative to the bulk of the distribution.

Overidentified model: A model that contains at least one less path than a just identified model.

Paired *t* test: A parametric test to compare two pairs of scores.

Pairwise deletion: In correlational analyses, cases (subjects) are excluded when they are missing one of the two variables being correlated.

Parameters: Characteristics of the population.

Parametric tests: Statistical tests based on assumptions that the sample is representative of the population and that the scores are normally distributed.

Partial correlation: A measure of the relationship between two variables after statistically controlling for the influence of some other variable(s) on both of the variables being correlated.

Path analysis: A causal model analytic technique using least squares regression.

Path coefficients: The magnitude of the influence of one variable on another in the path model.

Path model: A causal model.

Pearson product moment correlation: A formula used to calculate the correlation between two variables.

Percentile: Describes the relative position of a score.

Phi: A shortcut method of calculating Pearson's correlation coefficient when both variables are dichotomous.

Pie chart: A circle that is partitioned into percentage distributions of qualitative variables.

Pillai-Bartlett trace: Represents the sum of the explained variances.

Point estimate: A single number that serves as the estimate of the population parameter.

Polygon: A graph for interval or ratio-level variables that is the equivalent of the histogram but appears smoother. It is constructed by joining the midpoints of the top of each bar.

Point-Biserial coefficient: A shortcut method of calculating r when there is one dichotomous and one continuous variable.

Population: All members in a defined group.

Positive predictive value: The proportion of people with the disease who tested positive for the disease, that is, "true positives"; expressed as a percentage.

Posthoc tests: Tests of paired comparisons made when the overall test is significant.

Power: The likelihood of rejecting the null hypothesis.

Principal components analysis: A type of analysis that is based on the assumption that all measurement error is random and includes 1s in the diagonal of the correlation matrix that is analyzed.

Probability: A quantitative description of the likely occurrence of a particular event, conventionally expressed on a scale from 0 to 1.

Probability value (*p* value): In a statistical hypothesis test, the likelihood of getting the value of the statistic by chance alone.

Quartiles: The first quartile is the 25th percentile, the second is the 50th percentile, the third is the 75th percentile, and the fourth is the 100th percentile.

Quartimax rotation: A method of rotation in factor analysis that tends to produce a first, very general, factor with high loadings.

R: Multiple correlation.

R^2: Squared multiple correlation; the amount of variance accounted for in the dependent variable by a combination of independent variables.

R statistic: In logistic regression, the partial correlation.

Randomization: Assignment of individuals to groups by chance (ie, every subject has an equal chance of being assigned to a particular group).

Range: The difference between the maximum and minimum values in a distribution.

Ratio-level measurement: The highest level of measurement. In addition to equal intervals between data points, there is an absolute zero.

Raw data matrix: A matrix containing raw scores for each subject on each variable. The rows represent subjects, and the columns represent variables.

Receiver Operator Characteristic (ROC) Curve: graphic representation of the trade-off between false positive and false negative rates for every possible cut off value. The graph plots the false positive rate on the x-axis and the true positive rate ($1 -$ the false negative rate) on the y-axis. The area under the curve is of primary interest as it measures the correlation between the category predicted by the test and the true category into which the case falls.

Recursive model: The flow of causation in the model is unidirectional.

Redundancy: In canonical correlation, the percent of variance the canonical variates from the independent variables extract from the dependent variables and vice versa.

Reflect a variable: A form of recording a variable so that scores are reversed, that is, the highest score becomes the lowest, and so forth.

Regression: A statistical method that makes use of the correlation between two variables and the notion of a straight line to develop a prediction equation.

Regression coefficient (b): The rate of change in Y with a one-unit change in X.

Regression line: The line of best fit formed by the mathematical technique called the method of least squares.

Regression sum of squares: The variance that is accounted for by the variables in the equation.

Relative risk: The risk given one condition versus the risk given another condition.

Repeated measures analysis of variance: A method of analyzing within-cell designs in which subjects are measured more than once on the same variable or where subjects are exposed to all treatments, thus serving as their own controls.

Research problems: Questions that can be answered by collecting facts.

Residual: The difference between the actual and predicted scores; the variance that is not shared by the variables in the correlation; the unexplained or error variance.

Risk: The number of occurrences out of the total.

Roy's greatest characteristic root: An outcome statistic generated by multivariate analysis of variance and based on the first discriminate variate.

Sample size: Number of subjects included in the study.

Scatter diagram: A graph of pairs of scores for subjects.

Scheffé test: A conservative posthoc test; may be used with groups of equal or unequal size.

Scree test: A plot of eigenvalues.

Semipartial correlation: The correlation between two variables with the effect of another variable(s) removed from one of the variables being correlated.

Sensitivity: The proportion of people with disease who have a positive test result.

Shrinkage formula: An equation that provides an estimate of how much the multiple correlation coefficient is likely to shrink.

Significance level: Specifies the risk of rejecting the null hypothesis when it is true.

Significance test: A statistical calculation that assigns a probability to a statistical estimate; a small probability implies a significant result.

Simple structure: A criterion for factor rotation that seeks to maximize high and low loadings to reduce ambiguity.

Skewness: A measure of the shape of an asymmetrical distribution.

Spearman Rho: A shortcut formula for r when you have two sets of ranks.

Specification: The process of specifying or delineating the structural relationships among the component parts of a model.

Specificity: The proportion of people without the disease who have a negative test result.

Standard deviation: A measure of dispersion of scores around the mean. It is the square root of the variance.

Standard regression: All the independent variables are entered together.

Standard scores: z-scores; represent the deviation of scores around the mean in a distribution with a mean of zero and a standard deviation of 1.

Standardized canonical correlations: Similar to beta weights in regression. They are based on the standard scores of the variables and indicate the relative importance of each variable.

Statistics: The field of study that is concerned with obtaining, describing, and interpreting data; the characteristics of samples.

Stepwise regression: Variables are entered into the equation based on their measured relationship to the dependent variable. Methods include forward entry, backward removal, and a combination of forward and backward called stepwise.

Structural equation modeling: A method of testing theoretical models that analyzes covariances. It tests a measurement model and a theoretical model made up of measured and latent variables.

Structure coefficients: The correlations between the dependent and canonical variates. They are generally used for interpretation of results. Values of 0.30 or greater are considered meaningful.

Student Newman-Keuls: A posthoc test that is similar to Tukey's HSD, but the critical values do not remain constant.

Subjective probability: An individual's personal judgment of the likelihood of a particular event occurring.

Sum of squares: The sum of the squared deviations of each of the scores around a respective mean.

Tables: When data are organized into values or categories and then described with titles and captions, the result is a statistical table.

Tetrachoric: A coefficient that estimates r from the relationship between two dichotomized variables.

Theoretical model: A model of the hypothesized relationship between two latent variables.

Tolerance: A measure of collinearity. The proportion of the variance in a variable that is not accounted for by the other independent variables (1 −R2).

Transformation to normality: Altering data values in a skewed distribution to produce a normal or nearly normal distribution.

Trimmed mean: A statistical average calculated after removal of a certain percentage of extreme values from both ends of the distribution.

***t* test:** A parametric statistical test for comparing the means of two independent groups.

Tukey's honestly significant difference (HSD): The most conservative posthoc test.

Tukey's wholly significant difference: A posthoc test that is intermediate in conservatism between Newman-Keuls and Tukey's HSD.

Two-tailed test of significance: A test used with a nondirectional hypothesis, in which extreme values are assumed to occur in either tail of the distribution.

Type I error: Concluding that a significant difference or relationship exists when it does not.

Type II error: Concluding that there is no significant difference or relationship when there is.

Underidentified model: A nonrecursive model. It contains paths that are not undirectional.

Valid percent: The percentage with missing data excluded.

Variable: A measured characteristic that can take on different values.

Variance: A measure of the dispersion of scores around the mean. It is equal to the standard deviation squared.

Variance inflation factor: The reciprocal of tolerance.

Varimax rotation: Orthogonal rotation resulting in factors that are not correlated with each other.

Wald statistic: A value tested for significance in logistic regression.

Wilcoxon matched-pairs signed rank test: A nonparametric technique analogous to the paired *t* test. Used to compare paired measures.

Winsorized mean: A statistical average calculated after replacing the highest and lowest extreme values with the next-highest and next-lowest value.

Wilks' lambda: Represents the unexplained or error variance.

Within-groups variance: Variation of scores within the respective groups; represents the error term in analysis of variance.

Within-sample independence: Observations within the sample are independent of each other.

Within-subjects designs: Subjects serve as their own controls. Subjects are measured more than once on the same variable, or subjects are exposed to more than one treatment.

Y': The predicted score in a regression equation.

Zero-order correlation: The measured relationship between two variables.

z-scores: Standardized scores calculated by subtracting the mean from an individual score and dividing the result by the standard deviation; represents the deviation from the mean in a normal distribution.

Percent of Total Area of Normal Curve Between a z-Score and the Mean

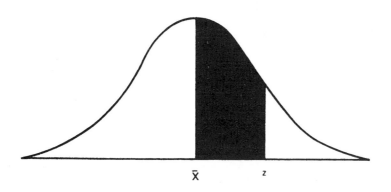

z	0.00	0.01	0.02	0.03	0.04	0.05	0.06	0.07	0.08	0.09
0.0	00.00	00.40	00.80	01.20	01.60	01.99	02.39	02.79	03.19	03.59
0.1	03.98	04.38	04.78	05.17	05.57	05.96	06.36	06.75	07.14	07.53
0.2	07.93	08.32	08.71	09.10	09.48	09.87	10.26	10.64	11.03	11.41
0.3	11.79	12.17	12.55	12.93	13.31	13.68	14.06	14.43	14.80	15.17
0.4	15.54	15.91	16.28	16.64	17.00	17.36	17.72	18.08	18.44	18.79
0.5	19.15	19.50	19.85	20.19	20.54	20.88	21.23	21.57	21.90	22.24
0.6	22.57	22.91	23.24	23.57	23.89	24.22	24.54	24.86	25.17	25.49
0.7	25.80	26.11	26.42	26.73	27.04	27.34	27.64	27.94	28.23	28.52
0.8	28.81	29.10	29.39	29.67	29.95	30.23	30.51	30.78	31.06	31.33
0.9	31.59	31.86	32.12	32.38	32.64	32.90	33.15	33.40	33.65	33.89

(Continued)

Appendix A (CONTINUED)

z	0.00	0.01	0.02	0.03	0.04	0.05	0.06	0.07	0.08	0.09
1.0	34.13	34.38	34.61	34.85	35.08	35.31	35.54	35.77	35.99	36.21
1.1	36.43	36.65	36.86	37.08	37.29	37.49	37.70	37.90	38.10	38.30
1.2	38.49	38.69	38.88	39.07	39.25	39.44	39.62	39.80	39.97	40.15
1.3	40.32	40.49	40.66	40.82	40.99	41.15	41.31	41.47	41.62	41.77
1.4	41.92	42.07	42.22	42.36	42.51	42.65	42.79	42.92	43.06	43.19
1.5	43.32	43.45	43.57	43.70	43.83	43.94	44.06	44.18	44.29	44.41
1.6	44.52	44.63	44.74	44.84	44.95	45.05	45.15	45.25	45.35	45.45
1.7	45.54	45.64	45.73	45.82	45.91	45.99	46.08	46.16	46.25	46.33
1.8	46.41	46.49	46.56	46.64	46.71	46.78	46.86	46.93	46.99	47.06
1.9	47.13	47.19	47.26	47.32	47.38	47.44	47.50	47.56	47.61	47.67
2.0	47.72	47.78	47.83	47.88	47.93	47.98	48.03	48.08	48.12	48.17
2.1	48.21	48.26	48.30	48.34	48.38	48.42	48.46	48.50	48.54	48.57
2.2	48.61	48.64	48.68	48.71	48.75	48.78	48.81	48.84	48.87	48.90
2.3	48.93	48.96	48.98	49.01	49.04	49.06	49.09	49.11	49.13	49.16
2.4	49.18	49.20	49.22	49.25	49.27	49.29	49.31	49.32	49.34	49.36
2.5	49.38	49.40	49.41	49.43	49.45	49.46	49.48	49.49	49.51	49.52
2.6	49.53	49.55	49.56	49.57	49.59	49.60	49.61	49.62	49.63	49.64
2.7	49.65	49.66	49.67	49.68	49.69	49.70	49.71	49.72	49.73	49.74
2.8	49.74	49.75	49.76	49.77	49.77	49.78	49.79	49.79	49.80	49.81
2.9	49.81	49.82	49.82	49.83	49.84	49.84	49.85	49.85	49.86	49.86
3.0	49.87									
3.5	49.98									
4.0	49.997									
5.0	49.99997									

(From Hald, A. [1952]. *Statistical tables and formulas.* New York: John Wiley & Sons. [Table 1].)

Distribution of χ^2 Probability

df	0.20	0.10	0.05	0.02	0.01	0.001
1	1.642	2.706	3.841	5.412	6.635	10.827
2	3.219	4.605	5.991	7.842	9.210	13.815
3	4.642	6.251	7.815	9.837	11.345	16.266
4	5.989	7.779	9.488	11.668	13.277	18.467
5	7.289	9.236	11.070	13.388	15.086	20.515
6	8.558	10.645	12.592	15.033	16.812	22.457
7	9.803	12.017	14.067	16.622	18.475	24.322
8	11.030	13.362	15.507	18.168	20.090	26.125
9	12.242	14.684	16.919	19.679	21.666	27.877
10	13.442	15.987	18.307	21.161	23.209	29.588
11	14.631	17.275	19.675	22.618	24.725	31.264
12	15.812	18.549	21.026	24.054	26.217	32.909
13	16.985	19.812	22.362	25.472	27.688	34.528
14	18.151	21.064	23.685	26.873	29.141	36.123
15	19.311	22.307	24.996	28.259	30.578	37.697
16	20.465	23.542	26.296	29.633	32.000	39.252
17	21.615	24.769	27.587	30.995	33.409	40.790
18	22.760	25.989	28.869	32.346	34.805	42.312
19	23.900	27.204	30.144	33.687	36.191	43.820
20	25.038	28.412	31.410	35.020	37.566	45.315

(Continued)

Appendix B (CONTINUED)

df	0.20	0.10	0.05	0.02	0.01	0.001
21	26.171	29.615	32.671	36.343	38.932	46.797
22	27.301	30.813	33.924	37.659	40.289	48.268
23	28.429	32.007	35.172	38.968	41.638	49.728
24	29.553	33.196	36.415	40.270	42.980	51.179
25	30.675	34.382	37.652	41.566	44.314	52.620
26	31.795	35.563	38.885	42.856	45.642	54.052
27	32.912	36.741	40.113	44.140	46.963	55.476
28	34.027	37.916	41.337	45.419	48.278	56.893
29	35.139	39.087	42.557	46.693	49.588	58.302
30	36.250	40.256	43.773	47.962	50.892	59.703

(From Fisher, R. A. [1970]. *Statistical methods for research workers* [14th ed.]. Darien, CT: Hafner Publishing. [Taken from Table III, pp. 112–113].)

Distribution of *t*

df	Level of Significance for One-Tailed Test					
	0.10	0.05	0.025	0.01	0.005	0.0005
	Level of Significance for Two-Tailed Test					
	0.20	0.10	0.05	0.02	0.01	0.001
1	3.078	6.314	12.706	31.821	63.657	636.619
2	1.886	2.920	4.303	6.965	9.925	31.598
3	1.638	2.353	3.182	4.541	5.841	12.941
4	1.533	2.132	2.776	3.747	4.604	8.610
5	1.476	2.015	2.571	3.365	4.032	6.859
6	1.440	1.943	2.447	3.143	3.707	5.959
7	1.415	1.895	2.365	2.998	3.499	5.405
8	1.397	1.860	2.306	2.896	3.355	5.041
9	1.383	1.833	2.262	2.821	3.250	4.781
10	1.372	1.812	2.228	2.764	3.169	4.587
11	1.363	1.796	2.201	2.718	3.106	4.437
12	1.356	1.782	2.179	2.681	3.055	4.318
13	1.350	1.771	2.160	2.650	3.012	4.221
14	1.345	1.761	2.145	2.624	2.977	4.140
15	1.341	1.753	2.131	2.602	2.947	4.073
16	1.337	1.746	2.120	2.583	2.921	4.015
17	1.333	1.740	2.110	2.567	2.898	3.965

(*Continued*)

Appendix C (CONTINUED)

	Level of Significance for One-Tailed Test					
	0.10	0.05	0.025	0.01	0.005	0.0005
	Level of Significance for Two-Tailed Test					
df	0.20	0.10	0.05	0.02	0.01	0.001
18	1.330	1.734	2.101	2.552	2.878	3.922
19	1.328	1.729	2.093	2.539	2.861	3.883
20	1.325	1.725	2.086	2.528	2.845	3.850
21	1.323	1.721	2.080	2.518	2.831	3.819
22	1.321	1.717	2.074	2.508	2.819	3.792
23	1.319	1.714	2.069	2.500	2.807	3.767
24	1.318	1.711	2.064	2.492	2.797	3.745
25	1.316	1.708	2.060	3.485	2.787	3.725
26	1.315	1.706	2.056	2.479	2.779	3.707
27	1.314	1.703	2.052	2.473	2.771	3.690
28	1.313	1.701	2.048	2.467	2.763	3.674
29	1.311	1.699	2.045	2.462	2.756	3.659
30	1.310	1.697	2.042	2.457	2.750	3.646
40	1.303	1.684	2.021	2.423	2.704	3.551
60	1.296	1.671	2.000	2.390	2.660	3.460
120	1.289	1.658	1.980	2.358	2.617	3.373
∞	1.282	1.645	1.960	2.326	2.576	3.291

(From Fisher, R. A. [1970]. *Statistical methods for research workers* [14th ed.]. Darien, CT: Hafner Publishing [Table IV, p. 176].)

The 5% and 1% Points for the Distribution of F

n_1 Degrees of Freedom (For Greater Mean Square)*

n_2	1	2	3	4	5	6	7	8	9	10	11	12	14	16	20	24	30	40	50	75	100	200	500	∞
1	161	200	216	225	230	234	237	239	241	242	243	244	245	246	248	249	250	251	252	253	253	254	254	254
	4,052	**4,999**	**5,403**	**5,625**	**5,764**	**5,859**	**5,928**	**5,981**	**6,022**	**6,056**	**6,082**	**6,106**	**6,142**	**6,169**	**6,208**	**6,234**	**6,258**	**6,286**	**6,302**	**6,323**	**6,334**	**6,352**	**6,361**	**6,366**
2	18.51	19.00	19.16	19.25	19.30	19.33	19.36	19.37	19.38	19.39	19.40	19.41	19.42	19.43	19.44	19.45	19.46	19.47	19.47	19.48	19.49	19.49	19.50	19.50
	98.49	**99.00**	**99.17**	**99.25**	**99.30**	**99.33**	**99.34**	**99.36**	**99.38**	**99.40**	**99.41**	**99.42**	**99.43**	**99.44**	**99.45**	**99.46**	**99.47**	**99.48**	**99.48**	**99.49**	**99.49**	**99.49**	**99.50**	**99.50**
3	10.13	9.55	9.38	9.12	9.01	8.94	8.88	8.84	8.81	8.78	8.76	8.74	8.71	8.69	8.66	8.64	8.62	8.60	8.58	8.57	8.56	8.54	8.54	8.53
	34.12	**30.82**	**29.46**	**28.71**	**28.47**	**27.91**	**27.67**	**27.49**	**27.34**	**27.23**	**27.13**	**27.05**	**26.92**	**26.83**	**26.69**	**26.60**	**26.50**	**26.41**	**26.35**	**26.27**	**26.23**	**26.18**	**26.14**	**26.12**
4	7.71	6.94	6.59	6.39	6.26	6.16	6.09	6.04	6.00	5.96	5.93	5.91	5.87	5.84	5.80	5.77	5.74	5.71	5.70	5.68	5.66	5.65	5.64	5.63
	21.20	**18.00**	**16.69**	**15.98**	**15.52**	**15.21**	**14.98**	**14.80**	**14.66**	**14.54**	**14.45**	**14.37**	**14.24**	**14.15**	**14.02**	**13.93**	**13.83**	**13.74**	**13.69**	**13.61**	**13.57**	**13.52**	**13.48**	**13.46**
5	6.61	5.79	5.41	5.19	5.05	4.95	4.88	4.82	4.78	4.74	4.70	4.68	4.64	4.60	4.56	4.53	4.50	4.46	4.44	4.42	4.40	4.38	4.37	4.36
	16.26	**13.27**	**12.06**	**11.39**	**10.97**	**10.67**	**10.45**	**10.27**	**10.15**	**10.05**	**9.96**	**9.89**	**9.77**	**9.68**	**9.55**	**9.47**	**9.38**	**9.29**	**9.24**	**9.17**	**9.13**	**9.07**	**9.04**	**9.02**
6	5.99	5.14	4.76	4.53	4.39	4.28	4.21	4.15	4.10	4.06	4.03	4.00	3.96	3.92	3.87	3.84	3.81	3.77	3.75	3.72	3.71	3.69	3.68	3.67
	13.74	**10.92**	**9.78**	**9.15**	**8.75**	**8.47**	**8.26**	**8.10**	**7.98**	**7.87**	**7.79**	**7.72**	**7.60**	**7.52**	**7.39**	**7.31**	**7.23**	**7.14**	**7.09**	**7.02**	**6.99**	**6.94**	**6.90**	**6.88**
7	5.59	4.74	4.35	4.12	3.97	3.87	3.79	3.73	3.68	3.63	3.60	3.57	3.52	3.49	3.44	3.41	3.38	3.34	3.32	3.29	3.28	3.25	3.24	3.23
	12.25	**9.55**	**8.45**	**7.85**	**7.46**	**7.19**	**7.00**	**6.84**	**6.71**	**6.62**	**6.54**	**6.47**	**6.35**	**6.27**	**6.15**	**6.07**	**5.98**	**5.90**	**5.85**	**5.78**	**5.75**	**5.70**	**5.65**	**5.65**
8	5.32	4.46	4.07	3.84	3.69	3.58	3.50	3.44	3.39	3.34	3.31	3.28	3.23	3.20	3.15	3.12	3.08	3.05	3.03	3.00	2.98	2.96	2.94	2.93
	11.26	**8.65**	**7.59**	**7.01**	**6.63**	**6.37**	**6.19**	**6.03**	**5.91**	**5.82**	**5.74**	**5.67**	**5.56**	**5.48**	**5.36**	**5.28**	**5.20**	**5.11**	**5.06**	**5.00**	**4.96**	**4.91**	**4.88**	**4.86**
9	5.12	4.26	3.86	3.63	3.48	3.37	3.29	3.23	3.18	3.13	3.10	3.07	3.02	2.98	2.93	2.90	2.86	2.82	2.80	2.77	2.76	2.73	2.72	2.71
	10.56	**8.02**	**6.99**	**6.42**	**6.06**	**5.80**	**5.62**	**5.47**	**5.35**	**5.26**	**5.18**	**5.11**	**5.00**	**4.92**	**4.80**	**4.73**	**4.64**	**4.56**	**4.51**	**4.45**	**4.41**	**4.36**	**4.33**	**4.31**
10	4.96	4.10	3.71	3.48	3.33	3.22	3.14	3.07	3.02	2.97	2.94	2.91	2.86	2.82	2.77	2.74	2.70	2.67	2.64	2.61	2.59	2.56	2.55	2.54
	10.04	**7.56**	**6.55**	**5.99**	**5.64**	**5.39**	**5.21**	**5.06**	**4.95**	**4.85**	**4.78**	**4.71**	**4.60**	**4.52**	**4.41**	**4.33**	**4.25**	**4.17**	**4.12**	**4.05**	**4.01**	**3.96**	**3.93**	**3.91**
11	4.84	3.98	3.59	3.36	3.20	3.09	3.01	2.95	2.90	2.86	2.82	2.79	2.74	2.70	2.65	2.61	2.57	2.53	2.50	2.47	2.45	2.42	2.41	2.40
	9.65	**7.20**	**6.22**	**5.67**	**5.32**	**5.07**	**4.88**	**4.74**	**4.63**	**4.54**	**4.46**	**4.40**	**4.29**	**4.21**	**4.10**	**4.02**	**3.94**	**3.86**	**3.80**	**3.74**	**3.70**	**3.66**	**3.62**	**3.60**
12	4.75	3.88	3.49	3.26	3.11	3.00	2.92	2.85	2.80	2.76	2.72	2.69	2.64	2.60	2.54	2.50	2.46	2.42	2.40	2.36	2.35	2.32	2.31	2.30
	9.33	**6.93**	**5.95**	**5.41**	**5.06**	**4.82**	**4.65**	**4.50**	**4.39**	**4.30**	**4.22**	**4.16**	**4.05**	**3.98**	**3.86**	**3.78**	**3.70**	**3.61**	**3.56**	**3.49**	**3.46**	**3.41**	**3.38**	**3.36**
13	4.67	3.80	3.41	3.18	3.02	2.92	2.84	2.77	2.72	2.67	2.63	2.60	2.55	2.51	2.46	2.42	2.38	2.34	2.32	2.28	2.26	2.24	2.22	2.21
	9.07	**6.70**	**5.74**	**5.20**	**4.86**	**4.62**	**4.44**	**4.30**	**4.19**	**4.10**	**4.02**	**3.96**	**3.85**	**3.78**	**3.67**	**3.59**	**3.51**	**3.42**	**3.37**	**3.30**	**3.27**	**3.21**	**3.18**	**3.16**
14	4.60	3.74	3.34	3.11	2.96	2.85	2.77	2.70	2.65	2.60	2.56	2.53	2.48	2.44	2.39	2.35	2.31	2.27	2.24	2.21	2.19	2.16	2.14	2.13
	8.86	**6.51**	**5.56**	**5.03**	**4.69**	**4.46**	**4.28**	**4.14**	**4.03**	**3.94**	**3.86**	**3.80**	**3.70**	**3.62**	**3.51**	**3.43**	**3.34**	**3.26**	**3.21**	**3.14**	**3.11**	**3.06**	**3.02**	**3.00**
15	4.54	3.68	3.29	3.06	2.90	2.79	2.70	2.64	2.59	2.55	2.51	2.48	2.43	2.39	2.33	2.29	2.25	2.21	2.18	2.15	2.12	2.10	2.08	2.07
	8.68	**6.36**	**5.42**	**4.89**	**4.56**	**4.32**	**4.14**	**4.00**	**3.89**	**3.80**	**3.73**	**3.67**	**3.56**	**3.48**	**3.36**	**3.29**	**3.20**	**3.12**	**3.07**	**3.00**	**2.97**	**2.92**	**2.89**	**2.87**
16	4.49	3.63	3.24	3.01	2.85	2.74	2.66	2.59	2.54	2.49	2.45	2.42	2.37	2.33	2.28	2.24	2.20	2.16	2.13	2.09	2.07	2.04	2.02	2.01
	8.53	**6.23**	**5.29**	**4.77**	**4.44**	**4.20**	**4.03**	**3.89**	**3.78**	**3.69**	**3.61**	**3.55**	**3.45**	**3.37**	**3.25**	**3.18**	**3.10**	**3.01**	**2.96**	**2.89**	**2.86**	**2.80**	**2.77**	**2.75**
17	4.45	3.59	3.20	2.96	2.81	2.70	2.62	2.55	2.50	2.45	2.41	2.38	2.33	2.29	2.23	2.19	2.15	2.11	2.08	2.04	2.02	1.99	1.97	1.96
	8.40	**6.11**	**5.18**	**4.67**	**4.34**	**4.10**	**3.93**	**3.79**	**3.68**	**3.59**	**3.52**	**3.45**	**3.35**	**3.27**	**3.16**	**3.08**	**3.00**	**2.92**	**2.86**	**2.79**	**2.76**	**2.70**	**2.67**	**2.65**
18	4.41	3.55	3.16	2.93	2.77	2.66	2.58	2.51	2.46	2.41	2.37	2.34	2.29	2.25	2.19	2.15	2.11	2.07	2.04	2.00	1.98	1.95	1.93	1.92
	8.28	**6.01**	**5.09**	**4.58**	**4.25**	**4.01**	**3.85**	**3.71**	**3.60**	**3.51**	**3.44**	**3.37**	**3.27**	**3.19**	**3.07**	**3.00**	**2.91**	**2.83**	**2.78**	**2.71**	**2.68**	**2.62**	**2.59**	**2.57**

df																								
19	4.38	3.52	3.13	2.90	2.74	2.63	2.55	2.48	2.43	2.38	2.34	2.31	2.26	2.21	2.15	2.11	2.07	2.02	2.00	1.96	1.94	1.91	1.90	1.88
	8.18	**5.93**	**5.01**	**4.50**	**4.17**	**3.94**	**3.77**	**3.63**	**3.52**	**3.43**	**3.36**	**3.30**	**3.19**	**3.12**	**3.00**	**2.92**	**2.84**	**2.76**	**2.70**	**2.63**	**2.60**	**2.54**	**2.51**	**2.49**
20	4.35	3.49	3.10	2.87	2.71	2.60	2.52	2.45	2.40	2.35	2.31	2.28	2.23	2.18	2.12	2.08	2.04	1.99	1.96	1.92	1.90	1.87	1.85	1.84
	8.10	**5.85**	**4.94**	**4.43**	**4.10**	**3.87**	**3.71**	**3.56**	**3.45**	**3.37**	**3.30**	**3.23**	**3.13**	**3.05**	**2.94**	**2.86**	**2.77**	**2.69**	**2.63**	**2.56**	**2.53**	**2.47**	**2.44**	**2.42**
21	4.32	3.47	3.07	2.84	2.68	2.57	2.49	2.42	2.37	2.32	2.28	2.25	2.20	2.15	2.09	2.05	2.00	1.96	1.93	1.89	1.87	1.84	1.82	1.81
	8.02	**5.78**	**4.87**	**4.37**	**4.04**	**3.81**	**3.65**	**3.51**	**3.40**	**3.31**	**3.24**	**3.17**	**3.07**	**2.99**	**2.88**	**2.80**	**2.72**	**2.63**	**2.58**	**2.51**	**2.47**	**2.42**	**2.38**	**2.36**
22	4.30	3.44	3.05	2.82	2.66	2.55	2.47	2.40	2.35	2.30	2.26	2.23	2.18	2.13	2.07	2.03	1.98	1.93	1.91	1.87	1.84	1.81	1.80	1.78
	7.94	**5.72**	**4.82**	**4.31**	**3.99**	**3.76**	**3.59**	**3.45**	**3.35**	**3.26**	**3.18**	**3.12**	**3.02**	**2.94**	**2.83**	**2.75**	**2.67**	**2.58**	**2.53**	**2.46**	**2.42**	**2.37**	**2.33**	**2.31**
23	4.28	3.42	3.03	2.80	2.64	2.53	2.45	2.38	2.32	2.28	2.24	2.20	2.14	2.10	2.04	2.00	1.96	1.91	1.88	1.84	1.82	1.79	1.77	1.76
	7.88	**5.66**	**4.76**	**4.26**	**3.94**	**3.71**	**3.54**	**3.41**	**3.30**	**3.21**	**3.14**	**3.07**	**2.97**	**2.89**	**2.78**	**2.70**	**2.62**	**2.53**	**2.48**	**2.41**	**2.37**	**2.32**	**2.28**	**2.26**
24	4.26	3.40	3.01	2.78	2.62	2.51	2.43	2.36	2.30	2.26	2.22	2.18	2.13	2.09	2.02	1.98	1.94	1.89	1.86	1.82	1.80	1.76	1.74	1.73
	7.82	**5.61**	**4.72**	**4.22**	**3.90**	**3.67**	**3.50**	**3.36**	**3.25**	**3.17**	**3.09**	**3.03**	**2.93**	**2.85**	**2.74**	**2.66**	**2.58**	**2.49**	**2.44**	**2.36**	**2.33**	**2.27**	**2.23**	**2.21**
25	4.24	3.38	2.99	2.76	2.60	2.49	2.41	2.34	2.28	2.24	2.20	2.16	2.11	2.06	2.00	1.96	1.92	1.87	1.84	1.80	1.77	1.74	1.72	1.71
	7.77	**5.57**	**4.68**	**4.18**	**3.86**	**3.63**	**3.46**	**3.32**	**3.21**	**3.13**	**3.05**	**2.99**	**2.89**	**2.81**	**2.70**	**2.62**	**2.54**	**2.45**	**2.40**	**2.32**	**2.29**	**2.23**	**2.19**	**2.17**
26	4.22	3.37	2.98	2.74	2.59	2.47	2.39	2.32	2.27	2.22	2.18	2.15	2.10	2.05	1.99	1.95	1.90	1.85	1.82	1.78	1.76	1.72	1.70	1.69
	7.72	**5.53**	**4.64**	**4.14**	**3.82**	**3.59**	**3.42**	**3.29**	**3.17**	**3.09**	**3.02**	**2.96**	**2.86**	**2.77**	**2.66**	**2.58**	**2.50**	**2.41**	**2.36**	**2.28**	**2.25**	**2.19**	**2.15**	**2.13**
27	4.21	3.35	2.96	2.73	2.57	2.46	2.37	2.30	2.25	2.20	2.15	2.13	2.08	2.03	1.97	1.93	1.88	1.84	1.80	1.76	1.74	1.71	1.68	1.67
	7.68	**5.49**	**4.60**	**4.11**	**3.79**	**3.56**	**3.39**	**3.26**	**3.14**	**3.06**	**2.98**	**2.93**	**2.83**	**2.74**	**2.63**	**2.55**	**2.47**	**2.38**	**2.33**	**2.25**	**2.21**	**2.16**	**2.12**	**2.10**
28	4.20	3.34	2.95	2.71	2.56	2.44	2.36	2.29	2.24	2.19	2.15	2.12	2.06	2.02	1.96	1.91	1.87	1.81	1.78	1.75	1.72	1.69	1.67	1.65
	7.64	**5.45**	**4.57**	**4.07**	**3.76**	**3.53**	**3.36**	**3.23**	**3.11**	**3.03**	**2.95**	**2.90**	**2.80**	**2.71**	**2.60**	**2.52**	**2.44**	**2.35**	**2.30**	**2.22**	**2.18**	**2.13**	**2.09**	**2.06**
29	4.18	3.33	2.93	2.70	2.54	2.43	2.35	2.28	2.22	2.18	2.14	2.10	2.05	2.00	1.94	1.90	1.85	1.80	1.77	1.73	1.71	1.68	1.65	1.64
	7.60	**5.42**	**4.54**	**4.04**	**3.73**	**3.50**	**3.33**	**3.20**	**3.08**	**3.00**	**2.92**	**2.87**	**2.77**	**2.68**	**2.57**	**2.49**	**2.41**	**2.32**	**2.27**	**2.19**	**2.15**	**2.10**	**2.06**	**2.03**
30	4.17	3.32	2.92	2.69	2.53	2.42	2.34	2.27	2.21	2.16	2.12	2.09	2.04	1.99	1.93	1.89	1.84	1.79	1.76	1.72	1.69	1.66	1.64	1.62
	7.56	**5.39**	**4.51**	**4.02**	**3.70**	**3.47**	**3.30**	**3.17**	**3.06**	**2.98**	**2.90**	**2.84**	**2.74**	**2.66**	**2.55**	**2.47**	**2.38**	**2.29**	**2.24**	**2.16**	**2.13**	**2.07**	**2.03**	**2.01**
32	4.15	3.30	2.90	2.67	2.51	2.40	2.32	2.25	2.19	2.14	2.10	2.07	2.02	1.97	1.91	1.86	1.82	1.76	1.74	1.69	1.67	1.64	1.61	1.59
	7.50	**5.34**	**4.46**	**3.97**	**3.66**	**3.42**	**3.25**	**3.12**	**3.01**	**2.94**	**2.86**	**2.80**	**2.70**	**2.62**	**2.51**	**2.42**	**2.34**	**2.25**	**2.20**	**2.12**	**2.08**	**2.02**	**1.98**	**1.96**
34	4.13	3.28	2.88	2.65	2.49	2.38	2.30	2.23	2.17	2.12	2.08	2.05	2.00	1.95	1.89	1.84	1.80	1.74	1.71	1.67	1.64	1.61	1.59	1.57
	7.44	**5.29**	**4.42**	**3.93**	**3.61**	**3.38**	**3.21**	**3.08**	**2.97**	**2.89**	**2.82**	**2.76**	**2.66**	**2.58**	**2.47**	**2.38**	**2.30**	**2.21**	**2.15**	**2.08**	**2.04**	**1.98**	**1.94**	**1.91**
36	4.11	3.26	2.86	2.63	2.48	2.36	2.28	2.21	2.15	2.10	2.06	2.03	1.98	1.93	1.87	1.82	1.78	1.72	1.69	1.65	1.62	1.59	1.56	1.55
	7.39	**5.25**	**4.38**	**3.89**	**3.58**	**3.35**	**3.18**	**3.04**	**2.94**	**2.86**	**2.78**	**2.72**	**2.62**	**2.54**	**2.43**	**2.35**	**2.26**	**2.17**	**2.12**	**2.04**	**2.00**	**1.94**	**1.90**	**1.87**
38	4.10	3.25	2.85	2.62	2.46	2.35	2.26	2.19	2.14	2.09	2.05	2.02	1.96	1.92	1.85	1.80	1.76	1.71	1.67	1.63	1.60	1.57	1.54	1.53
	7.35	**5.21**	**4.34**	**3.86**	**3.54**	**3.32**	**3.15**	**3.02**	**2.91**	**2.82**	**2.75**	**2.69**	**2.59**	**2.51**	**2.40**	**2.32**	**2.22**	**2.14**	**2.08**	**2.00**	**1.97**	**1.90**	**1.86**	**1.84**
40	4.08	3.23	2.84	2.61	2.45	2.34	2.25	2.18	2.12	2.07	2.04	2.00	1.95	1.90	1.84	1.79	1.74	1.69	1.66	1.61	1.59	1.55	1.53	1.51
	7.31	**5.18**	**4.31**	**3.83**	**3.51**	**3.29**	**3.12**	**2.99**	**2.88**	**2.80**	**2.73**	**2.66**	**2.56**	**2.49**	**2.37**	**2.29**	**2.20**	**2.11**	**2.05**	**1.97**	**1.94**	**1.88**	**1.84**	**1.81**
42	4.07	3.22	2.83	2.59	2.44	2.32	2.24	2.17	2.11	2.06	2.02	1.99	1.94	1.89	1.82	1.78	1.73	1.68	1.64	1.60	1.57	1.54	1.51	1.49
	7.27	**5.15**	**4.29**	**3.80**	**3.49**	**3.26**	**3.10**	**2.96**	**2.86**	**2.77**	**2.70**	**2.64**	**2.54**	**2.46**	**2.35**	**2.26**	**2.17**	**2.08**	**2.02**	**1.94**	**1.91**	**1.85**	**1.80**	**1.78**
44	4.06	3.21	2.82	2.58	2.43	2.31	2.23	2.16	2.10	2.05	2.01	1.98	1.92	1.88	1.81	1.76	1.72	1.66	1.63	1.58	1.56	1.52	1.50	1.48
	7.24	**5.12**	**4.26**	**3.78**	**3.46**	**3.24**	**3.07**	**2.94**	**2.84**	**2.75**	**2.68**	**2.62**	**2.52**	**2.44**	**2.32**	**2.24**	**2.15**	**2.06**	**2.00**	**1.92**	**1.88**	**1.82**	**1.78**	**1.75**

Appendix D (CONTINUED)

n_1 Degrees of Freedom (For Greater Mean Square)*

n_2	1	2	3	4	5	6	7	8	9	10	11	12	14	16	20	24	30	40	50	75	100	200	500	∞
46	4.05	3.20	2.81	2.57	2.42	2.30	2.22	2.14	2.09	2.04	2.00	1.97	1.91	1.87	1.80	1.75	1.71	1.65	1.62	1.57	1.54	1.51	1.48	1.46
	7.21	**5.10**	**4.24**	**3.76**	**3.44**	**3.22**	**3.05**	**2.92**	**2.82**	**2.73**	**2.66**	**2.60**	**2.50**	**2.42**	**2.30**	**2.22**	**2.13**	**2.04**	**1.98**	**1.90**	**1.86**	**1.80**	**1.76**	**1.72**
48	4.04	3.19	2.80	2.56	2.41	2.30	2.21	2.14	2.08	2.03	1.99	1.96	1.90	1.86	1.79	1.74	1.70	1.64	1.61	1.56	1.53	1.50	1.47	1.45
	7.19	**5.08**	**4.22**	**3.74**	**3.42**	**3.20**	**3.04**	**2.90**	**2.80**	**2.71**	**2.64**	**2.58**	**2.48**	**2.40**	**2.28**	**2.20**	**2.11**	**2.02**	**1.96**	**1.88**	**1.84**	**1.78**	**1.73**	**1.70**
50	4.03	3.18	2.79	2.56	2.40	2.29	2.20	2.13	2.07	2.02	1.98	1.95	1.90	1.85	1.78	1.74	1.69	1.63	1.60	1.55	1.52	1.48	1.46	1.44
	7.17	**5.06**	**4.20**	**3.72**	**3.41**	**3.18**	**3.02**	**2.88**	**2.78**	**2.70**	**2.62**	**2.56**	**2.46**	**2.39**	**2.26**	**2.18**	**2.10**	**2.00**	**1.94**	**1.86**	**1.82**	**1.76**	**1.71**	**1.68**
55	4.02	3.17	2.78	2.54	2.38	2.27	2.18	2.11	2.05	2.00	1.97	1.93	1.88	1.83	1.76	1.72	1.67	1.61	1.58	1.52	1.50	1.46	1.43	1.41
	7.12	**5.01**	**4.16**	**3.68**	**3.37**	**3.15**	**2.98**	**2.85**	**2.75**	**2.66**	**2.59**	**2.53**	**2.43**	**2.35**	**2.23**	**2.15**	**2.06**	**1.96**	**1.90**	**1.82**	**1.78**	**1.71**	**1.66**	**1.64**
60	4.00	3.15	2.76	2.52	2.37	2.25	2.17	2.10	2.04	1.99	1.95	1.92	1.86	1.81	1.75	1.70	1.65	1.59	1.56	1.50	1.48	1.44	1.41	1.39
	7.08	**4.98**	**4.13**	**3.65**	**3.34**	**3.12**	**2.95**	**2.82**	**2.72**	**2.63**	**2.56**	**2.50**	**2.40**	**2.32**	**2.20**	**2.12**	**2.03**	**1.93**	**1.87**	**1.79**	**1.74**	**1.68**	**1.63**	**1.60**
65	3.99	3.14	2.75	2.51	2.36	2.24	2.15	2.08	2.02	1.98	1.94	1.90	1.85	1.80	1.73	1.68	1.63	1.57	1.54	1.49	1.46	1.42	1.39	1.37
	7.04	**4.95**	**4.10**	**3.62**	**3.31**	**3.09**	**2.93**	**2.79**	**2.70**	**2.61**	**2.54**	**2.47**	**2.37**	**2.30**	**2.18**	**2.09**	**2.00**	**1.90**	**1.84**	**1.76**	**1.71**	**1.64**	**1.60**	**1.56**
70	3.98	3.13	2.74	2.50	2.35	2.23	2.14	2.07	2.01	1.97	1.93	1.89	1.84	1.79	1.72	1.67	1.62	1.56	1.53	1.47	1.45	1.40	1.37	1.35
	7.01	**4.92**	**4.08**	**3.60**	**3.29**	**3.07**	**2.91**	**2.77**	**2.67**	**2.59**	**2.51**	**2.45**	**2.35**	**2.28**	**2.15**	**2.07**	**1.98**	**1.88**	**1.82**	**1.74**	**1.69**	**1.62**	**1.56**	**1.53**
80	3.96	3.11	2.72	2.48	2.33	2.21	2.12	2.05	1.99	1.95	1.91	1.88	1.82	1.77	1.70	1.65	1.60	1.54	1.51	1.45	1.42	1.38	1.35	1.32
	6.96	**4.88**	**4.04**	**3.56**	**3.25**	**3.04**	**2.87**	**2.74**	**2.64**	**2.55**	**2.48**	**2.41**	**2.32**	**2.24**	**2.11**	**2.03**	**1.94**	**1.84**	**1.78**	**1.70**	**1.65**	**1.57**	**1.52**	**1.49**
100	3.94	3.09	2.70	2.46	2.30	2.19	2.10	2.03	1.97	1.92	1.88	1.85	1.79	1.75	1.68	1.63	1.57	1.51	1.48	1.42	1.39	1.34	1.30	1.28
	6.90	**4.82**	**3.98**	**3.51**	**3.20**	**2.99**	**2.82**	**2.69**	**2.59**	**2.51**	**2.43**	**2.36**	**2.26**	**2.19**	**2.06**	**1.98**	**1.89**	**1.79**	**1.73**	**1.64**	**1.59**	**1.51**	**1.46**	**1.43**
125	3.92	3.07	2.68	2.44	2.29	2.17	2.08	2.01	1.95	1.90	1.86	1.83	1.77	1.72	1.65	1.60	1.55	1.49	1.45	1.39	1.36	1.31	1.27	1.25
	6.84	**4.78**	**3.94**	**3.47**	**3.17**	**2.95**	**2.79**	**2.65**	**2.56**	**2.47**	**2.40**	**2.33**	**2.23**	**2.15**	**2.03**	**1.94**	**1.85**	**1.75**	**1.68**	**1.59**	**1.54**	**1.46**	**1.40**	**1.37**
150	3.91	3.06	2.67	2.43	2.27	2.16	2.07	2.00	1.94	1.89	1.85	1.82	1.76	1.71	1.64	1.59	1.54	1.47	1.44	1.37	1.34	1.29	1.25	1.22
	6.81	**4.75**	**3.91**	**3.44**	**3.14**	**2.92**	**2.76**	**2.62**	**2.53**	**2.44**	**2.37**	**2.30**	**2.20**	**2.12**	**2.00**	**1.91**	**1.83**	**1.72**	**1.66**	**1.56**	**1.51**	**1.43**	**1.37**	**1.33**
200	3.89	3.04	2.65	2.41	2.26	2.14	2.05	1.98	1.92	1.87	1.83	1.80	1.74	1.69	1.62	1.57	1.52	1.45	1.42	1.35	1.32	1.26	1.22	1.19
	6.76	**4.71**	**3.88**	**3.41**	**3.11**	**2.90**	**2.73**	**2.60**	**2.50**	**2.41**	**2.34**	**2.28**	**2.17**	**2.09**	**1.97**	**1.88**	**1.79**	**1.69**	**1.62**	**1.53**	**1.48**	**1.39**	**1.33**	**1.28**
400	3.86	3.02	2.62	2.39	2.23	2.12	2.03	1.96	1.90	1.85	1.81	1.78	1.72	1.67	1.60	1.54	1.49	1.42	1.38	1.32	1.28	1.22	1.16	1.13
	6.70	**4.66**	**3.83**	**3.36**	**3.06**	**2.85**	**2.69**	**2.55**	**2.46**	**2.37**	**2.29**	**2.23**	**2.12**	**2.04**	**1.92**	**1.84**	**1.74**	**1.64**	**1.57**	**1.47**	**1.42**	**1.32**	**1.24**	**1.19**
1000	3.85	3.00	2.61	2.38	2.22	2.10	2.02	1.95	1.89	1.84	1.80	1.76	1.70	1.65	1.58	1.53	1.47	1.41	1.36	1.30	1.26	1.19	1.13	1.08
	6.66	**4.62**	**3.80**	**3.34**	**3.04**	**2.82**	**2.66**	**2.53**	**2.43**	**2.34**	**2.26**	**2.20**	**2.09**	**2.01**	**1.89**	**1.81**	**1.71**	**1.61**	**1.54**	**1.44**	**1.38**	**1.28**	**1.19**	**1.11**
∞	3.84	2.99	2.60	2.37	2.21	2.09	2.01	1.94	1.88	1.83	1.79	1.75	1.69	1.64	1.57	1.52	1.46	1.40	1.35	1.28	1.24	1.17	1.11	1.00
	6.64	**4.60**	**3.78**	**3.32**	**3.02**	**2.80**	**2.64**	**2.51**	**2.41**	**2.32**	**2.24**	**2.18**	**2.07**	**1.99**	**1.87**	**1.79**	**1.69**	**1.59**	**1.52**	**1.41**	**1.36**	**1.25**	**1.15**	**1.00**

5% = roman type, 1% = boldface type

*Numerator.

+Denominator.

(From Snedecor, G. W. [1938]. *Statistical methods*. Ames, Iowa: Collegiate press. [Table 10–3, pp. 184–187].)

Critical Values of the Correlation Coefficient

df	Level of Significance for One-Tailed Test			
	.05	.025	.01	.005
	Level of Significance for two-Tailed Test			
	.10	.05	.02	.01
1	.988	.997	.9995	.9999
2	.900	.950	.980	.990
3	.805	.878	.934	.959
4	.729	.811	.882	.917
5	.669	.754	.833	.874
6	.622	.707	.789	.834
7	.582	.666	.750	.798
8	.549	.632	.716	.765
9	.521	.602	.685	.735
10	.497	.576	.658	.708
11	.476	.553	.634	.684
12	.458	.532	.612	.661
13	.441	.514	.592	.641
14	.426	.497	.574	.623
15	.412	.482	.558	.606
16	.400	.468	.542	.590
17	.389	.456	.528	.575

(*Continued*)

Appendix E (CONTINUED)

df	Level of Significance for One-Tailed Test			
	.05	.025	.01	.005
	Level of Significance for two-Tailed Test			
	.10	.05	.02	.01
18	.378	.444	.516	.561
19	.369	.433	.503	.549
20	.360	.423	.492	.537
21	.352	.413	.482	.526
22	.344	.404	.472	.515
23	.337	.396	.462	.505
24	.330	.388	.453	.496
25	.323	.381	.445	.487
26	.317	.374	.437	.479
27	.311	.367	.430	.471
28	.306	.361	.423	.463
29	.301	.355	.416	.456
30	.296	.349	.409	.449
35	.275	.325	.381	.418
40	.257	.304	.358	.393
45	.243	.288	.338	.372
50	.231	.273	.322	.354
60	.211	.250	.295	.325
70	.195	.232	.247	.303
80	.183	.217	.256	.283
90	.173	.205	.242	.267
100	.164	.195	.230	.254
125		.174		.228
150		.159		.208
200		.138		.181
300		.113		.148
400		.098		.128
500		.088		.115
1000		.062		.081

(From Fisher, R. A. [1970]. *Statistical methods for research workers* [14th ed.]. Darien, CT: Hafner Publishing Co. [Table V. A., p. 211].)

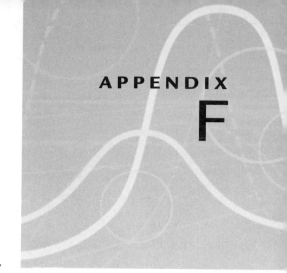

Transformation of *r* to *z*_r

r	z_r	r	z_r	r	z_r	r	z_r	r	z_r
.000	.000	.200	.203	.400	.424	.600	.693	.800	1.099
.005	.005	.205	.208	.405	.430	.605	.701	.805	1.113
.010	.010	.210	.213	.410	.436	.610	.709	.810	1.127
.015	.015	.215	.218	.415	.442	.615	.717	.815	1.142
.020	.020	.220	.224	.420	.448	.620	.725	.820	1.157
.025	.025	.225	.229	.425	.454	.626	.733	.825	1.172
.030	.030	.230	.234	.430	.460	.630	.741	.830	1.188
.035	.035	.235	.239	.435	.466	.635	.750	.835	1.204
.040	.040	.240	.245	.440	.472	.640	.758	.840	1.221
.045	.045	.245	.250	.445	.478	.645	.767	.845	1.238
.050	.050	.250	.255	.450	.485	.650	.775	.850	1.256
.055	.055	.255	.261	.455	.491	.655	.784	.855	1.274
.060	.060	.260	.266	.460	.497	.660	.793	.860	1.293
.065	.065	.265	.271	.465	.504	.665	.802	.865	1.313
.070	.070	.270	.277	.470	.510	.670	.811	.870	1.333
.075	.075	.275	.282	.475	.517	.675	.820	.875	1.354
.080	.080	.280	.288	.480	.523	.680	.829	.880	1.376
.085	.085	.285	.293	.485	.530	.685	.838	.885	1.398
.090	.090	.290	.299	.490	.536	.690	.848	.890	1.422
.095	.095	.295	.304	.495	.543	.695	.858	.895	1.447
.100	.100	.300	.310	.500	.549	.700	.867	.900	1.472
.105	.105	.305	.315	.505	.556	.705	.877	.905	1.499

(Continued)

Appendix F (CONTINUED)

r	z_r	r	z_r	r	z_r	r	z_r	r	z_r
.110	.110	.310	.321	.510	.563	.710	.887	.910	1.528
.115	.116	.315	.326	.515	.570	.715	.897	.915	1.557
.120	.121	.320	.332	.520	.576	.720	.908	.920	1.589
.125	.126	.325	.337	.525	.583	.725	.918	.925	1.623
.130	.131	.330	.343	.530	.590	.730	.929	.930	1.658
.135	.136	.335	.348	.535	.597	.735	.940	.935	1.697
.140	.141	.340	.354	.540	.604	.740	.950	.940	1.738
.145	.146	.345	.360	.545	.611	.745	.962	.945	1.783
.150	.151	.350	.365	.550	.618	.750	.973	.950	1.832
.155	.156	.355	.371	.555	.626	.755	.984	.955	1.886
.160	.161	.360	.377	.560	.633	.760	.996	.960	1.946
.165	.167	.365	.383	.565	.640	.765	1.008	.965	2.014
.170	.172	.370	.388	.570	.648	.770	1.020	.970	2.092
.175	.177	.375	.394	.575	.655	.775	1.033	.975	2.185
.180	.182	.380	.400	.580	.662	.780	1.045	.980	2.298
.185	.187	.385	.406	.585	.670	.785	1.058	.985	2.443
.190	.192	.390	.412	.590	.678	.790	1.071	.990	2.647
.195	.198	.395	.418	.595	.685	.795	1.085	.995	2.994

(From Hinkle, D. E., Wiersma, W., & Jurs, S. G. [1998]. Applied statistics for the behavioral sciences [4th ed.]. [Appendix C.6, p. 645]. Boston: Houghton Mifflin. Used by permission.)

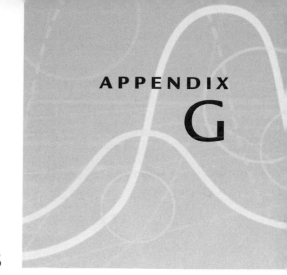

Survey for Exercises

BOSTON COLLEGE SCHOOL OF NURSING
A SURVEY FOR NU744

This questionnaire is designed to gather data for use in a course on statistics. The data will be used *only* to help students learn how to use the computer to manage and analyze data. Thank you for your help.

Code Number ☐

1. Gender	Male	0
	Female	1
2. Age in years		☐
3. Marital status	Never married	1
	Married	2
	Living with significant other	3
	Separated	4
	Widowed	5
	Divorced	6
4. Education (in years)		☐
5. Smoking history	Never smoked	0
	Quit smoking	1
	Still smoking	2
6. Current work status	Unemployed	0
	Part-Time	1
	Full-Time	2
7. Political affiliation	Republican	1
	Democrat	2
	Independent	3

8. Depressed state of mind

Rarely	1
Sometimes	2
Often	3
Routinely	4

9. Exercise

Rarely	1
Sometimes	2
Often	3
Routinely	4

10. Eat 3 regular meals a day

Rarely	1
Sometimes	2
Often	3
Routinely	4

11. How satisfied are you with your current weight? (circle one)

Very
Dissatisfied

1	2	3	4	5	6	7	8	9	10

Very
Satisfied

12. How satisfied were you with your weight when you were 18?

Very
Dissatisfied

1	2	3	4	5	6	7	8	9	10

Very
Satisfied

13. Please rate your overall state of health on the following scale (circle one number)

Very
Ill

1	2	3	4	5	6	7	8	9	10

Very
Healthy

14. How happy, satisfied, or pleased have you been with your quality of life during the past month? (Circle the number for the one answer that comes closest to the way you are feeling.)

extremely happy, could not be more satisfied or pleased	6
very happy most of the time	5
generally satisfied, pleased	4
sometimes fairly satisfied, sometimes fairly unhappy	3
generally dissatisfied, unhappy	2
very dissatisfied, unhappy most of the time	1

15. How happy, satisfied, or pleased were you with your quality of life when you were 18? (Circle the number for the one answer that comes closest to the way you were feeling.)

extremely happy, could not be more satisfied or pleased	6
very happy most of the time	5
generally satisfied, pleased	4
sometimes fairly satisfied, sometimes fairly unhappy	3
generally dissatisfied, unhappy	2
very dissatisfied, unhappy most of the time	1

16. If you were given a tax-free gift of $500,000, and you had only five days to choose one specific way to use it, which of the following would you pick:

    1. invest it with a brokerage firm.

    2. buy a vacation home at a place of my choice.

    3. pay off my existing mortgage; or, if I don't own a primary residence, buy one of my choice outright.

    4. donate the whole amount to a charity of my choice.

17. You are planning your winter vacation. Of the following, which place would you choose to visit?

    1. a beachfront condo in Hawaii

    2. a chalet in the Swiss Alps

    3. a luxury hotel at Disney World in Florida

    4. an ocean cruise through the Caribbean Islands

INVENTORY OF PERSONAL ATTITUDES

The following pages contain a series of *statements and their opposites*. Notice that the statements extend from one extreme to the other. Where would you place yourself on this scale? Place a circle on the number that is *most true for you at this time*. Do not put your circles between numbers.

1. During most of the day my energy level is

   very high .... very low

1	2	3	4	5	6	7

2. When there is a great deal of pressure being placed on me

   I remain calm .... I get tense

1	2	3	4	5	6	7

3. As a whole, my life seems

   dull .... vibrant

1	2	3	4	5	6	7

4. May daily activities are

   a source of satisfaction .... not a source of satisfaction

1	2	3	4	5	6	7

5. I experience anxiety

   all the time .... never

1	2	3	4	5	6	7

6. I have come to expect that every day will be

   new and different .... exactly the same

1	2	3	4	5	6	7

7. I am fearful

   all the time .... never

1	2	3	4	5	6	7

8. When I think deeply about life

I feel there is a purpose to it					I do not feel there is any purpose to it	
1	2	3	4	5	6	7

9. I feel that my life so far has

not been productive					been productive	
1	2	3	4	5	6	7

10. When I have made a mistake

I feel extreme dislike for myself					I continue to like myself	
1	2	3	4	5	6	7

11. I feel that the work* I am doing

is of no value					is of great value	
1	2	3	4	5	6	7

12. I wish I were different than who I am.

agree strongly					disagree strongly	
1	2	3	4	5	6	7

13. At this time, I have

clearly defined goals for my life					no clearly defined goals for my life	
1	2	3	4	5	6	7

14. I find myself worrying that something bad is going to happen to me or those I love

all the time						never
1	2	3	4	5	6	7

15. In a stressful situation,

I can concentrate easily					I cannot concentrate easily	
1	2	3	4	5	6	7

16. When I need to stand up for myself

I cannot do it					I can do it quite easily	
1	2	3	4	5	6	7

17. I feel less than adequate in most situations.

agree strongly					disagree strongly	
1	2	3	4	5	6	7

18. I react to problems and difficulties

with a great deal of frustration					with no frustration	
1	2	3	4	5	6	7

19. When sad things happen to me or other people

I cannot feel positive about life					I continue to feel positive about life	
1	2	3	4	5	6	7

20. When I think about what I have done with my life, I feel

worthwhile						worthless
1	2	3	4	5	6	7

21. My present life

does not satisfy me						satisfies me
1	2	3	4	5	6	7

22. In really difficult situations

I feel able to respond in positive ways						I feel unable to respond in positive ways
1	2	3	4	5	6	7

23. I feel joy in my heart

never						all the time
1	2	3	4	5	6	7

24. When I need to relax

I experience a peacefulness free of thoughts and worries						I experience no peace, only thoughts and worries
1	2	3	4	5	6	7

25. I feel trapped by the circumstances of my life.

agree strongly						disagree strongly
1	2	3	4	5	6	7

26. When I am in a frightening situation

I panic						I remain calm
1	2	3	4	5	6	7

27. When I think about my past

I feel no regrets						I feel many regrets
1	2	3	4	5	6	7

28. Deep inside myself

I do not feel loved						I feel loved
1	2	3	4	5	6	7

29. I worry about the future

never						all the time
1	2	3	4	5	6	7

30. When I think about the problems that I have

I do not feel hopeful about solving them						I feel very hopeful about solving them
1	2	3	4	5	6	7

* *The definition of work is not limited to income-producing jobs. It includes childcare, housework, studies, and volunteer services.*

Bibliography

Agresti, A., & Finlay, B. (1997). *Statistical methods for the social sciences.* Upper Saddle River, NJ: Prentice-Hall.

Allison, P. (2001). *Missing data.* Thousand Oaks, CA: Sage.

American Psychological Association (APA). (2001). *Publication manual of the American Psychological Association* (5th ed.). Washington, DC: American Psychological Association.

Anderson, M. A., & Helms, L. B. (1998). Extended care referral after hospital discharge. *Research in Nursing & Health, 21*(5), 385–394.

Anderson, R. A., Hsieh, P-C, & Su, H-F. (1998). Resource allocation and resident outcomes in nursing homes: Comparisons between the best and the worst. *Research in Nursing & Health, 21*(4), 297–313.

Appel, S. J., Harrell, J. S., & Deng, S. (2002). Racial and socioeconomic differences in risk factors for cardiovascular disease among southern rural women. *Nursing Research, 51*(3), 140–147.

Aroian, K. J., Norris, A. E., Tran, T. V., & Schappler-Morris, N. (1998). Development and psychometric evaluation of the Demands of Immigration Scale. *Journal of Nursing Measurement, 6*(2), 175–194.

Aroian, K. J., Schappler-Morris, N., Neary, S., Spitzer, A., & Tran, T. V. (1997). Psychometric evaluation of a Russian language version of the Resilience Scale. *Journal of Nursing Measurement, 5*(2), 151–164.

Asher, A. B. (1983). *Causal modeling* (2nd ed.). Sage University Papers: Quantitative Applications in the Social Sciences Series, 3. Newbury Park, CA: Sage.

Bachand, D. A., & Beard, M. T. (1995). Structural equation modeling. In M. T. Beard (Ed.), *Theory construction and testing* (pp. 220–230). Lisle, IL: Tucker Publishing, Inc.

Bennet, J. A., Stewart, A. L., Kayser-Jones, J., & Glaser, D. (2002). The mediating effect of pain and fatigue on level of functioning in older adults. *Nursing Research, 51*(4), 254–265.

Bentler, P. M. (1992). *EQS structural equations program manual.* Los Angeles: BMDP Statistical Software.

Bentler, P. M., & Bonnett, D. G. (1980). Significance tests and goodness of fit in the analysis of covariance structures. *Psychological Bulletin, 88*(3), 588–606.

Bollen, K. A. (1989). *Structural equations with latent variables.* New York: John Wiley & Sons.

Bollen, K. A., & Long, J. S. (1993). Introduction. In K. A. Bollen & J. S. Long (Eds.), *Testing structural equation models* (pp. 1–9). Thousand Oaks, CA: Sage.

Borenstein, M., Rothstein, H., & Cohen, J. (1997). Power and precision [Software Program]. Teaneck, NJ: Biostat. found at http://wwwpowerandprecision.com.

Bournaki, M-C. (1997). Correlates of pain-related responses to venipunctures in school-age children. *Nursing Research, 46*(3), 147–154.

Brooten, D. (1988) *Early hospital discharge and nurse specialist followup.* Program grant, funded by the National Center for Nursing Research, PO1-NR1859.

Brooten, D. (1991). *Nurse home care for high-risk pregnant women. Outcomes and cost.* Grant funded by National Institute for Nursing Research, NR-02867.

Brooten, D., Naylor, M., York, R., Brown, L., Roncoli, M., Hollingsworth, A., Cohen, S., Arnold, L., Finkler, S., Munro, B., & Jacobsen, B. (1995). Effects of nurse specialist transitional care on patient outcomes and cost: Results of five randomized trials. *American Journal of Managed Care, 1*(1), 45–51.

Browne, M. W., MacCullum, R. C., Kim, C.-T., Andersen, B. L., & Glaser, R. (2002). When fit indices and residuals are incompatible. *Psychological Methods, 7*(4), 403–421.

Burns, N., & Grove, S. K. (2001). *The practice of nursing research: Conduct, critique and utilization* (4th ed.). Philadelphia: W. B. Saunders.

Byrne, B. B. (1994). *Structural equation modeling with EQS and EQS/Windows: Basic concepts, applications, and programming.* Thousand Oaks, CA: Sage.

Capasso, V. A. (2000). *Arterial and diabetic wound healing: The cost and efficacy of two wound treatments.* Unpublished doctoral diss., Boston College.

Carmines, E. G., & McIver, J. P. (1983). An introduction of the analysis of models with unobserved variables. *Political Methodology, 9*(1), 51–102.

Champion, J. D., Piper, J., Shain, R. N., Perdue, S. T., & Newton, E. R. (2001). Minority women with sexually transmitted diseases: Sexual abuse and risk for pelvic inflammatory disease. *Research in Nursing & Health, 24*(1), 38–43.

Chatfield, C. (1988). *Problem solving: A statistician's guide.* London: Chapman and Hall.

Chou, C-P., & Bentler, P. M. (1995). Estimates and tests in structural equation modeling. In R. H. Hoyle (Ed.), *Structural equation modeling: Concepts, issues, and applications* (pp. 37–55). Thousand Oaks, CA: Sage.

Cleveland, W. S. (1985). *The elements of graphing data.* Belmont, CA: Wadsworth.

Cohen, J. (1983). The cost of dichotomization. *Applied Psychologial Measurement, 7,* 249–253.

Cohen, J. (1987). *Statistical power analysis for the behavioral sciences* (Rev. ed.). Hillsdale, NJ: Lawrence Erlbaum Associates.

Cohen, J. (1988). *Statistical power analysis for the behavioral sciences* (2nd ed.). Hillsdale, NJ: Lawrence Erlbaum Associates.

Cohen, J. (1990). Things I have learned (so far). *American Psychologist, 45,* 1304–1312.

Cohen, J. & Cohen, P. (1983) *Applied multiple regression/correlation analysis for the behavioral sciences* (2nd ed.). Hillsdale, N.J.: Lawrence Erlbaum Associates.

Curley, M., Razmus, I., Roberts, K., & Wypij, D. (2003). Predicting pressure ulcer risk in pediatric patients: The Braden Q scale. *Nursing Research, 52*(1): 22–31.

Curran, P. J., Bollen, K. A., Paxton, P., Kirby, J., & Chen, F. (2002). Chi-square distribution in mispecified structural equation models: Results from a Monte Carlo Simulation. *Multivariate Behavioral Research, 37*(1), 1–36.

Daniel, W. W. (1987). *Biostatistics: A foundation for analysis in the health sciences* (4th ed.). New York: John Wiley & Sons.

Davidson, F. (1996). *Principles of statistical data handling.* Thousand Oaks, CA: Sage.

Derdiarian, A. K., & Lewis, S. (1986). The D-L test of agreement: A stronger measure of interrater reliability. *Nursing Research, 35,* 375–378.

DeVellis, B. (2003). *Scale development* (2nd ed). Newbury Park, CA: Sage.

Ehrenberg, A. S. C. (1977). Rudiments of numeracy. *Journal of the Royal Statistical Society A, 140* (part 3), 277–297.

Elwood, M. (1998). Critical appraisal of epidemiological studies and clinical trials (2nd ed.). Oxford. Oxford University Press.

Essex-Sorlie, D. (1995). *Medical statistics & epidemiology first edition.* Norwalk, CT: Appleton & Lange.

Fan, X., & Wang, L. (1998). Effects of potential confounding factors on fit indices and parameter estimates for true and misspecified models. *Educational and Psychological Measurement, 58*(5), 701–735.

Ferguson, D. A., & Horwood L. J. (1984). Life events and depression in women: A structural equation model. *Psychological Medicine, 14*(4), 881–889.

Ferketich, S., & Muller, M. (1990). Factor analysis revisited. *Nursing Research, 39,* 59–62.

Fishbein, M., & Ajzen, I. (1975). *Belief, attitude, intention, and behavior: An introduction to theory and research.* Reading, MA: Addison-Wesley.

Fisher, L. D., & van Belle, G. (1993). *Biostatistics: A methodology for the health sciences.* New York: John Wiley & Sons.

Fisher, R. A. (1970). *Statistical methods for research workers* (14th ed.). Darien, CT: Hafner Publishing Co.

Fleury, J. (1998). The index of self-regulation: Development and psychometric analysis. *Journal of Nursing Measurement, 6*(1), 3–17.

Fox, J. (1984). *Linear statistical models and related methods with applications to social research.* New York: John Wiley & Sons.

Fox, J. (1997). *Applied regression analysis, linear models, and related methods.* Thousand Oaks, CA: Sage.

Freedman, D., Pisani, R., Purves, R., & Adhikari, A. (1991). *Statistics* (2nd ed.). New York: W. W. Norton.

Freund, J. E. (1988). *Modern elementary statistics* (7th ed.). Englewood Cliffs, NJ: Prentice Hall.

Fry, S., & Duffy, M. (2000). *Ethics and human rights in nursing practice: A study of New England Registered nurses.* Chestnut Hill, MA: Nursing Ethics Network & The Center for Nursing Research, Boston College.

Funk, M., Ostfeld, A. M., Chang, V. M., & Lee, F. A. (2002). Racial differences in the use of cardiac procedures in patients with acute myocardial infarction. *Nursing Research, 51*(3), 148–157.

Gardner, P. L. (1975). Scales and statistics. *Review of Educational Research, 45,* 43–57.

Glass, G. V., & Hopkins, K. D. (1996). *Statistical methods in education and psychology* (3rd ed.). Boston: Allyn and Bacon.

Gonzalez, R., & Griffen, D. (2001). Testing parameters in structural equation modeling: Every "one" matters. *Psychological Methods, 6* (3), 258–269.

Gould, S. J. (1985). The median isn't the message. *Discover, 6,* 40–42.

Grimes-Holsinger, V. (2002). Comparing the effect of a skills checklist on teaching time required to achieve independence in administration of infusion medication. *Journal of Infusion Nursing, 25*(2), 109–120.

Hackett, T. P., & Cassem, N. H. (1969). Factors contributing to delay in responding to the signs and symptoms of acute myocardial infarction. *American Journal of Cardiology, 24,* 651–658.

Hahn, G. J., & Meeker, W. Q. (1991). *Statistical intervals—A guide for practitioners.* New York: John Wiley & Sons.

Hair, J. F., Anderson, R. E., Tatham, R. L., & Black, W. C. (1998). *Multivariate data analysis* (5th ed.). Upper Saddle River, NJ: Prentice-Hall.

Hald, A. (1952). *Statistical tables and formulas.* New York: John Wiley & Sons.

Hancock, G. R., & Freeman, M. J. (2001). Power and sample size for the root mean error of approximation test of not close fit in structural equation modeling. *Educational and Psychological Measurement, 61*(5), 741–758.

Harvey, R., Roth, E., Yarnold, P. Durham, J., & Green, D. (1992). Deep vein thrombosis in stroke: The use of plasma d-dimer level as a screening test in the rehabilitation setting. *Stroke, 27*(9): 1516–1520.

Hawkins, J. W., Pearce, C. W., Kearney, M. H., Munro, B. H., Haggerty, L. A., Dwyer, J., Higgins, L. P., Aber, C. S., & Mahony, D. (1996). *Abuse, women's self-care, and pregnancy out comes.* Funded by the National Institute for Nursing Research, National Institutes of Health AREA grant 1 R15 NRO4246-01.

Hayduk, L. A. (1996). *LISREL issues, debates, and strategies.* Baltimore: Johns Hopkins University Press.

Heise, D. R. (1969). Problems in path analysis and causal inference. In E. F. Borgatta & G. W. Bohrnstedt (Eds.), *Sociology methodology 1969.* San Francisco: Jossey-Bass.

Henkel, R. E. (1986). *Tests of significance.* Beverly Hills, CA: Sage.

Henton, F. E., Hays, B. J., Walker, S. N., & Atwood, J. R. (2002). Determinants of Medicare home healthcare service use among Medicare recipients. *Nursing Research, 51*(6), 355–362.

Hertzog, C. (1989). Using confirmatory factor analysis for scale development and validation. In M. P. Lawton & A. R. Hertzog (Eds.),. *Social research methods for gerontology* (pp. 281–306). New York: Bagwool Publishing.

Hildebrand, D. K. (1986). *Statistical thinking for behavioral scientists.* Boston: Duxbury Press.

Hinkle, D. E., Wiersma, W., & Jurs, S. G. (1998). *Applied statistics for the behavioral sciences* (4th ed.). Boston, MA: Houghton-Mifflin.

Hojat, M., Nasca, T. J., Cohen, M. J. M., Fields, S. K., Rattner, S. L., Griffiths, M., Ibarra, D., de Gonzalez, A. A., Torres-Ruiz, A., Ibarra, G., & Garcia, A. (2001). Attitudes toward physician-nurse collaboration: A cross-cultural study of male and female physicians and nurses in the United States and Mexico. *Nursing Research, 50*(2),123–128.

Horowitz, J. (1998). *Promoting healthy responsiveness between depressed mothers and their infants.* Funded by March of Dimes Birth Defects Foundation, 12-FY98-0014.

Hosmer, D. W., & Lemeshow, S. (1989). *Applied logistic regression.* New York: John Wiley & Sons.

Hoyle, R. H. (1995). *Structural equation modeling: Concepts, issues, and applications.* Thousand Oaks, CA: Sage.

Hoyle, R. H., & Panter, A. T. (1995). Writing about structural equation models. In R. H. Hoyle (Ed.), *Structural equation modeling: Concepts, issues, and applications* (pp. 158–176). Thousand Oaks, CA: Sage.

Hu, L-T., & Bentler, P. M. (1995). Evaluating model fit. In R. H. Hoyle (Ed.), *Structural equation modeling: Concepts, issues, and applications* (pp. 76–99). Thousand Oaks, CA: Sage.

Ingelfinger, J. A., Mosteller, F., Thibodeau, L. A., & Ware, J. H. (1994). *Biostatistics in clinical medicine* (3rd ed.). New York: McGraw-Hill.

Jacobsen, B. S. (1981). Know thy data. *Nursing Research, 30,* 254–255.

Jacobsen, B. S., & Lowery, B. J. (1992). Further analysis of the psychometric properties of the Levine Denial of Illness Scale. *Psychosomatic Medicine, 54,* 372–381.

Jacobsen, B. S., & Meininger, J. C. (1985). The designs and methods of published nursing research: 1956–1983. *Nursing Research, 34,* 306–312.

Janz, N., & Becker, M. (1984). The Health Belief Model: A decade later. *Health Education Quarterly, 11*(1), 1–47.

Jöreskog, K. G., & Sörbom, D. (1988). *LISREL 7: A guide to the program and applications.* Chicago: SPSS, Inc.

Kaplan, D. (1995). Statistical power in structural equation modeling. In R. H. Hoyle (Ed.), *Structural equation modeling: Concepts, issues, and applications.* Thousand Oaks, CA: Sage.

Kaplan, D., & Wenger, R. N. (1993). Asymptomatic independence and separability in covariance structure models. *Multivariate Behavioral Research, 28*(4), 483–498.

Kass, J. D., Friedman, R., Leserman, J., Caudill, M., Zuttermeister, P. C., & Benson, H. (1991). An inventory of positive psychological attitudes with potential relevance to health outcomes: Validation and preliminary testing. *Behavioral Medicine, Fall,* 121–129.

Kenny, D. (1979). *Correlation and causality.* New York: John Wiley & Sons.

Klockars, A. J., & Sax, G. (1991). *Multiple comparisons.* Series: Quantitative Applications in the Social Sciences, #61, Newbury Park, CA: Sage.

Knapp, T. R. (1990). Treating ordinal scales as interval scales: An attempt to resolve the controversy. *Nursing Research, 39,* 121–123.

Knapp, T. R. (1993). Treating ordinal scales as ordinal scales. *Nursing Research, 42,* 184–186.

Knapp, T. R. (1998). *Quantitative nursing research*. Thousand Oaks, CA: Sage.

Knapp, T. R., & Brown, J. K. (1995). Ten measurement commandments that often should be broken. *Research in Nursing & Health, 18,* 465–469.

Kneipp, S., & McIntosh, M. (2001). Handling missing data in nursing research with multiple imputation. *Nursing Research, 50*(6),384–389.

Koopmans, L. H. (1987). *Introduction to contemporary statistics* (2nd ed.). Boston: Duxbury Press.

Kotz, S., & Stroup, D. F. (1983). *Educated guessing: How to cope in an uncertain world*. New York: Marcel Dekker.

Kraemer, H. (1992). *Evaluating medical tests: Objective and quantitative guidelines*. Newbury Park, CA: Sage.

Kraemer, H., & Thiemann, S. (1987). *How many subjects?* Newbury Park, CA: Sage.

Kurlowicz, L. (1998). Perceived self-efficacy, functional ability, and depressive symptoms in older elective surgery patients. *Nursing Research, 47*(4), 219–226.

Lake, E. T. (2002). Development of the Practice environment Scale of the Nursing Work Index. *Research in Nursing and Health, 25,* 176–188.

LaMontagne, L. L., Hepworth, J. T., Cohen, F., & Salisbury, M. H. (2003). Cognitive-behavioral intervention effects on adolescents' anxiety and pain following spinal fusion surgery. *Nursing Research, 52*(3), 183–190.

Leamer, E. E. (1978). *Specification searches*. New York: John Wiley & Sons.

Lenoci, J. M., Telfair, J., Cecil, H., & Edwards, R. R. (2002). Self-care in adults with sickle cell disease. *Western Journal of Nursing Research, 24,* 228–245.

Little, R. J. A., & Rubin, D. B. (1987). *Statistical analysis with missing data*. New York: John Wiley & Sons.

Little, R. J. A., & Rubin, D. B. (1989). The analysis of social science data with missing values. *Sociological Methods & Research, 18,* 292-326.

Little, R. J. A., & Rubin, D. B. (2002). *Statistical analysis with missing data (2nd ed.)*. New York: John Wiley & Sons.

Long, J. S. (1988). *Confirmatory factor analysis. A preface to LISREL*. Beverly Hills, CA: Sage.

Lybrand, M., Medoff-Cooper, B., & Munro, B. H. (1990). Periodic comparisons of specific gravity using urine from a diaper and collecting bag. *American Journal of Maternal/Child Nursing, 15*(4), 238–239.

MacCallum, R. C., Browne, M. W., & Suawara, H. M. (1996). Power analysis and determination of sample size for covariance structure modeling. *Psychological Methods, 1*(2), 130–149.

Mallik, M., & Rafferty, A. (2000). Diffusion of the concept of patient advocacy. *Journal of Nursing Scholarship, 32*(4), p. 402.

Manias, E. (1998). Australian nurses' experiences and attitudes in the "Do Not Resuscitate" decision. *Research in Nursing & Health, 21*(5), 429–441.

Marsh, H. W., Balla, J. R., & Hau, K.-T. (1996). An evaluation of incremental fit indices: A clarification of mathematical and empirical properties. In G. A. Marcoulides & R. E. Schumacker (Eds.), *Advanced structural equation modeling: Issues and techniques* (pp. 315–353). Mahwah, NJ: Lawrence Erlbaum Associate.

Maxwell, S. E., & Delaney, H. D. (1990). *Designing experiments and analyzing data: A model comparison perspective*. Pacific Grove, CA: Brooks/Cole Publishing Company.

McCullagh, M., Lusk, Sally L., & Ronis, D. L. (2002). Factors influencing use of hearing protection among farmers. *Nursing Research, 51*(1), 33–39.

McGovern, P. G., Pankow, J. S., Shahar, E., Doliszny, K. M., Folsom, A. R., Blackburn, H., & Luepker, R. V. (1996). Recent trends in acute coronary heart disease. *New England Journal of Medicine, 34*(14), 887.

McLaughlin, F. E., & Marascuilo, L. A. (1990). *Advanced nursing and health care research: Quantification approaches*. Philadelphia: W. B. Saunders.

Mertler, C., & Vannatta, R. (2002). *Advanced and multivariate statistical methods practice application and interpretation (2nd ed.)*. Los Angeles, CA: Pyrczak Publishing.

Miller, A. M., & Chandler, P. J. (2002). Acculturation, resilience, and depression in midlife women from the former Soviet Union. *Nursing Research, 51*(1), 26-32.

Moore, D. S. (1991). *Statistics: Concepts and controversies* (3rd ed.). New York: W. H. Freeman.

Morgan, S., Reichert, T., & Harrison, T. (2002). *From numbers to words: Reporting statistical results for the social sciences*. Boston: Allyn and Bacon.

Mueller, R. O. (1996). Confirmatory factor analysis. In *Basic principles of structural equation modeling: An introduction to LISREL and EQS* (pp. 62–128). New York: Springer-Verlag.

Murphy, K., & Myers, B. (1998). *Statistical power analysis: A simple and general model for traditional and modern hypothesis tests*. Mahwah, NJ: Lawrence Erlbaum Associates.

Musil, C., Warner, C., Yobas, P., & Jones, S. (2002). A comparison of imputation techniques for handling missing data. *Western Journal of Nursing Research, 24*(7), 815–829.

Muthén, B. O. (1993). Goodness of fit with categorical and other non-normal variables. In K. A. Bollen & J. S. Long (Eds.), *Testing structural equation models* (pp. 205–234). Thousand Oaks, CA: Sage.

NCSS. (2002). PASS. Kaysville, Utah: NCSS Statistical Software. Retrieved March 15, 2003, from http://www.ncss.com.

Newton, R., & Rudestam, K. (1999). *Your statistical consultant: Answers to your data analysis questions*. Thousand Oaks, CA: Sage.

Norris, A. E., & Devine, P. G. (1992). Linking pregnancy concerns to pregnancy risk avoidant action: The role of construct accessibility. *Personality and Social Psychology Bulletin, 18*(2), 118–192.

Norris, A. E., & Ford, K. (1995). Condom use by low-income African-American and Hispanic youth with a well-known partner: Integrating the Health Belief Model, Theory of Reasoned Action, and Construct Accessibility Model. *Journal of Applied Social Psychology, 25*(20), 1801–1830.

Norusis, M. J. (1993). *SPSS professional statistics 6.1*. Chicago, IL: SPSS.

Norusis, M. J. (2002). *SPSS 11.0 guide to data analysis*. Upper Saddle River, NJ: Prentice-Hall.

Nunnally, J. C., & Bernstein, I. H. (1994). *Psychometric theory* (3rd ed.). New York: McGraw-Hill.

Ott, L., & Mendenhall, W. (1990). *Understanding statistics* (5th ed.). Boston: PWD-Kent Publishing.

Owens, S. V., & Froman, R. D. (1998). Uses and abuse of the analysis of covariance. *Research in Nursing & Health, 21*(6), 557–562.

Parshall, M. B. (2002). Psychometric characteristics of dyspnea descriptor ratings in Emergency Department patients with exacerbated Chronic Obstructive Pulmonary Disease. *Research in Nursing and Health, 25,* 331–344.

Patrician, P. (2002). Multiple imputation for missing data. *Research in Nursing & Health, 25,* 76–84.

Pedhazur, E. J. (1997). *Multiple regression in behavioral research, explanation and prediction* (3rd ed.). Orlando, FL: Harcourt Brace.

Pedhazur, E. J., & Schmelkin, L. P. (1991). *Measurement, design, and analysis: An integrated approach*. Hillsdale, NJ: Lawrence Erlbaum Associate.

Pender, N. J. (1987). *Health promotion in nursing practice* (2nd ed). Norwalk, CT: Appleton & Lange.

Piantadosi, S. (1997). *Clinical trials: A methodologic perspective*. New York: John Wiley & Sons.

Powell, R. W., McSweeney, M. B., & Wilson, C. E. (1983). X-ray calcifications as the only basis for breast biopsy. *Annals of Surgery, 197,* 555–559.

Random.org. (1998). Retrieved March 11, 2003 from: http://www.random.org.

Remington, R. (2002). Calming music and hand massage with agitated elderly. *Nursing Research, 51(5),* 317–323.

Research Randomizer, v.3.0. (2003). Retrieved March 11, 2003 from: http://www.randomizer.org.

Riegelman, R. K. (1981). *Studying a study and testing a test: How to read the medical literature.* Boston: Little, Brown, & Co.

Rigdon, E. E. (1994). Demonstrating the effects of unmodeled random measurement error. *Structural Equation Modeling, 1(4),* 375–380.

Robinson, J. H. (1995). Grief responses, coping processes, and social support of widows: Research with Roy's model. *Nursing Science Quarterly, 8(4),* 158–164.

Rubin, D. (1987). *Multiple imputation for nonresponse in surveys.* New York: Wiley.

Rudestam, K., & Newton, R. (1992). *Surviving your dissertation: A comprehensive guide to content and process.* Newbury Park, CA: Sage.

Saris, W. E., & Satorra, A. (1993). Power evaluations in structural equation models. In K. A. Bollen & J. S. Long (Eds.), *Testing structural equation models* (pp. 181–204). Thousand Oaks, CA: Sage.

Schaie, K. W., & Hertzog, C. (1985). Measurement in the psychology of adulthood and aging. In J. E. Birren & K. W. Schaie (Eds.), *Handbook of the psychology of aging* (2nd ed., pp. 61–92). New York: Van Nostrand Reinhold.

Schmid, C. F. (1983). *Statistical graphics: Design principles and practices.* New York: John Wiley & Sons.

Schroeder, M. A. (1990). Diagnosing and dealing with multicollinearity. *Western Journal of Nursing Research, 12(2),* 175–187.

Skinner, B. F. (1972). *Cumulative record: A selection of papers* (3rd ed.). New York: Appleton-Century-Crofts, Meredith Corporation.

Smith-Campbell, B. (2000). Access to health care: Effects of public funding on the uninsured. *Journal of Nursing Scholarship, 32(3),* 298.

Smithson, M. (2003). *Confidence intervals.* Thousand Oaks, CA: Sage.

Snedecor, G. W. (1938). *Statistical methods.* Ames, Iowa: Collegiate Press.

Spielberger, C. D. (1983). *Manual for the State-Trait Anxiety Inventory.* Palo Alto, CA: Consulting Psychologists Press.

SPSS, Inc. (1999a). *SPSS Advanced models 10.0.* Chicago, IL: SPSS Inc.

SPSS, Inc. (1999b). *SPSS Base 10.0 applications guide.* Chicago, IL: SPSS Inc.

SPSS, Inc. (1999c). *SPSS Base 10.0 user's guide.* Chicago, IL: SPSS Inc.

SPSS, Inc. (1999d). *SPSS regression models 10.0.* Chicago, IL: SPSS Inc.

SPSS Inc. (2002). SamplePower, 2.0. Chicago: SPSS Inc. Retrieved March 15, 2003, from: http://www.spss.com.

Stevens, S. S. (1946). On the theory of scales of measurement. *Science, 102,* 677–680.

Stevens, S. S. (1968). Measurement, statistics, and the schemapiric view. *Science, 161,* 849–856.

Strommel, M., Wang, S., Given, C. W., & Given, B. (1992). Confirmatory factor analysis (CFA) as a method to assess measurement equivalence. *Research in Nursing & Health, 15(5),* 399–405.

Sulzbach, L. M., Munro, B. H., & Hirshfeld, Jr., J. W. (1995). A randomized clinical trial of the effect of bed position after PTCA. *American Journal of Critical Care, 4(3),* 221–226.

Swinney, J. E. (2002). African Americans with cancer: The relationships among self-esteem, locus of control, and health perception. *Research in Nursing & Health, 25(5),* 371–382.

Tabachnick, B. G., & Fidell, L. S. (2001). *Using multivariate statistics* (4th ed.). New York: HarperCollins College Publishers.

Tanguma, J. (2001). Effects of sample size on the distribution of selected fit indices: A graphical approach. *Educational and Psychological Measurement, 61(5),* 759–776.

Templin, T., & Peters, R. (2002). Rules for calculating degrees of freedom in structural equation modeling. Paper presented at the annual meeting of the Midwest Nursing Research Society, Chicago, March 2002.

Third National Health and Nutrition Examination Survey, 1988–1994. (1996). NHANES III Laboratory Data File (CD-ROM). U.S. Department of Health and Human Services (DHHS). Documentation Number 76200. Hyattsville, MD: Centers for Disease Control.

Thurstone, L. L. (1947). *Multiple-factor analysis.* Chicago: University of Chicago Press.

Tombes, M. B., & Gallucci, B. (1993). The effects of hydrogen peroxide rinses on the normal oral mucosa. *Nursing Research, 42*(6), 332–337.

Toothaker, L. E. (1993). *Multiple comparison procedures.* Series: Quantitative Applications in the Social Sciences, #89. Newbury Park, CA: Sage.

Tran, T. V., & Aroian, K. J. (1999). Assessing public health and health care needs of elderly Russian immigrants. Unpublished raw data.

Tucker, L. A., & Maxwell, K. (1992). Effects of weight training on the emotional well-being and body image of females: predictors of greatest benefit. *American Journal of Health Promotion, 6*(6), 338–344.

Tufte, E. R. (1983). *The visual display of quantitative information.* Cheshire, CT: Graphics Press.

Tukey, J. W. (1969). Analyzing data: Sanctification or detective work? *American Psychologist, 24,* 83–91.

Tukey, J. W. (1977). *Exploratory data analysis.* Reading, MA: Addison-Wesley.

Tulman, L. R., & Jacobsen, B. S. (1989). Goldilocks and variability. *Nursing Research, 38,* 377–379.

Ulrich, C. M., Soeken, K. L., & Miller, N. (2003). Ethical conflict associated with managed care. *Nursing Research, 52*(3), 168–175.

U.S. Department of Health and Human Services (DHHS). (1996). National Center for Health Statistics. *Third National Health and Nutrition Examination Survey, 1988–1994,* NHANES III Laboratory Data File (CD-ROM). Public Use Data File Documentation Number 76200. Hyattsville, MD: Centers for Disease Control and Prevention.

Vaughan, E. D. (1998). *Statistics: Tools for understanding data in the behavioral sciences.* Upper Saddle River, NJ: Prentice-Hall.

Verran, J. A., & Ferketich, S. L. (1987). Testing linear model assumptions: Residual analysis. *Nursing Research, 36*(2), 127–129.

Vessey, J. (2000). Development of the CATS: Child-Adolescent Teasing Scale. Funded by the National Institute of Nursing Research, R01 NR04838.

Von Eye, A., & Clogg, C. (Eds.). (1994). *Latent variables analysis: Applications for developmental research.* Thousand Oaks, CA: Sage.

Wagnild, G. M., & Young, H. M. (1993). Development and psychometric evaluation of the Resilience Scale. *Journal of Nursing Measurement, 1*(2), 165–178.

Wallgren, A., Wallgren, B., Persson, R., Jorner, U., & Haaland J. (1996). *Graphing statistics & data creating better charts.* Thousand Oaks, CA: Sage.

Wang, L., Fan, X., & Willson, V. L. (1996). Effects of nonnormal data on parameter estimates and fit indices for a model with latent and manifest variables: An empirical study. *Structural Equation Modeling, 3*(3), 228–247.

Wang, S., Yu, M., Wang, C., & Huang, C. (1999). Bridging the gap between the pros and cons in treating ordinal scales as interval from an analysis point of view. *Nursing Research, 48*(4), 226–229.

Weisberg, H. F. (1992). *Central tendency and variability.* Series: Quantitative Applications in the Social Sciences, #83. Newbury Park, CA: Sage.

West, S. G., Finch, J. F., & Curran, P. J. (1995). Structural equation models with non-normal variables: Problems and remedies. In R. H. Hoyle (Ed.), *Structural equation modeling: Concepts, issues, and applications* (pp. 56–75). Thousand Oaks, CA: Sage.

Wikoff, R. L., & Miller, P. (1991). Canonical analysis in nursing research. Methodology Corner. *Nursing Research, 40*(6), 367–370.

Williams, G. C., Gagne, M., Ryan, R. M., & Deci, E. L. (2002). Facilitating autonomous motivation for smoking cessation. *Health Psychology, 21*(1), 40–40.

Winer, B. J. (1971). *Statistical principles in experimental design* (2nd ed.). New York: McGraw-Hill.

Wood, R. Y. (1997). The development & testing of video breast health kits for older women. National Cancer Institute Small Business Innovation Research (SBIR) Phase II R43 CA 63935-02.

Wood, R. Y., Duffy, M. E., Morris, S. J., & Carnes, J. E. (2002). The effect of an educational intervention on promoting breast self-examination in older African American and Caucasian women. *Oncology Nursing Forum, 29*(7), 1081–1090.

Wothke, W. (1996). Models for multitrait-multimethod matrix analysis. In G. A. Marcoulides & R. E. Schumacker (Eds.), *Advanced structural equation modeling: Issues and techniques* (pp. 7–56). Mahwah, NJ: Lawrence Erlbaum Associate.

Wright, S. (1934). The method of path coefficients. *Annals of Mathematical Statistics, 5*(September), 161–215.

Wu, Y. B., & Slakter, M. J. (1990). Increasing the precision of data analysis: Planned comparisons versus omnibus tests. Methodology Corner. *Nursing Research, 39*(4), 251–253.

Wynd, C. A. (2002). Testicular self-examination in young adult men. *Journal of Nursing Scholarship, 34*(3), 251–255.

Youngblut, J. M., Brooten, D., Singer, L. T., Standing, T., Lee, H., and Rodgers, W. L. (2001). Effects of maternal employment and prematurity on child outcomes in single parent families. *Nursing Research, 50*(6), 346–355.

Index

Page numbers followed by "t" indicate table; those followed by "f" indicate figure.